中医药智能计算

浙江大学成果汇编

未来计算编委会 编

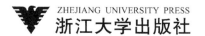

浙江大学出版社

未来计算编委会

主 编
吴朝晖

编 委
（按拼音排序）

陈华钧　邓水光　顾宗华　姜晓红
李　红　李石坚　李　莹　刘海风
马　德　潘　纲　潘之杰　尚永衡
唐华锦　吴　健　尹建伟　郑国轴

《中医药智能计算》编写工作组

吴朝晖　陈华钧　姜晓红　吴　健　李　红　陈　翎

目　录

绪论　中医药和人工智能

　　中医药是具有鲜明民族特色的传统医药学体系,反映了中华民族数千年来对生命、健康和疾病的认知和传统医药知识的传承。习近平总书记于 2019 年 10 月对中医药工作做出重要指示指出,中医药学包含着中华民族几千年的健康养生理念及其实践经验,是中华文明的一个瑰宝,凝聚着中国人民和中华民族的博大智慧。在 2020 年的新冠疫情抗击过程中,中医药治疗也发挥了核心作用。据国家中医药管理局数据,全国中医药参与治疗比例超过 92%。积极推动中医药在传承创新中高质量发展,对于传承中华文明瑰宝和增进人民健康福祉都具有重要意义。

　　当代科技发展的一个重要特征是以大数据、云计算、人工智能等为代表的信息科学与计算机技术向各个传统学科广泛而深入渗透,通过交叉融合,孕育形成新的技术领域,催生新的应用模式。将新兴的信息技术引入中医药,可以辅助研究中医药信息的运动规律,阐明和理解大量数据所包含的意义,发展信息驱动的中医药学理论与方法学,并支撑中医药临床、科研、教育、管理等各个方面迅速进步发展。

　　浙江大学在中医药信息及大数据、人工智能等技术在中医药领域的应用研究可以追溯到 20 世纪 90 年代中期,至今已有二十余年历史。从早期开展中医药科技文献电子化起步,逐步围绕中医药科学数据库共建共享、中医药知识工程、中医药数据挖掘与知识发现、中医药云平台与服务计算技术等多个方面取得了一系列丰硕的研究成果。

　　早在 1996 年,浙江大学计算机系与中国中医研究院建立合作关系,在国家中医药管理局的持续支持下,开展中医药科学数据库共建共享平台的建设,在国际上最早引入联邦数据库技术,建成了由近百个数据库组成的中医药联邦数据集成搜索与共建共享平台。

　　知识工程是人工智能的重要技术基石。浙江大学中医药智能计算研究团队自 2000 年起将知识表示、本体工程以及语义网技术引入中医药领域,并与中国中医研究院合作构建了国际上首个基于本体论的中医药一体化语言系统(2001);此后,进一步基于中医药本体技术构建了首个中医药语义搜索引擎(2003)、基于本体的中医药语义文献标引平台(2004)和中医药本体工程平台(2006)等多个新型实用的系统,极大地提升了中医药知识搜索与文献检索的效率和质量。2006 年,有关中医药知识工程和语义搜索引擎的工作获得国际语义网会议 ISWC 2006 年最佳论文奖,并于 2008 年被国际万维网联盟 W3C 选为语义互联网十大最佳实践。

　　数据挖掘与知识发现技术可以用于从海量的数据中发现与挖掘潜在的规律和知识。浙江大学先后研制了中药复方组成规律的关联规则发现系统(2001)、中医药文献挖掘与分析系统(2004)、中医方剂数据挖掘模式和算法库(2006)等多个中医药知识发现系统;逐步围绕知识抽取质量问题开展了中医药知识发现可靠性研究(2008),结合大数据技术开展了基于 MapReduce 的中医药并行数据挖掘(2008),结合语义网及 Linked Open Data 技术开展了中医药语义关系抽取和关联发现研究(2010),并构建了 DartSpora 中医药知识发现平台(2012)。2012 年 Elsevier 出版的英文专著《现代计算技术与中医药信息处理》(*Modern Computational Approaches to Traditional Chinese Medicine*)系统性总结了浙江大学在这个领域的研究成果和工作。

数据与应用的服务化和云化可以为信息的传播与触达提供便利,极大地提升中医药信息与知识服务的能力和效率。浙江大学早期将网格与服务计算技术引入中医药领域,构建了基于 SOA 和 OGSA 网格架构的中医药数据库网格系统(2004),并在 Springer 出版英文专著《语义网络:模型、方法和运用》(*Semantic Grid:Model,Methodology,and Applications*)。自 2008 年起,浙江大学进一步将云计算和知识服务等技术引入中医药领域,分别持续构建了方药知识服务、中医临床知识服务、中医养生知识服务等多个中医药知识服务系统。2013 年,浙江大学牵头的"基于语义图的知识服务技术及中医药应用"项目获得高等学校科学研究优秀成果奖(科学技术)技术发明一等奖。

近年来,合作团队进一步结合知识图谱、深度学习等新兴人工智能技术开展了临床、养生、药材、方剂、中药制造等多个中医药知识图谱的建设,开展了自动化关系抽取、知识图谱推理、知识图谱问答等多项技术的中医药应用研究,并将深度学习、图表示学习等技术方法进一步应用于中医药大数据的挖掘与分析。2017 年出版专著《中医药知识工程》,2019 年出版专著《知识图谱:方法、应用与实践》。此外,团队还在中医药信息标准方面开展了大量工作。2017 年,浙江大学牵头向国际标准化组织(ISO)提交了《中医制药过程工艺语义框架》标准提案,该标准已于 2020 年 1 月正式出版发布。

在不断变革的新科技时代,复兴的人工智能技术必将更加全面和深入地影响中医药事业和产业发展的方方面面。更准确地把握这些技术变革的方向与趋势,并深入结合中医药现代化的需要,开展中医药和人工智能的应用研究,将有力推动中医药走向世界,为建设健康中国和健康世界贡献中国智慧和力量。

第1章　中医药科学数据库共建共享

中医在许多中国人日常健康医疗中扮演了重要的角色。千百年的中医药实践和研究积累了大量文字记录。辛亥革命之前,国内的中医古籍出版就达到了大约 13 万册,每年在全世界的期刊上发表成百上千篇关于中医治疗的科研工作的论文,例如在 1984—2005 年期间共计发表超过 60 万篇中医药期刊论文。这些都是宝贵的中医药信息。鉴于其巨大的体量,科学的中医药信息管理方法显得非常重要。只有运用科学的中医药信息管理方法,才能进一步促进这些信息得到有效且便捷的使用,尽可能体现出这些信息的价值。

现代计算机数据库技术以及搜索引擎技术为各个领域的数据整合和数据共享提供了有效的技术手段。中医药智能计算研究团队发现,尽管中医药领域留存了海量信息,但数据孤岛现象严重,且数据形式各异,缺乏有效的组织手段。因此我们着力研究了中医药科学数据库的共建共享,致力于建立一个中医药领域的公开共享且完善齐全的数据库,并提供有效的查询检索结果,让用户便捷而准确地获取到所需的中医药相关知识。

在中医药科学数据库共建共享研究中,我们着重从以下几个方面进行了研究。

(1)中医药数据共建体系研究

主要目的为形成一个互联、互通、归一化的中医药数据共建体系。重点研究了文献的自动标注,提出并开发了中医药文献自动标引系统,见文献[1-2]。设计开发了基于语义的中医药数据采集及应用平台,研究了面向领域关系数据库全文检索的优化设计,开发了基于语义标注的离线数据加工平台 DartAnnotation、研究管理平台 TCMManager、数据共建平台 DartMani,见文献[3-8]。提出并实现了本体模式和关系数据库模式的语义映射方法,研究了分布式图数据库的存储、基于图论的大数据存储架构,见文献[9-11]。开发了基于本体的网络数据工作平台 NetData,实现了基于 SOAP 的网络数据库,见文献[12-13]。

[1] 周孟霞. 基于规则学习的中医药文献自动标引系统[D]. 杭州:浙江大学,2004.

主要研究了中医药文献自动标引,提出并开发了一个基于规则学习的主题自动标引系统,该系统从文献的题名中抽取并识别主题模式,有效地解决了医学科技文献的自动标引中涉及的主题词和副主题词的组配问题。

[2] Wu Z,Chen H,Jiang X. Modern Computational Approaches to Traditional Chinese Medicine[M]. Elsevier,2012.

主要研究了如何在传统中医药应用中融合分散的数据,以帮助有效地进行数据检索以及知识发现。提出了针对传统中医药信息和知识的数据化方法,解决了为临床决策、药物发现以及教育提供智能资源的应用难题。

[3] 陶金火. 基于语义的中医药数据采集工程及应用平台[D]. 杭州：浙江大学，2011.

主要研究了基于语义的中医药数据采集工程及应用平台,提出了一种采用语义本体配置元数据对中医药数据模型和存储逻辑进行配置的方法,以及一种语义关系图标注算法,用以辅助数据采集,实现了一体化中医药数据采集平台,以语义配置信息为系统配置元数据,将不同专题的数据集成到一个统一的平台中采集,解决了中医药领域数据采集系统数量太多、彼此之间相互孤立、无法相互连接访问、组件重用性较低、可维护性差、数据采集智能化程度偏低等应用难题。

[4] 张慧敏. 面向领域的关系数据库全文检索系统的优化设计[D]. 杭州：浙江大学，2008.

主要研究了面向领域的关系数据库全文检索系统的优化设计,提出 DartSearch V3 所要解决的问题和系统的架构设计,解决了海量数据及数据孤岛严重阻碍数据有效共享的难题。

[5] 吴振宇. 基于语义标注的中医药数据加工平台[D]. 杭州：浙江大学，2007.

主要研究了针对中医药领域的专题数据库开发的平台,提出了建立基于语义标注的离线数据加工平台 DartAnnotation 和开发中医药虚拟研究管理平台 TCMManager。DartAnnotation 和 TCM-Manager 分别解决了目前在线数据加工平台无法基于中医药本体离线数据加工以及整体化的问题。

[6] 裴君. DartConsole：数据库网格管理平台的设计与实现[D]. 杭州：浙江大学，2005.

从动态开放的网格环境下数据资源共享与协同管理的应用需求背景出发,综合了现有的 Internet 下的数据资源的信息共享与整合管理的解决方案,提出了一套面向数据库资源的管理方案,即 DartConsole 数据库网格管理模型,解决了如下问题：统一的数据库资源访问、动态数据库网格环境的监控及性能管理、基于 VO 的数据库网格环境的安全管理等。

[7] 范宽. 基于语义本体的中医药科学数据共建工程[D]. 杭州：浙江大学，2006.

主要研究了中医药科学数据建设的特点,开发了基于自定义元数据的通用数据共建平台 DartMani 1.0 和基于本体的中医药科学数据共建平台 DartMani 2.0,解决了中医药科学数据共建中存在的保存和最大限度使用数据两方面难题。

[8] Chen H，Wu Z，Mao Y. RDF-based ontology view for relational schema mediation in semantic web[C]//KES，2005，LNAI 3682：873-879.

主要研究了语义 Web 应用程序如何定义关系模型和 RDF 模型之间的映射,提出了一种基于视图的方法,使用基于 RDF 的本体来调解关系模式。通过该方法,发现 RDF 空白节点在定义语义映射和表示关系模式的不完整部分中起到重要作用。

[9] 吴朝晖，周春英，王恒，等. 本体模式与关系数据库模式之间语义映射信息的编辑方法：200710156361.5[P]. 2010-02-17.

提出了一种本体模式与关系数据库模式之间语义映射信息的编辑方法,通过对本体模式与关系数据库模式的分析,定义从异质异构的关系数据库模式到本体模式的语义映射,实现了复杂关系数据库模式,提供了自动化的配置。

[10] 郭健. 对等结构的 NoSQL 存储在图数据库上的应用研究[D]. 杭州：浙江大学，2013.

主要研究了对等结构的 NoSQL 存储在图数据库上的应用,介绍了以 CAP 定力为代表的分布式系统的理论基础以及对等结构的 NoSQL 大规模数据存储系统的方案,讨论了分布式图数据库 Titan

的存储后端扩展技术方案。

[11]陈云路.基于图论的空间大数据仓库的实现[D].杭州:浙江大学,2014.

将空间信息数据整体分类为遥感影像数据和传统文件数据两类,介绍了大数据仓库架构及基于图论的大数据存储架构、I/O加速缓存优化层、多维度空间信息数据发布模块、基于空间信息和网络协议的数据监控等系列模块设计,描述了大数据仓库的代码实现情况、测试结果以及传统关系型与非关系型数据库的性能比较结果。

[12] 范宽,吴朝晖,陈华钧.基于本体的网络数据工作平台 NetData[J]. 计算机科学,2006,33(9):85-88.

基于语义网和数据库网格技术,设计实现了基于本体的网络数据工作平台 NetData,支持地理上分布的研究人员在网上实现协同数据库和本体构建工作。整个平台由三部分组成:语义支持模块,包括语义本体、知识库、语义引擎;RDF 数据生成模块,包括 RDF 解释表达器、RDF 检索器、RDF 生成、RDF 仓库;存储层接口模块。

[13] 周雪忠,陆伟,吴朝晖. 基于 SOAP 的 Web Databases 实现[J].计算机科学,2002,29(8):151-153.

使用 SOAP(简单对象访问协议)——一种将 HTTP 和 XML 结合在一起的协议,以实现 Internet 数据库,讨论了 SOAP 中间件技术基础结构。

(2)中医药数据共享理论与方法研究

主要目的是形成一个中医药信息共享体系。重点研究了中医药共享体系的设计和实现,数据库资源的集成与共享,异构数据库语义模式集成,异构数据的集成与共享,科学数据库的集成与共享,数据质量的提升,元数据交换协议的标准化,中文模糊自动补全纠正打字错误,以及从域的链接数据中发现社会社区等。提出了中医药数据共享平台的架构设计,开发实现了 Dart 数据库网格系统,见文献[14-15]。研究了语义 Web 层完成模式的集成,实现了基础 DartGrid V3 的 Web 查询处理系统,基于 SPARQL 的分布式语义查询优化算法,以及融合多维度的数据质量提升方法,见文献[16-20]。实现了基于语义的浏览器 Semantic Browser,基于汉字音形的错别字纠正算法,从链接数据中发现域中包含的社会社区结构的聚类方法,见文献[21-23]。

[14] 王俊健.中医药共享平台与 Mashup[D].杭州:浙江大学,2010.

主要研究了中医药共享系统的设计和实现,提出了新的面向中医药数据共享平台的架构设计,主要包括数据层、本体层、服务层、逻辑层和展现层,解决了 DartGrid 中各个独立共享系统的开发零散、搜索结果缺乏语义关联、界面展示不够丰富等问题。

[15] Wu Z,Chen H,Mao Y,et al. Dart database grid:A dynamic,adaptive,RDF-mediated,transparent approach to database integration for semantic web[C]// 7th Asia-Pacific Web Conference(APWeb'2005),2005:1053-1057.

主要介绍了由浙江大学网格研究中心开发的 Dart 数据库网格系统。该系统是基于语义网标准和 Globus 网络工具集开发的,目的是提供一种动态、自适应、以 RDF 为媒介的透明的(DART)方法实现语义网数据库集成。该方法已应用于中医药数据库资源的集成和共享。

[16]裴君,吴朝晖,徐昭.基于 OWL 本体论映射的数据库网格语义模式集成研究[J]. 计算机科

学,2005,32(5):4-7.

主要研究了基于本体的异构数据库语义模式集成技术。首先将数据库关系模式转化为 RDF/OWL 语义描述实现局部映射,再建立局部数据语义与全局共享本体之间的联系,实现全局映射。即通过本体显性表达异构数据库模式的语义,在语义 Web 层完成模式的集成。实现了统一语义层次上的共享和查询,特有的分层结构也使得跨库/单库环境中进行语义查询变得更加灵活。

[17] 谢聘超. 基于语义的数据库全文检索系统[D]. 杭州:浙江大学,2006.

主要研究了异质异构数据的集成与共享,开发了基于 DartGrid V3 的 Web 查询处理系统,将语义技术与全文检索引擎相结合,解决了 DartGrid V1 的稳定性和性能不够好的问题,加快了数据查询。

[18] Wu Z. DartGrid:A semantic grid and application for Traditional Chinese Medicine [C]// International Conference on the Principles and Practice of Multi-Agent Systems(PRIMA' 2006),2006:7-9.

基于语义网和网格技术,提出了一种动态、自适应、以 RDF 为媒介的、透明的 DartGrid 方法来快速构建语义网应用,为实现快速的跨域异构数据库的集成、分类、搜索、浏览、检索提供解决方案。

[19] 唐晶明. 基于 SPARQL 的分布式语义查询处理[D]. 杭州:浙江大学,2007.

主要研究了异质异构数据的集成与共享背景下的语义查询问题,提出了基于 SPARQL 的分布式语义查询优化算法,并介绍了具体的实现过程。最终开发了数据库全文检索引擎和 Web 查询处理系统,有效地解决了中医药领域科学数据库的集成与共享。

[20] Feng Y,Wu Z,Chen H,et al. Data quality in Traditional Chinese Medicine[C]//2008 International Conference on BioMedical Engineering and Informatics. IEEE,2008,1:255-259.

主要研究了中医领域中的数据质量问题,提出了考察中医数据质量的三个关键维度,包括粒度、表示一致性和完整性,提出了从这三个维度来提高中医领域数据质量的方法,解决了领域特异性下的数据质量问题。

[21] Mao Y,Wu Z,Xu Z,et al. Interactive semantic-based visualization environment for Traditional Chinese Medicine information[C]//7th Asia-Pacific Web Conference (APWeb' 2005),2005:950-959.

主要研究了利用语义网交换中药信息的元数据交换协议的标准化问题,提出了一套设计原则,描述了一种新颖的基于语义的信息浏览器 Semantic Browser,解决了针对诸如 TCM 之类的数据密集型领域共享和管理大规模信息的问题。

[22] Feng Y,Chen H,Sheng H. A Chinese fuzzy autocompletion approach[C]//2010 IEEE International Conference on Information Reuse & Integration(IRI'2010),IEEE,2010:355-358.

主要研究了中文模糊自动补全纠正打字错误的问题,提出了一种新型的考虑汉字音形的模糊匹配算法,解决了中文打字自动纠错的问题,成功应用于中药应用程序中。

[23] 曹凌,陈华钧. 基于域驱动的链接数据的社区发现研究与实现[J]. 计算机应用与软件,2011,28(5):78-81.

主要研究了如何从域中的链接数据来发现特定的属性,提出了一种能够从域的链接数据中发现社会社区的聚类方法,该方法从链接数据中发现域中包含的社会社区结构,帮助人们更好地了解域及域中人。

(3)从数据库到知识库

主要目的是探索怎样进一步基于中医药数据库,提供智能搜索、语义大数据处理、中医药百科等知识层面的应用服务及应用。提出了基于隐语义的中医药文献搜索引擎,实现了中文搜索引擎的模糊自动补全,见文献[24-25]。与中国中医研究院中医药信息研究所联合开发了 Web 数据库全文搜索引擎 FTSS_TCM,见文献[26]。实现了基于超链数据的中医药语义查询系统,提出了新颖的查询重写算法以及基于本体的语义搜索结果排序算法,见文献[27-31]。开发了一种简化的基于语义推理规则的中医发热病理论的诊断系统,面向语义 Web 查询推理的知识网格服务体系,基于 Hadoop 的语义大数据分布式推理框架,一个面向中医药领域的三维虚拟原型世界,见文献[32-34]。研究了生物信息学技术对中医和西医的相互促进作用,中医养生知识管理的现状和发展思路,以及中医药知识共享系统——中医百科系统,见文献[35-38]。总结了知识发现在中医药领域的若干探索,提出了 DartGrid Ⅱ 查询优化器的设计,实现了一组支持关系数据库集成和基于语义的信息浏览的语义工具等,见文献[39-41]。

[24] 冯叶磊. 基于隐语义的中医药文献搜索引擎[D]. 杭州:浙江大学,2011.

主要研究了针对中医文献的搜索引擎,提出了基于隐语义的中医文献搜索引擎,为海量文献数据提供了平台,解决了数据库中的文献和万维网上的文献的应用难题。

[25]陈华钧,冯叶磊,姜晓红,等. 基于广义后缀树的中文搜索引擎模糊自动补全方法:201110003711.0[P]. 2013-06-05.

依据中文语境中以字为单位的特点,利用广义后缀树能够高效地保存词库中所有词的后缀,根据相似度权重,在计算机上实现了中文搜索引擎的模糊自动补全,增强了计算机中文自动补全的功能和适用性。

[26]陆伟,周雪忠,吴朝晖. 基于 XML 的 Web 数据库全文搜索引擎[C]// 中国中医药信息研究会第二届理事大会暨学术交流会议论文汇编,2003.

主要讨论了由浙江大学和中国中医研究院中医药信息研究所联合开发的 Web 数据库全文搜索引擎 FTSS_TCM。FTSS_TCM 采用 XML 和 Web 技术相结合的方法,成功解决了 Internet 环境下数据通信受防火墙等网络安全设备影响的问题。

[27] 盛浩. 基于超链数据的中医药语义查询系统[D]. 杭州:浙江大学,2011.

主要研究了利用语义本体、语义查询等技术手段在海量中医药学科信息中的应用,提出了基于超链数据的中医药语义查询系统,解决了在中医药领域有效组织、共享和利用数据的应用难题。

[28] Chen H，Wu Z，Mao Y. Rewriting queries using views for RDF-based relational data integration[C]//17th IEEE International Conference on Tools with Artificial Intelligence (ICTAI'05),IEEE,2005:5-264.

主要研究了通过目标 RDF 本体回答查询的问题,设计了一种新颖的查询重写算法,解决了使用 RDF 集成关系数据时表示关系数据的不完整语义问题。

[29] Chen H，Wu Z，Wang H，*et al*. RDF/RDFS-based relational database integration

［C］//22nd International Conference on Data Engineering（ICDE'06），IEEE，2006：94-94.

主要研究了通过 RDF/RDFS 本体回答查询的问题，正式定义了查询语义并设计了一种新颖的查询重写算法，应用于中国中医科学院的 70 个关系数据库。

［30］Chen H，Wu Z，Mao Y，et al. DartGrid：A semantic infrastructure for building database Grid applications［J］. Concurrency and Computation：Practice and Experience，2006，18（14）：1811-1828.

主要设计实现了一个语义网格系统 DartGrid，为快速构建数据库网格应用提供语义基础设施和网格服务，包括一组基于 RDF 的语义服务工具：语义浏览器、语义映射工具、本体服务、语义查询服务和语义注册服务。提出了一种基于 RDF 视图的关系模式介导方法，实现了基于视图的语义查询重写算法。用 DartGrid 实现了一个真实的中医药语义网格应用系统。

［31］杨克特，陈华钧. 面向特定领域的语义搜索结果排序算法［J］. 计算机应用与软件，2011，28（12）：172-174.

主要提出了面向中医药领域的基于本体的语义搜索结果排序算法。该算法主要考虑了本体的重要性，并结合用户查询和本体之间的匹配度，对搜索的结果做了一个优化排序。

［32］Gu P，Chen H. Knowledge-driven diagnostic system for Traditional Chinese Medicine ［C］//Joint International Semantic Technology Conference，2011：258-267.

主要研究了中医识别疾病的语义化建模问题，提出了一种简化的基于语义推理规则的中医发热病理论诊断系统。该系统利用基于医学本体的语义推理能力，解决了基于医学知识进行基本的临床诊断的应用难题。

［33］陈曦，陈华钧，顾珮嵚，等. 一种基于 Hadoop 的语义大数据分布式推理框架［J］. 计算机研究与发展，2013，50（S2）：103-113.

主要研究了大规模语义数据之间的语义关联与信息关联，提出了一种基于 Hadoop 的语义大数据分布式推理框架，并且设计了相应的基于属性链（property chain）的原型推理系统，高效地发现海量语义数据中潜在的有价值的信息，解决了传统推理引擎在进行大规模语义数据推理时存在的计算性能和可扩展性不足的问题。

［34］于彤，陈华钧，王超，等. 中医药三维虚拟世界构建研究［J］. 中国数字医学，2013（10）：73-75.

主要提出了一个面向中医药领域的三维虚拟原型世界。它为中医药领域知识的获取、保护和共享提供了有效手段，为该领域的学术交流和医患互动提供了理想的平台。

［35］Gu P，Chen H. Modern bioinformatics meets Traditional Chinese Medicine［J］. Briefings in Bioinformatics，2014，15（6）：984-1003.

主要研究了生物信息学技术对中医和西医的相互促进作用，总结了生物学技术应用于中药研究取得的重要成就，解决了生物医学上处理快速增长的生物医学数据及异构性的难题。

［36］Zhou X，Wu Z，Lu W. TCMMDB：A distributed multidatabase query system and its key technique implemention［C］//2001 IEEE International Conference on Systems，Man and Cybernetics. e-Systems and e-Man for Cybernetics in Cyberspace（Cat. No. 01CH37236），IEEE，2001，2：1095-1100.

主要研究了分布式数据库中的多数据库合作问题,提出了一种分布式多数据库查询系统的通用体系结构 TCMMDB(中药多数据库),解决了分布式查询计划生成、分布式查询同步和 TCMMDB 中的分布式错误处理等多个应用难题。

[37] 于彤,崔蒙,高宏杰,等. 中医养生知识管理的现状和发展思路[J]. 中国数字医学,2016,11(4):73-75.

通过文献检索、互联网浏览等方式,对中医养生领域的知识资源进行调研,分析知识管理的现状并提出未来的发展思路。

[38] 于彤,贾李蓉,刘丽红,等. 语义维基技术在中医药领域的应用研究[C]// 第一届中国中医药信息大会论文集,2014.

主要介绍了语义维基技术,以及通过该技术构建的中医药知识共享系统——中医百科系统。该系统基于中医药领域本体实现中医药领域知识的整合,为网络用户提供百科全书式的知识服务。

[39] 吴朝晖,封毅. 数据库中知识发现在中医药领域的若干探索(Ⅱ)[J]. 中国中医药信息杂志,2005,12(11):92-95.

主要介绍了数据库中知识发现在中医药领域的若干探索,介绍了中医药领域对知识发现的需求,以及知识发现的基本模型和发展趋势,并进行了多种应用的探索,包括方剂配伍规律研究、基于功效的中医药聚类分析、中医药数据预处理以及面向中医药数据库的知识发现平台研究等。

[40] Zheng X,Chen H,Wu Z,*et al*. Query optimization in database grid[C]// International Conference on Grid and Cooperative Computing,2005:486-497.

DarGrid Ⅱ 是一个已实现的数据库网格系统,其目标是为集成 Web 上的数据库资源提供语义解决方案。与传统的分布式数据库相比,数据库网格中的查询优化出现了更多的挑战。本文提出了 DartGrid Ⅱ 查询优化器的设计,并提出了一种启发式、动态、并行的查询优化方法来处理数据库网格中的查询。

[41] Zheng X Q,Chen H J,Wu Z H,*et al*. Dynamic query optimization approach for semantic database grid[J]. Journal of Computer Science and Technology,2006,21(4):597-608.

主要研究了 DartGrid Ⅱ 中查询优化器的设计,提出了一种启发式、动态和并行查询优化方法来处理数据库网格中的查询,实现了一组支持关系数据库集成和基于语义的信息浏览的语义工具。

1.1　代表性学术论文全文

本节选取了中医药科学数据库共建共享方向的 2 篇代表性学术论文“RDF/RDFS-Based Relational Database Integration”和“Modern Bioinformatics Meets Traditional Chinese Medicine” 全文(分别于 2006 年和 2013 年发表于国际会议论文集 ICDE 及国际期刊 *Briefings in Bioinformatics*)。

RDF/RDFS-Based Relational Database Integration

Huajun Chen, Zhaohui Wu, Heng Wang, Yuxin Mao

首发于 *ICDE*，2006：94-106

Abstract

We study the problem of answering queries through a RDF/RDFS ontology, given a set of view-based mappings between one or more relational schemas and this target ontology. Particularly, we consider a set of RDFS semantic constraints such as *rdfs：subClassof*, *rdfs：subPropertyof*, *rdfs：domain*, *and rdfs：range*, which are present in RDF model but neither XML nor relational models. We formally define the query semantics in such an integration scenario, and design a novel query rewriting algorithm to implement the semantics. On our approach, we highlight the important role played by RDF Blank Node in representing incomplete semantics of relational data. A set of semantic tools supporting relational data integration by RDF is also introduced. The approach have been used to integrate 70 relational databases at China Academy of Traditional Chinese Medicine.

1 Introduction

The Semantic Web aims to provide a common semantic framework allowing data to be shared and reused across application, enterprize, and community boundaries. It is based on the Resource Description Framework (RDF), which is a language for representing web information in a minimally constrained, flexible, but meaningful way so that web data can be exchanged and integrated without loss of semantics. Most of existing data, however, is stored in relational databases. Therefore, for semantic web to be really useful and successful, great efforts are required to offer methods and tools to support integration of heterogeneous relational databases using RDF model. This paper is devoted to address this problem. Specifically, it concerns the problem of answering queries through a RDF ontology, given a set of semantic mappings between one or more relational schemas and the RDF ontology.

Essentially, it is the old problem of uniformly querying many disparate data sources through one common virtual interface. A typical approach, called answering query using view [5,7], is to describe data sources as precomputed views over a mediated schema, and reformulate the user query, posed over the mediated schema into queries that refer directly to source schemas by query rewriting.

While most of the preceding work has been focused on the relational case [5,8], and recently the XML case [9,10], we consider the case of RDF-based relational data integration. In particular, we consider a set of extra RDFS semantic constraints set on the mediated schema such as *rdfs：subClassof*, *rdfs：subPropertyof*, *rdfs：domai*, and *rdfs：range*, which are present in RDF model but neither XML nor relational models. These constraints are of great importance in web data integration. Take an example：suppose there is a statement in the RDF ontology saying[①]：*foaf：schoolHomepage rdfs：subPropertyOf foaf：homepage*. Given a semantic mapping from a column of a relational table to the property *foaf：schoolHomepage*, and a semantic query

---

① N3 notation is used to represent RDF statements.

referring the property *foaf*:*homepage* the rewriting algorithm should automatically infer that can be used to generate rewritings for *Q*. On the other hand, if a triple like :*aaa foaf*:*schoolHomepage*: *bbb* is generated as a query result, the system should automatically infer that the triple :*aaa foaf*:*homepage*: *bbb* is also a query result. In other words, *rdfs*:*subPropertyOf* sets an extra constraints on the mediated schema, and enables the query rewriting to infer more results.

Another motivation of our work is the *big model and small model problem*. In the case of semantic web, shared ontologies are normally designed to cover a whole domain, and are normally *big*, *complete models*. Take the *Traditional Chinese Medicine* (TCM) domain as an example, the number of the RDF classes of current TCM ontology [14] developed by China Academy of TCM has reached to 100,000. However, the legacy relational databases are often designed for local user, and are normally *small*, *incomplete models*. In fact, it is often difficult to find a direct mapping from the relational schema (small model) to the RDF ontology (big model) because of the incompleteness of legacy relational data. We take the advantages of *RDF Blank Node construct to help define the semantic mappings*. *Our experi*ences in TCM application shows that the RDF Blank Node is very useful in representing incomplete semantics of relational data when it is mapped to the RDF ontology. However, the formal analysis in Section 3.2 shows that introducing Blank Node to define semantic mappings makes query computation hard. As our work reveals, there is a tradeoff between the mapping flexibility and the computational complexity of query processing. The main contribution can be summarized as below.

1) Formal Aspects of Answering Queries Using Views

We formally and precisely specify what it means to answer a RDF query, given a set of view based mappings between the source relational schemas and RDF ontology. We define a *Target RDF Instance* that satisfies all the requirements with respect to the given views and RDFS semantic constraints, and take the query semantics to be the result of evaluating the query on this *Target RDF Instance*. In addition, we highlight the important role played by RDF Blank Node in representing incomplete or hidden semantics of relational data when defining semantic mapping.

2) RDF Query Rewriting Algorithm

An RDF-inspired query rewriting algorithm is implemented according to the formal query semantics. It rewrites RDF queries into a set of source SQL queries. Evaluating the union of these SQL queries has essentially the same effect as running the RDF query on the *Target RDF Instance*. This algorithm extends earlier relational and XML techniques for rewriting queries using views, with consideration of the features of RDF model.

3) A Set of Semantic Tools and their Application in Traditional Chinese Medicine

A set of semantic tools is developed. For examples, the *Visual Semantic Query Tool* enables users to visually construct RDF queries, and the *Visual Semantic Mapping Tool* enables users to speed up the process of defining view-based mapping. The query system has been deployed at China Academy of Traditional Chinese Medicine to integrate 70 TCM relational databases.

This paper is laid out as follows: Section 2 formally discusses the problem of answering queries using views for RDF/RDFS-based relational data integration. Section 3 presents the RDF rewriting algorithm.

Section 4 introduces the implementation of some semantic tools and the application in Traditional Chinese Medicine.

2 Answering Queries Using View

2.1 RDF Views

We start with a simple mapping case. Suppose both W3C and *Zhejiang University* (abbreviated as ZJU) have a legacy employee database, and we want to integrate them using the FOAF ontology[②], so that we can uniformly query these two databases by formulating RDF queries upon the FOAF ontology. The mapping scenario in Figure 1 illustrates two source relational schemas, a part of the FOAF ontology, and two mappings between them. Graphically, the mappings are described by the arrows that go between the mapped schema elements. The extra RDFS semantic constraints state that both foaf: school Homepage and foaf: account Service Homepage are sub property of foaf: homepage, and both foaf: Online Chat Account and foaf: Online Ecommerce Account are subclass of foaf: Online Account. Mappings are often defined as views in conventional data integration systems. With our approach, each relational table in the source is defined as a view over the RDF ontologies. Such views are called as RDF Views. For formal discussion, RDF views are expressed in a Datalog like notation. The upper part of Figure 2 illustrates the examples of RDF views corresponding to semantic mappings in Figure 1. A typical RDF view consists of two parts. The left part is called the view head, and is a relational predicate. The right part is called the view body, and is a set of RDF triples. In general, the body can be viewed as a RDF query over the RDF ontology, and it defines the semantics of the relational predicate from the perspective of RDF ontology.

Being similar to conventional view definitions expressed in Datalog, there are two kinds of variables for RDF view. The variables appearing in the view head is often called distinguished variable. The variables appearing only in the view body but not in the view head are called existential variables.

Definition 1. RDF View. A typical RDF View is like the form: $R(\bar{X})^- : G(\bar{X}, \bar{Y})$; where:

(1) $R(\bar{X})$ is called the head of the view, and R is a relational predicate.

(2) $G(\bar{X}, \bar{Y})$ is called the body of the view, and G is a set of RDF triples with some nodes replaced by variable names.

(3) The $\bar{X}, \bar{Y}$ contain either variables or constants. The variables in $\bar{X}$ are called distinguished variables, and the variables in $\bar{Y}$ are called existential variables.

2.2 RDF Queries

Next, we pay some attention on the types of RDF queries dealt with in this paper. The following example $Q1$ is specified in terms of foaf ontology.

Q1: SELECT ?en ?em ?eh ?y2 ?an ?ah where

?y1 rdf:type foaf:Person.

?y1 foaf:name ?en. ?y1 foaf:mbox ?em. OPTIONAL ?y1 foaf:homepage ?eh.

?y1 foaf:holdsAccount ?y2.

---

② The Friend of a Friend (FOAF) project: http://www.foaf-project.org.

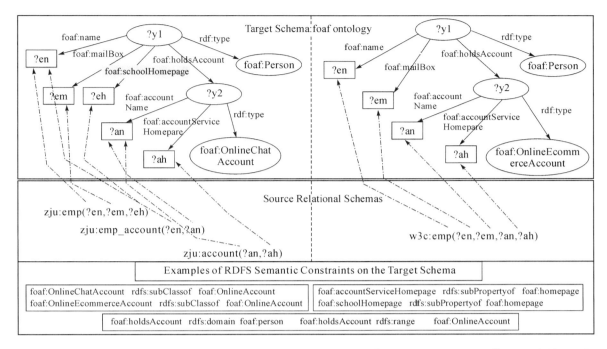

Figure 1　Semantic mapping from relational tables to RDF ontology. "?en,?em,?eh,?an,?ah" are variables and represent, respectively, "employee name", "employee email", "employee homepage at school", "account name", "account service homepage". "?y1,?y2" are existential variables.

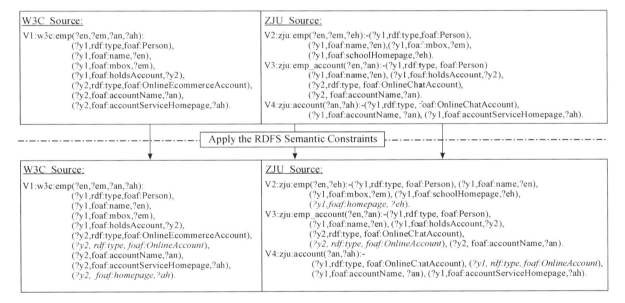

Figure 2　RDF views examples. Upper part is the set of original views, lower part is the set of views after applying RDFS semantic constraints(see Section 3.2). The newly added triples are italicized.

?y2 rdf:type foaf:OnlineAccount.

?y2 foaf:accountName ?an.

?y2 foaf:homepage ?ah.

The query is written in SPARQL③ query language. The query semantics is to find out the person name (?en), the mail box (?em), the homepage (?eh), his/her online account(?y2), the account name (?an), the homepage of the account service (?ah). We note that there is an *Optional Block* in *Q*1. According to the SPARQL specification, the *OPTIONAL* predicate specifies that if the optional part does not lead to any solutions, the variables in the optional block can be left unbound. As can be seen in Section 4, *OPTIONAL* predicate has an effect on the possible number of valid query writings that the algorithm can yield.

2.3 The Problem

The fundamental problem we want to address is: *given a set of source relational instances I such as in Figure 3, and a set of RDF views such as V1, V2 in Figure 2, plus a set of RDFS semantic constraints such as rdfs : subClassof in Figure 1, what should the answers to a target RDF query such as Q1 be?*

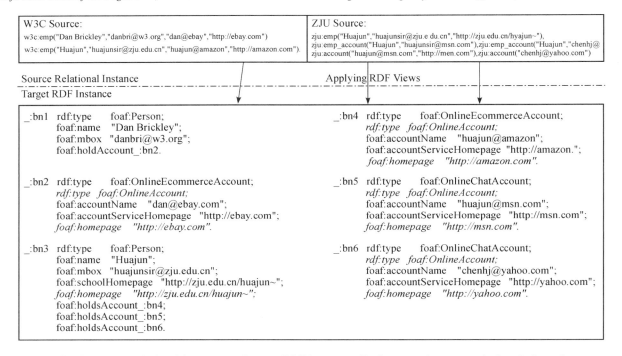

Figure 3 **The source relational instances and target RDF instances. In the target instance, _ : bn1, _ : bn2, and so on, are all newly generated blank node IDs. The italicized triples are generated because of the RDFS semantic constraints. The triples are represented in N3 notation.**

One possible approach that has been extensively studied in the relational literatures, is to consider the target instance, which is yielded by applying the view definitions onto the source instances, as an incomplete databases [7]. Often a number of possible databases *D* are consistent with this incomplete database. Then the query semantics is to take the intersection of *Q*(*D*) over all such possible *D*. This intersection is called the set of the certain answers [7].

This approach can not be applied directly to our case, since we need to consider extra semantic

③　W3C SPARQL: http://www. w3. org/TR/rdf-sparql-query.

constraints on the target schema. We take a similar but somewhat different approach, which is more RDF-inspired. In general, we define the semantics of target query answering by constructing a *Target RDF Instance* *G* based on the view definitions and RDFS semantic constraints. We then define the result of answering a target RDF query *Q*1 using the views to be the result of evaluating *Q*1 directly on *G*. In detail, two phases are involved in the construction process:

1）Applying constraints onto RDF views

Before constructing *G*, an extra inference process is firstly applied onto the RDF views. As the example in Figure 2 illustrated, five extra triples are added into the view definitions by applying the RDFS constraints in Figure 1. For instance, applying the constraint (*foaf:accountServiceHomepage rdfs:subPropertyof foaf:homepage*) to the triple (*?y2 foaf:accountServiceHomepage ?ah*) will yield a new triple (*?y2 foaf:homepage ?ah*).

2）Applying RDF views onto source instances

Next, relational instances are transformed into RDF instances according to extended RDF views. In other words, for each tuple in the source relational instance, a set of RDF triples is added in the target instance such that the RDF views are satisfied with. Figure 3 illustrates the examples of relational instance and target instance. The evaluation of *Q*1 on the target instance produces the tuples in Table 1.

Table 1　Query answers after evaluating *Q*1 on the Target RDF Instance in Figure 3. Note for Dan Brickley the variable ?eh is left unbound, namely, is nullable, but other variables MUST have a binding

Person.name	Person.mail-box	Person.homepage	Account	Account.name	Account.homepage
Dan Brickley	danbri@w3.org	NULL	_:bn2	dan@ebay	http://ebay.com
Huajun	huajunsir@zju.edu.cn	http://zju.edu.cn/huajun	_:bn4	huajun@amazon.com	http://amazon.com
Huajun	huajunsir@zju.edu.cn	http://zju.edu.cn/huajun	_:bn5	huajun@msn.com	http://msn.com
Huajun	huajunsir@zju.edu.cn	http://zju.edu.cn/huajun	_:bn6	huajun@yahoo.com	http://yahoo.com

One important notion is the *skolem functions* introduced to generate *blank node IDs* in target instance. As can be seen in Figure 3, corresponding to each existential variable $?y \in \overline{Y}$ in the view, a new blank node ID is generated in the target instance. As examples, _:bn1, _:bn2 are both newly generated blank node IDs corresponding to the variables $?y1$, $?y2$ in *V*1. This treatment of the existential variable is in accordance with the RDF semantics, since blank nodes can be viewed as existential variables[④]. In general, each RDF class in the target ontology is associated with a unique Skolem Function that can generate blank node ID at that type. For instances, the RDF classes in Figure 1 are associated with the following skolem functions respectively:

*foaf:Person SF*1(*?en*), *foaf:OnlineAccount SF*2(*?an*).

The choice of function parameters depends on the constraints users who want to set on the target schema. For example, *SF*1(*?en*) sets a constraint that says:"if two instances have same value for property foaf:name, then they are equivalent and the same blank node ID is generated for both". This is somewhat similar to the

---

④　W3C RDF Semantics：http://www.w3.org/TR/rdf-mt.

Primary Key Constraint, and is useful for merging instances stemming from different sources. Take the example in Figure 3 again, for person name "Huajun", the same blank node ID_: bn3 is generated for both W3C and ZJU sources.

Note: RDF Blank Node and Incomplete Semantics. *For many legacy databases, the data semantics are often not represented explicitly enough. Take the w3c: emp table as an example, it implies the semantics that says "for each person, there is an online account whose account name is…". The "There is an…" semantics is lost. This kind of semantics can be well captured by RDF Blank Node, since blank nodes are treated as simply indicating the existence of a thing, without identifying that thing. Indeed, it is the case of incomplete semantics. The incomplete problem* [15] [16] *has been considered as an important issue with related to view-based data integration system, and it is more acute for semantic web applications because web is open-ended system. Indeed, the Target RDF Instance can be viewed as an incomplete databases in which the Blank Nodes can be viewed as existential variables. This make it somewhat similar to the conditional table* [16] *introduced in database literature to model incomplete databases. From this point of view, we argue that blank node is an important representation construct for data integration in semantic web.*

We finally give the formal specification of the query semantics. We adopt this semantics as a formal requirement on answering queries using views for RDF/RDFS-based relational data integration. We will show in the next section how to implement this semantics, without materializing the *Target RDF Instance*, but instead by query rewriting. Moreover, this query semantics is also different from the certain answer [7] in relational literatures for two practical reasons: a) The query answer can contain *NULL*, because of the OPTIONAL predicate used in RDF query, b) The query answer can contain newly generated blank node IDs which can be viewed as existential variables.

Theorem 1 is about the fundamental complexity of the query answering problem. The result and the proof⑤ reveal that although blank nodes offer us great flexibility in defining semantic mappings, but it also makes the query computation harder. Therefore, there is a tradeoff between the mapping flexibility and the computational complexity.

Definition 2. Query Semantics. Let Q be a RDF query, then the set of the query answer of q with respect to a set of relational source instance I, a set of RDF views V, plus a set of RDFS semantic constraints C, denoted by $answer_{v,c}: (Q, I)$, is the set of all tuples t such that $t \in Q(G)$ where G is the Target RDF Instance.

Theorem 1. Let $\sum_v$ be a set of RDF view definitions, I be a view instance, C is a set of RDFS semantic constraints, Q be a RDF query, then the problem of computing the query answer with respect to $\sum_v, I, C, Q$ is NP-Complete.

3 RDF Query Rewriting

In most of cases, there is no full permission to access source instances, and thus query rewriting is required. In this section, a query rewriting algorithm satisfying with the query semantics defined in previous

---

⑤ The formal proof is available upon e-mail request.

section is presented.

3.1　Preprocessing Views

Before rewriting, the RDF views must be preprocessed. The purpose is two fold. Firstly, the *RDFS Constraints* are applied onto views, so that more types of query can be answered by using the extended views. Secondly, the view definitions are turned into a set of smaller rules called *Class Mapping Rules*, so that the RDF query expressions can be more directly substituted by relational terms.

Applying constraints has been introduced in Section 3.2. This extra inference process is valuable because it enables the rewriting algorithm to answer more types of query. For example, without this process, $Q1$ can not be answered by rewriting using the views, because the query terms *foaf:OnlineAccount* and *foaf:homepage* do not appear in any view definitions at all. Generating class mappings rules is somewhat complex. The algorithm is illustrated in the left part of Figure 5. In general, the algorithm can be divided into three steps.

1) Grouping Triples

The algorithm starts by looking at the body of views, and groups the triples by subject name, i.e., a separate group is created for each set of triples having same subject name. For example, three triple groups are created for $V1$ as illustrated in Figure 4. In the first group, three triples share the same subject name $?y1$ which will be replaced by the skolem function name SF1 $(?en)$ in next step.

2) Skolemizing Triples

Next, the algorithm replaces all existential variables $?yn \in Y$ with corresponding Skolem Function Names. As introduced in Section 3.2, we associate each RDF class with a unique Skolem Function to generate blank node IDs for that class. For example, the $?y1$, $?y2$ in $V1$ are replaced by skolem function name $SF1(?en)$, $SF2(?pn)$ respectively.

```
rule 1--w3c:emp(?en,?em,?an):-
     (SF1(?en),rdf:type,foaf:Person),
     (SF1(?en),foaf:name,?en),(?y1,foaf:mbox,?em),
     (SF1(?en),foaf:holdsAccount,SF2(?an))
rule 2--w3c:acc(?an,?ah):-
     (SF2(?an),rdf:type,foaf:OnlineEcommerceAccount),
     (SF2(?an),rdf:type,foaf:OnlineAccount),
     (SF2(?an),foaf:accountName,?an),
     (SF2(?an),foaf:accountServiceHomepage,?ah),
     (SF2(?an),foaf:homepage,?ah)
rule 3--zju:emp(?en,?em,?eh):-
     (SF1(?en),rdf:type,foaf:Person),
     (SF1(?en),foaf:name,?en),(SF1(?en),foaf:mbox,?em),
     (SF1(?en),foaf:schoolHomepage,?eh),
     (SF1(?en),foaf:homepage,?eh)
rule 4--zju:emp_accoun(?an):-
     (SF1(?en),rdf:type,foaf:Person),
     (SF1(?en),foaf:name,?en),
     (SF1(?en),foaf:holdsAccount,SF2(?an))
rule 5--zju:emp_accoun(?an):-
     (SF2(?an),rdf:type,foaf:OnlineChatAccount),
     (SF2(?an),rdf:type,foaf:OnlineAccount),
     (SF2(?an),foaf:accountName,?an)
rule 6--zju:account(?an,?ah):-
     (SF2(?an),rdf:type,foaf:OnlineChatAccount),
     (SF2(?an),rdf:type,foaf:OnlineAccount),
     (SF2(?an),foaf:accountName,?an),
     (SF2(?an),foaf:accountServiceHomepage,?ah),
     (SF2(?an),foaf:homepage,?ah)
```

```
rule 3_4--zju:emp(?en,?eh),zju:em_account(?en,?an)
     (SF1(?en),rdf:type,foaf:Person),
     (SF1(?en),foaf:name,?en),(SF1(?en),foaf:mbox,?em),
     (SF1(?en),foaf:schoolHomepage,?eh),
     (SF1(?en),foaf:homepage,?eh),
     (SF1(?en),foaf:holdsAccount,SF(?an))
rule 5_6--account(?an,?ah):-
     (SF2(?an),rdf:type,foaf:OnlineChatAccount),
     (SF2(?an),rdf:type,foaf:OnlineAccount),
     (SF2(?an),foaf:accountName,?an),
     (SF2(?an),foaf:accountServiceHomepage,?ah),
     (SF2(?an),foaf:homepage,?ah)
```

Figure 4　Examples of class mapping rules.

3) Constructing Class Mapping Rules

Next, for each triple group, a new class mapping rule is created. The rule head is the original relational predicate, and the rule body is set of the triples of that group.

4) Merging Class Mapping Rules

At last, some mapping rules are merged. There are two cases when rules need to be merged. One is the

Algorithm 1: Class Mapping Rule Generation

1. Input:set of RDF view V
2. Initialize mapping rules list M;
3. For each v in V
4. Group the triples in v.body by subject name;
5. Replace variables in v with corresponding skolem function names;
6. Let L be the set of triple groups of v.body;
7. For each triple group g in L
8. create a new mapping rule m;
9. m.head=v.head
10. m.body=g;
11. add m to M
12. End For
13. End For
14. Merge rules if necesary;
15. Output:mapping rule list M;

Algorithm 2: Query Transformation

1. Input:target query q, set of mapping rules M
2. Initialize rewriting list Q;
3. Group the triples in q.body by subject name;
4. Replace variables in q.body with corresponding skolem function name;
5. Let L be the set of triple groups of q.body;
6. For each triple group g in L
7. Let A M=the set of mapping rules applicable to g;
8. For each q in Q;
9. remove q from Q;
10. For each rule m in A M
11. For each OPTIONAL triple t in g
12. Let x be the variable in t and x in q.head;
13. q.head=q.head[x/x=null];
14. End For
15. q=q[g/m.head];
16. Add q' to Q;
17. End For
18. End For
19. End For
20. Output: rewriting list Q

Figure 5   The algorithms. We use "q＝q[a/b]" to denote replacing all occurrence of "a" in "q" with "b", and use "q. head" and "q. body" to denote the head and body of q.

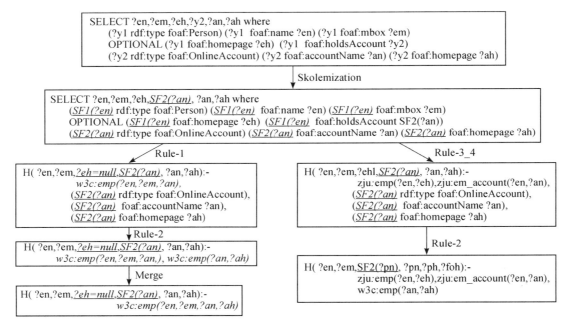

Figure 6   The query rewriting example. The final rewriting is expressed using Datalog like notation which can be easily transformed into a SQL query.

case of redundant rule. For example, rule5 and rule6 will be merged as rule5_6 because rule5 is a redundant rule. Another case is: if there is a referential constraints between two relational tables within a source, then their rules will be merged. For example, rule3 and rule4 will be merged into the rule3_4 because there are referential constraints between zju:emp(?en,?eh) and zju:em_account(?en,?an).

3. 2   Query Rewriting

In this phase, the algorithm transforms the input query using the newly generated mapping rules, and outputs a set of valid rewritings. The algorithm is illustrated in the right part of Figure 5. Being similar to generating class mappings rules, the rewriting algorithm starts by looking at the body of the query and group the triples by subject name, then replace all variables ?yn with corresponding Skolem Function Names. Next, it begins to look for rewritings for each triple group by trying to find an *applicable mapping rule*. If it finds one, it replaces the triple group by the head of the mapping rule, and generate a new partial rewriting. After all triple groups have been replaced, a candidate rewriting is yielded. If a triple t in $Q1$ is OPTIONAL and no triple in the mapping rule is mapped to t, the variable in t is set to NULL as default value. Figure 6 illustrates the rewriting process for query $Q1$. Because of space limitation, only two candidate rewritings are illustrated.

Definition 3. Triple Mapping. Given two triples $t1$, $t2$, $t1$ is said to map with $t2$, if there is a variable mapping φ from $\mathrm{Vars}(t1)$ to $\mathrm{Vars}(t2)$ such that $t2 = \varphi(t1)$. $\mathrm{Vars}(t1)$ denotes the set of variables in $t1$.

Definition 4. Applicable Class Mapping Rule. Given a triple group g of a query Q, a mapping rule m is a Applicable Class Mapping Rules with respect to g, if there is a triple mapping φ that maps every *non-optional* triple in g to a triple in m.

Theorem 2. Soundness. Let $\sum_v$ be a set of RDF Views. For query Q over the RDF ontology, the rewriting algorithm generates a set of rewriting R such that: whenever I is a source instance, G is the *Target RDF Instance* with respect to I and $\sum_v$, then $R(I) \subseteq Q(G)$.

Theorem 3. Completeness. Let $\sum_v$ be a set of RDF Views. For every query Q over the RDF ontology, let P be a query rewriting such that $R(I) \subseteq Q(G)$, and R is the rewriting generated by the algorithm, we have: whenever I is a source instance, G is a *Target RDF Instance* with respect to I and $\sum_v$, then $P(I) \subseteq R(I)$.

Theorems 2 and 3 are statements of the correctness of the algorithm. The formal proofs are available in the full version of this paper. Finally, we give an analysis on the complexity of the algorithm. Let n be the number of triple groups in $Q1$, let m be the number of mapping rules, it is not difficult to see that the rewriting can be done in time $O(m^n)$. The worst case experiment in the next section reflects the correctness of this proposition. We note that all rewriting algorithms are limited in cases where the number of resulting rewritings is especially large since a complete algorithm must produce an exponential number of rewritings. In general, the problem of query rewriting using views is NP-Complete [6]. In Section 4, we show although the computational problem is theoretically hard, the algorithm still works well in most of practical cases in our TCM application.

3.3　Experimental Evaluations

The goal of our experiment is to validate that our algorithm can scale up to deal with large mapping complexity. We consider two general classes of relational schema: chain schema and star schema. In these two case, we consider queries and views that have the same shape and size. Moreover, we also consider the worst case in which two parameters are looked upon: a) the number of triple groups of query, b) the number of sources. The whole system is implemented in Java and all experiments are performed on a PC with a single 1.8GHz P4 CPU and 512MB RAM, running Windows XP(SP2) and JRE 1.4.1.

1) Chain Scenario

In a chain schema, there is a line of relational tables that are joined one by one with each other. The chain scenario simulates the case where multiple interlinked relational tables are mapped to a target RDF

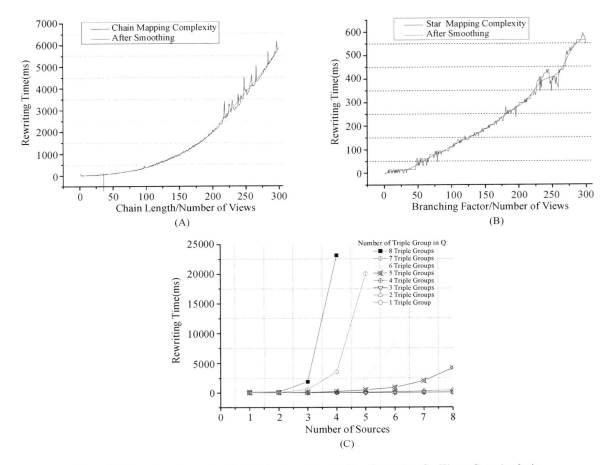

Figure 7   Experiment results. A. Chain Scenario, B. Star Scenario, C. Worst Case Analysis.

ontology with large number of levels (depth). The panel A of Figure 7 shows the performance in the chain scenario with the increasing length of the chain and also the number of views. The algorithm can scale up to 300 views under 10 seconds.

2) Star Scenario

In a star schema, there exists a unique relational tables that is joined with every other tables, and there are no joins between the other tables. The star scenario simulates the case where source relational tables are mapped to a target RDF graph with large branching factor. The panel B of Figure 7 shows the performance in the star scenario with the increasing branching factor of the star and also the number of views. The algorithm can easily scale up 300 views under 10 seconds. The experiments illustrate that the algorithm works better in star scenario.

3) Worst Case Analysis

The worst case happens when for each RDF class, there are a lot of class mapping rules generated for them, and the number of triple groups in the query is also large. In this case, for each triple group of the query, there are a lot of applicable mapping rules. Thus, there would be many rewritings, since virtually all combinations produce valid rewritings, and complete algorithm is forced to form an exponential number rewritings. In the experiment illustrated in C in Figure 7, we set up 10 sources, and for each source, 8 chained tables are mapped to 8 RDF classes respectively. The figure shows the cost of rewriting increases quickly as the number of triple groups and number of sources increases. As can be seen, in the case of 8 groups, the cost reaches 25 seconds with only 4 sources.

4　Implementation and Application

The DartGrid [11,12] system uses the techniques described in the previous sections to provide a uniform RDF query interface to sets of relational data sources.

Normal users interact with DartGrid through a *Semantic Browser* [13] that enables users to visually construct RDF queries. Figure 8 illustrates an example from our TCM application, which showcases how users can step by step specify a RDF query. In the first step, the user selects the *TCM Prescription* class and its three properties: *name*, *dosage*, and *preparationMethod*. In the second step, the user selects the *Disease* class and three properties *name*, *symptom*, and *pathogeny*. At last he inputs a constraint which specifies that the name of the *Disease* is "*influenza*". Take all, the semantic of this query is to query out *TCM Prescriptions* that can cure influenza.

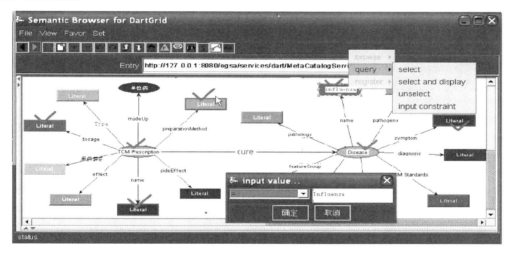

Figure 8　Visually construct a RDF query. Two RDF classes are involved, TCM-Prescription and Disease. For readability, we translate Chinese terms into English ones.

To speed up the process of defining RDF views, a *Visual Semantic Mapping* tool is developed. As Figure 9 displays, users can use the registration panel (the right part of the Figure 9) to view relational schema definitions, and use the semantic browsing panel (the left part of the Figure 9) to view RDF ontologies. Then users specify which RDF classes one table should be mapped to and which RDF property one column should be mapped to. Finally, the tool automatically generates a RDF view and submits it to a semantic registry.

The system has been deployed at China Academy of Traditional Chinese Medicine and currently provides access to over 70 databases including TCM herbal medicine databases, TCM compound formula databases, clinical symptom databases, traditional Chinese drug database, traditional Tibetan drug database, TCM product and enterprize databases, and so on. The current TCM ontology includes 28 RDF classes, 255 RDF properties, 9 *rdfs*: *subClassof* constraints, and 25 *rdfs*: *subPropertyof* constraints. We found the *rdfs*:

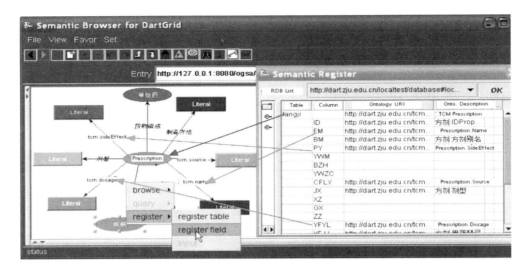

Figure 9   Visual Semantic Mapping Tool. The left is RDF ontology, and the right is a source relational table. User can visually specify the mappings from relational schema to RDF ontology.

subPropertyof is very useful in practice. Indeed, about 30% of the 70 TCM databases share some similar properties with each other. Blank nodes are commonly used, and we found it is very useful in case of non-normalized table. Although introducing blank nodes adds complexity to the query processing system, practical evaluation by our users shows that the system works well in most of practical use cases. However, practical scalability still needs to be tested if the number of databases become larger.

5   Related Work

In the context of semantic web research, a lot of research concerns mapping RDF with the relational model. Some of them deal with the issue of using RDBMS as RDF triple storage, such as Jena or Sesame's relational storage component. This issue is not touched upon in this paper. Some Others deal with the issue of integrating relational data using RDF, such as D2RMap [4], KAON REVERSE, D2RQ [1] and RDF Gateway①. However, none of them consider the issue of RDFS semantic constraints, and the formal aspects such as query semantics, query complexity is not considered. Another issue they did not consider is the incompleteness of legacy database. For example, both of D2RQ and RDF Gateway define a declarative language to describe mappings. However, the mappings, as they defined, are simple and equivalent mappings: it consists of statements asserting that some portion of relational data is equivalent to some portion of the RDF data. In contrast, the RDF views that we consider involves incomplete mappings, where each statement asserts that a relational source is an incomplete, partial view of the big model. Piazza [2] considers the mapping of XML-to-XML and XML-to-RDF. Francois [3] considers the problem of answering query using views for semantic web, but his approach is more description-logic-oriented.

6   Summary and Future Work

This paper studies the problem of answering RDF queries using RDF views over incomplete relational

---

① RDF Gateway: http://www.intellidimension.com.

databases under RDFS semantic constraints. We define a *Target RDF Instance* that satisfies all the requirements with respect to the given views and RDFS semantic constraints such as rdfs：subClassof, rdfs：subPropertyof, rdfs：domain, and rdfs：range, which are present in RDF model but neither XML nor relational models, and take the semantics of query answering to be the result of evaluating the query on this *Target RDF Instance*. With our approach, we highlight the important role played by the *RDF Blank Nodes* in representing incomplete semantics of relational data. A set of semantic tools and the application in the TCM domain is also reported. Some of future work is：extension to a more expressive RDF-based query languages such as OWL, and how to make mappings evolve if the ontology evolves.

References

[1] Christian Bizer. D2RQ system. Poster at ISWC2004.

[2] Alon Y. Halevy *et al*. Peer Data Management Systems：Infrastructure for the Semantic Web. WWW2003.

[3] Francois Goasdoue. Answering Queries using Views：a KRDB Perspective for the Semantic Web. ACM Transaction on Internet Technology. June 2003, P1-22.

[4] Chris Bizer, Freie. D2R MAP A Database to RDF Mapping Language. WWW2003.

[5] A. Y. Halevy. Answering queries using views：A survey. Journal of VLDB,2001；10(4), 75-102.

[6] A. Y. Levy, A. O. Mendelzon, Y. Sagiv, and D. Srivastava. Answering queries using views. In PODS, 1995.

[7] Serge Abiteboul. Complexity of Answering Queries Using Materialized Views. PODS1998, 254-263.

[8] Rachel Pottinger, Alon Y. Halevy. MiniCon：A Scalable Algorithm for Answering Queries Using Views. Journal of VLDB, 2001, 10(2-3),182-198.

[9] Cong Yu and Lucian Popa. Constraint-based XML Query Rewriting for Data Integration. SIGMOD2004,371-382.

[10] A. Deutsch and V. Tannen. MARS：A system for publishing XML from mixed and redundant storage. VLDB2003.

[11] Zhaohui Wu, Huajun Chen, *et al*. DartGrid：Semanticbased Database Grid. Lecture Notes in Computer Science. v3036, pp. 59-66,2004.

[12] Zhaohui Wu, Huajun Chen, *et al*. DartGrid II：A Semantic Grid Platform for ITS, IEEE Intelligent Systems, Vol.20, No.3, Jun. 2005.

[13] Mao Yuxin, Wu Zhaohui, Chen Huajun. Semantic Browser：An intelligent client for Dart-Grid, Lecture Notes in Computer Science 3036：470-473, 2004.

[14] Zhou Xuezhong, Wu Zhaohui. Ontology development for Unified Traditional Chinese Medical Language System, Journal of AI in Medicine 32(1)：15-27,2004.

[15] R. vander Meyden. Logical Approaches to Incomplete Information：A Survey. In Logics for Databases and Information Systems, p307-356. Kluwer, 1998.

[16] Imielinski T., W. Lipski Jr. Incomplete Information in Relational Databases. J. ACM 31：4,1984,pp.761-791.

Modern Bioinformatics Meets Traditional Chinese Medicine

Peiqin Gu, Huajun Chen

首发于 *Briefings In Bioinformatics*, 2013, 15(6):984-1003

Abstract

Traditional Chinese medicine (TCM) is gaining increasing attention with the emergence of integrative medicine and personalized medicine, characterized by pattern differentiation on individual variance and treatments based on natural herbal synergism. Investigating the effectiveness and safety of the potential mechanisms of TCM and the combination principles of drug therapies will bridge the cultural gap with Western medicine and improve the development of integrative medicine.

Dealing with rapidly growing amounts of biomedical data and their heterogeneous nature is two important tasks among modern biomedical communities. Bioinformatics, as an emerging interdisciplinary field of computer science and biology, has become a useful tool for easing the data deluge pressure by automating the computation processes with informatics methods. Using these methods to retrieve, store and analyze the biomedical data can effectively reveal the associated knowledge hidden in the data, and thus promote the discovery of integrated information.

Recently, these techniques of bioinformatics have been used for facilitating the interactional effects of both Western medicine and TCM. The analysis of TCM data using computational technologies provides biological evidence for the basic understanding of TCM mechanisms, safety and efficacy of TCM treatments. At the same time, the carrier and targets associated with TCM remedies can inspire the rethinking of modern drug development.

This review summarizes the significant achievements of applying bioinformatics techniques to many aspects of the research in TCM, such as analysis of TCM-related '-omics' data and techniques for analyzing biological processes and pharmaceutical mechanisms of TCM, which have shown certain potential of bringing new thoughts to both sides.

Keywords

bioinformatics; traditional Chinese medicine; systems biology; herbal synergism; linked life data

1 Introduction

Traditional Chinese medicine (TCM) is a unique Chinese health care system of ancient medical practice that covers a broad range of medical theories and practices that are based on ancient Chinese philosophy, including *Yin-Yang* theory, five-phase theory, herbal medicine and acupuncture [1]. It has played an important role in health maintenance for the people of Asia for thousands of years, and is becoming frequently used in Western countries [2]. TCM is also a part of the pantheon of traditional systems of medicine used in Asia that includes Siddha and Ayurveda, which are mainly practiced in India. Its therapies and treatment have been proven to have better effects on some fatal diseases such as malaria [3], benefiting the global health care with auxiliary therapies. In Eastern countries, TCM has a good reputation for improving the health of individuals and preventing or healing diseases, not to mention the great advantages in early intervention, combination therapies and personalized medicine for chronic diseases. In Western countries, the efficacy of herbal medicine and acupuncture has been recognized [4]. The uniqueness of the TCM system is derived from the philosophical logic behind the daily practices, which accumulates thousands of years of empirical studies and provides a unique view of the relationships between the human body and the universe. Compared with modern medicine, the underlying knowledge of TCM is rather vague because its major corpus was written in ancient natural language; however, academic and industrial agents [5] all around the world, including the Chinese government [6], have been trying to find scientific evidence that could support a deeper understanding of the mysterious Eastern medicine using modern technologies [7].

The fundamental components of TCM are different from modern medicine, and those functional units form a microecosystem of balancing forces. Thus, the conventional reduction approach in biology research cannot effectively draw useful conclusions out of the holism of TCM [8]. The main challenge for researchers is how to discover the physical existence of these units and explain the mechanisms of coherently related parts as a whole system. A systematic model of TCM components and their interrelations would be helpful to explain the physical foundation of TCM theories, just like the anatomy in Western medicine (WM), yet the model has not been proposed. Take Qi for an example; it is currently impossible to detect the physical existence of the driving forces like Qi, and therefore the understanding of the mechanisms is difficult. As the biological model of the human body is fairly clear, discovering the association relationships between modern biology (e.g. genes, proteins, molecules) and TCM entities (e.g. Qi, syndrome, herb) may uncover the biological foundation and effectiveness of TCM.

Meanwhile, from the perspective of modern medicine, understanding the functional mechanisms of the whole organism has become more popular, with increasing attention on integrative medicine [9] and personalized medicine [10]. Taking TCM as one of their parts, integrative medicine and personalized medicine emphasize wellness and healing of the entire person and deliver personalized therapeutic solutions to every individual patient rather than disease-target therapies. Systems biology—a biology-based inter-disciplinary field that has emerged as an alternative and promising method for exploring the complex systems of life using a more holistic perspective (instead of traditional reductionism)—proposes novel solutions for integrative medicine and personalized medicine involving TCM [11, 12].

2　Problems and Challenges

TCM and WM are obviously different medical systems, both of which provide support for disease diagnosis, treatment and health prevention. Research on possible relevance between these two large medical systems is likely to solve the following problems:

- Understanding the biological foundation of TCM. As we mentioned, explaining the biological foundation and core mechanisms of TCM based on the discovery of genes, proteins and molecules is gaining increasing interest among academic communities. The basic idea is to find the genetic, proteomic, cellular, molecular targets or associated biological pathways related to the three important parts of TCM: basic theories, diagnosis and treatment principles and herbal drugs. The biological findings can help researchers understand the mechanisms of TCM.

- Modern drug development inspired by TCM. Different from Western herbal medicine, in which herbs are often delivered singly or combined into small formulas of herbs with the same function, Chinese herbalists usually prescribe combined drug therapies of multiple herbs to treat a disease.

For some fatal diseases, Chinese herbal medicine has slower, but better, effects. These diseases are assumed to have complex causes and multiple targets. Investigating TCM-inspired multicomponent herbal drugs can be a future direction of multitarget drug development for effective personalized medicine.

The accumulation of a massive amount of biomedical data makes data- and knowledge-intensive computation technologies more important. Bioinformatics techniques [13], including computer science, mathematical and engineering methods, are broadly used to generate useful biological knowledge and to discover association relationships in biological data, e. g. inferring gene association networks [14]. Those methods include patternrecognition, data mining, machine-learning algorithms and visualization [15].

Combining systems biology with bioinformatics to probe the mystery of TCM potentially bridges the methodological gap between TCM and modern medicine, providing the scientific evidence to support simplification of the complexity of TCM, which can verify the value of TCM in modern medicine. These techniques serve as a driving force for the translation of TCM formulas and pathological mechanisms into practice.

In this review, we survey the available sources and bioinformatics methods that have been applied to these two concerned problems and subsequent subproblems (as shown in Figure 1), and present a vision regarding the use of semantically linked biomedical data in the future.

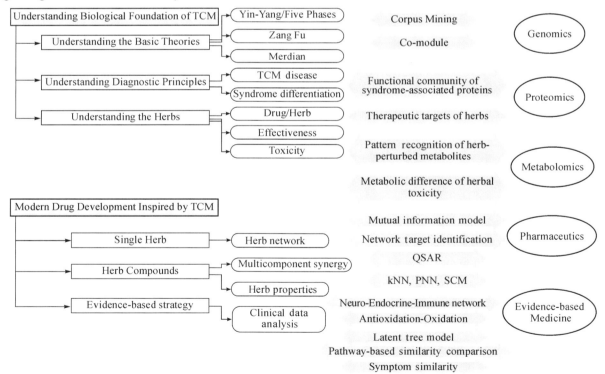

Figure 1   The research problems and applied bioinformatics solutions in Traditional Chinese Medicine.

3　TCM Meets Systems Biology

Pathological disorders can be regarded as a reaction of the human body to changes of the environment, including virus, bacteria, physical damage and internal pathological changes such as cancer. The cause and the reaction usually involve the structure and dynamics of cellular and organismal function. To understand biology at the system level, systems biology [16], an emerging field that focuses on complex interactions within biological systems, is characterized by using a holistic approach to model biological systems. It is gaining interest from academic communities and enables us to collect comprehensive data and gain system-level understanding of biological systems. A systems biological approach typically includes observing (measuring) data from different sub-categories, e. g. "-omics", physical parameters, developmental parameters, along with the various chemometric methods to extract information such as correlations and similarities between biological entities (e.g. genes, proteins, molecules).

The goals of the systems biology-based medicine potentially overlap with the holistic and integrative view of TCM, as they both aim toward personalized medicine. In the past decade, the question of whether systems biology can unify TCM and modern medicine has become an issue of growing concern. For example, to understand the Chinese medicinal concept of *Qi* in the perspective of systems biology, research suggested that the transmission of *Qi* along the meridians is based on molecules that travel via an intercellular communication system [17], in which nitric oxide is considered as a prime candidate for such a signaling molecule in the meridian system. The mechanotransduction properties of nitric oxide elicitation [18], recently modeled comprehensively, may provide important insights in this research.

Although TCM and modern medicine understand the living systems based on different criteria, there are similar disease patterns (e. g. insomnia), and the metabolites of herb-perturbed bodies can be studied and analyzed using screening to figure out the chemical compounds of the herbs and their possible targets, as demonstrated in Figure 2. Advances like this example in systems biology have enabled the discovery of biomarkers and provided the basis for the development of new targeted drugs, potentially facilitating "the right therapy for the right patient", which fits the goal of TCM. A broad range of biological technologies [19] and computer models [20], e.g. genomics, proteomics and metabolomics, that come along with systems biology, can identify biomarkers of a particular disease or herbal drugs within the set of genes, proteins and metabolites of a given organism.

This diagram illustrates the following points: (i) Syndrome refers to a pattern of disharmony that is characterized by a collection of symptoms, which can be regarded as a certain profile along with one or more diseases. (ii) Identifying the mutant genotypes responsible for certain genetic diseases can create the links between genes and TCM entities, e.g. syndromes, symptoms and drugs. (iii) With the development of proteomics and metabolomics, the contributing compounds in Chinese herbs can be filtered and studied.

3.1　TCM meets genomics

Genetic information [21] is likely to elucidate the mechanisms underlying the fundamental biological processes perturbed in human diseases and regulated pathways affected by herb intervention. The combined genome-wide expression analysis with methods of systems biology can identify the functional gene networks

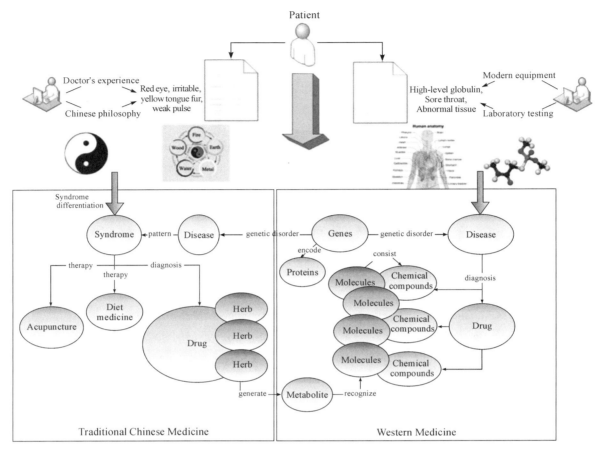

Figure 2　Interconnections and differences of TCM and WM from doctors' and biologists' perspective.

for the sets of clinical symptoms that comprise the major information for pattern classification related to pathological and treatment patterns in TCM [22]. With the accumulation of biological data, data about genetic regulated diseases and the corresponding herbal therapies are growing. In recent years, many herbal medicines have been reported to be associated with various symptoms or diseases and may exhibit a variety of effects through regulation of a wide range of gene expressions or protein activities.

1）Discovering TCM-gene relationships from corpus learning

Hidden knowledge about the association relationships between genes and TCM entities implicitly exist in varieties of textual corpus. Those associations come from isolated small biological experiments all over the world. Through corpus analysis, pieces of association information can be gathered and integrated to support high-level data analysis.

The most popular TCM information database, *TCMGeneDIT* [23], collected information from public databases, including TCM herb database HULU, TCM-ID, NCBI Entrez Gene and medical subject headings vocabulary, to form a unique database that offers diverse association information related to TCM and participating genes. The collected terms of TCM names, gene names, medical subject headings vocabulary diseases and TCM ingredients were used to annotate the literature corpus obtained from the literature database PubMed using entity annotation. Useful co-occurrence and corresponding confidence values can then be observed through association discovery and rule-based extraction during corpus analysis. The final results contain association groups as (TCM, gene), (TCM, disease), (TCM, gene, disease), (TCM, ingredient), (TCM, effect) and (gene, ingredient). The creation of such a database could facilitate the understanding of therapeutic mechanisms involving TCM and gene interactions, which would further be used to inspire modern clinical research.

Wu *et al*. [24] also applied a text mining approach to uncover the functional relationships from PubMed literature. They used a bootstrapping method to extract disease names from TCM-related articles, and then extracted the relationship of symptom complex (SC) and disease based on disease names and SC terminological database. Here, SC refers to a holistic concept reflecting the dynamic, functional, temporal and spatial morbid status of the human body. The term co-occurrence is used to identify the disease-gene and SC-gene relationships within the articles. It is suggested that the related genes of the same SC will have some functional interactions. In all, 1100 SC-disease relationships were collected, e. g. 72 related genes of kidney YangXu SC were filtered, such as chronic renal failure. In TCM, syndromes play an important role in disease diagnosis; it is reasonable to guess that the related genes of the same syndrome may also have some biological functional relationships. Similar work has been done to find syndrome-gene relations [25].

2) Novel representation of drug-gene-disease patterns

Genes share notable patterns with respect to diseases, syndromes and even drugs. Zhao *et al*. [26] proposed an alternative approach to define drug-gene-disease relationships, called *co-module*, to characterize closely related drugs, diseases and genes. A co-module consists of a gene module and those drugs and diseases associated with it. They implemented a Bayesian partition method to identify drug-gene-disease co-modules underlying the gene closeness data. In a gene closeness profile, a gene whose products are more highly interconnected in the network with drug targets or disease-gene products, receives a higher closeness score with respect to that drug or disease. Given these gene closeness data, one can find important genes interconnected with drug targets or disease-related genes. Though not directly mentioned in the article, the approach of discovering co-modules should be useful or highlight the genetic basis of TCM diseases and drugs.

3) TCM patterns of clinical manifestations based on gene profiles

Genome-wide expression analysis in *in vivo* studies can also be used with methods of systems biology to identify the functional gene networks for clinical patterns in TCM. In TCM, cold and hot patterns are two opposite properties that are used to identify and categorize the universe of things, such as food, diseases, etc., classify symptoms and conduct treatment. The clinical manifestations of a specific disease can be clustered into these two patterns before blood samples, and the genes significantly related to hot and cold patterns can be identified to study the mechanism of pathogenesis and diagnosis criteria of TCM. This approach has recently been implemented in a study of rheumatoid arthritis [27], a systemic autoimmune disease with unknown cause and various treatment methods. Through factor analysis and correlation analysis, the genes were used to search protein interaction information from protein interaction databases and literature data, and consequently several significant pathways were found to be related to TCM patterns.

From the aforementioned work, we have found that the associations between genome and TCM entities including diseases, syndromes, drugs and patterns have already existed in a broad range of literature, databases and patient samples, which are available for textural analysis and association discovery. The associations discovered can be analyzed to infer advanced relations, such as protein pathways related to diseases, and the molecular basis of TCM clinical patterns. In all, we proposed a basic workflow of such data processing jobs, as shown in Figure 3. Recently, a new scientific field of toxicogenomics has been proposed to investigate the toxicity and reactions based on the integration of genomics and toxicology, which is another important concern regarding the safety of the natural products used in TCM herbal medicine [28].

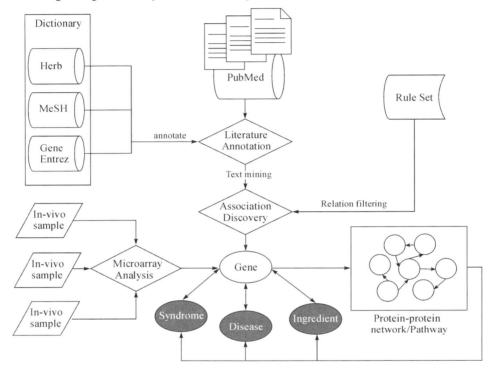

Figure 3   Bioinformatics workflow in the study of genome-related TCM.

3. 2   TCM meets proteomics

As proteins are vital parts of living organisms, proteomics gives us a better understanding of an organism by studying the structures and functions of proteins. In a model organism, proteomics [29] aims to identify and quantify the cellular levels of each protein that is encoded by the genome, through studying protein biomarkers, identifying gene-modified proteins and establishing protein-protein interactions. One aim of systems biology is to model the whole cell by integrating such protein-protein interactions [30], which can likely be aided by using the whole physiome approaches of ancient systems of medicine such as TCM. It can be used to link genomics and metabolism, leading to an integrated understanding of the entire organism. In addition, the ability to detect expressed proteins has enormous potential for early diagnostics and intervention at curable stages of disease and multitarget drug development.

With the broad use of systems biology technologies, the adoption of the proteomics technologies can potentially leverage the study of pharmacological effects and their action mechanisms of TCM [31]. For example, using proteomics approaches, it was found that the Siwu decoction, which is an ancient TCM therapy for enriching blood tonic, could regulate the protein expression of the bone marrow of blood-deficient mice [32]. Fundamentally, proteomics can benefit the research in TCM in two ways: (i) Proteomics could provide a platform for studying the cellular basis of diagnostic principles of TCM. In modern therapeutics, individual variance concerning expression profiles of proteins is of great importance in TCM syndrome variance. (ii) Proteomics technologies can be used to screen the target molecules of the action of TCM, isolate and characterize new active components, as well as analyze toxic substances from TCM. Using proteomic approaches to identify therapeutic targets, to evaluate the effects of new drugs and to explore the functional mechanism of the effects of new drugs may meet the shortcomings of the conventional methodology being applied in the current studies.

1) Identifying functional community of syndrome-associated proteins

Syndrome ("Zheng" in Chinese) is an essential part of TCM theory, which refers to a characteristic profile of all clinical manifestations (e.g. symptoms) that can be identified by TCM practitioners as an important criterion during diagnosis. All these characteristics of TCM syndromes might be related to various proteins with different contents, functions, structures and interactions of proteins expressed for different syndrome behaviors, and the changes of proteins before and after treatment with single herb or formulas could be analyzed. Understanding of the characteristic changes in proteomics associated with a specific syndrome will facilitate syndrome identification and novel diagnostic approaches that will potentially lead to personalized health care strategies [33].

A practical way to investigate the proteome basis of syndrome is to study syndrome in the context of the expressed proteins of a specific disease, for example, coronary heart disease (CHD). According to experimental survey [34], blood stasis syndrome in TCM plays an important role in CHD patients. In clinical analysis, WM specifications and diagnosis criterion of the syndrome were both studied given blood samples of patient profiles. The case group and the control group were analyzed using traditional bioinformatics methods to obtain significant proteins related to the specific disease. As there are no standardized models of disease-syndrome, one way to study the associations between certain syndromes and proteomes is through pattern discovery over prior data of related proteins and symptoms. Mutual information between each pair of variables (e.g. proteins, symptoms) can be studied, and the set that has the high correlative value of variables will be considered significant. Thus, this approach can generate a bunch of identified patterns of closely related proteins and symptoms, and the validation results showed that discovering a protein-symptom pattern helps understand the molecular basis of syndrome.

2) Finding potential therapeutic targets of Chinese herbs

The components of Chinese herbal medicine, either a single herb or formulas, are complex chemical systems, and each component binds to its own target receptor. Typical proteomics technologies such as 2D electrophoresis with mass spectrometry can reveal statistically significant changes in the intensity of proteins, which will provide clues for studying the cellular mechanisms of Chinese herb medicine.

Salvia miltiorrhiza (SAME) ("Dan Shen" in Chinese) has been widely used for the treatment of cardiovascular and cerebrovascular diseases in Chinese herbal medicine, yet little is known about its cellular mechanisms except for the effect of relieving oxidative stress. Thus, in 2010, a research group from Taiwan [35] investigated the protein-protein inter-action network related to the herb SAME using pathway analysis, to identify transcriptional factors in its cellular mechanisms. To evaluate the effect of salvianolic acid B (the main compound of SAME) on A10 cells, differential protein expression in Hcy-induced A10 cells with or without SAME treatment was uploaded into MetaCore bioinformatics software for network analysis. Basically, the analysis algorithm attempted to deduce scoring processes regulated by differentially expressed proteins, and to find the shortest path in a protein network of the smallest possible number of direct interactions between differentially expressed proteins. The protein interaction network results indicated that proteins expressed after SAME treatment were primarily involved in regulating oxidation, the apoptotic process and cytoskeletal rearrangement. Other than that, SAME was related to the inhibition of reactive oxygen species levels, as well as modulation of several transcriptional factors such as c-Fos, C-Myc and p53. The study provided proteomic and pathway evidence that SAME exhibits a protective effect by inhibiting oxidative stress-induced damage.

Figure 4 demonstrates the common workflow of applying these computational methods to the analysis of symptom, syndrome, disease and related proteins. The principal task of today's drug discovery process is to identify the biotargets that are related to diseases, clinical profiles, herbs or drugs. Proteomics appreciates the individual differences that are characterized by distinct profiles during disease development and drug response, and the interaction network or pathways among proteins show great value for exploring the potential value of TCM, including disease patterns and herbal medicine. The future of proteomics combined with TCM will enhance the development of drug discovery and personalized therapy.

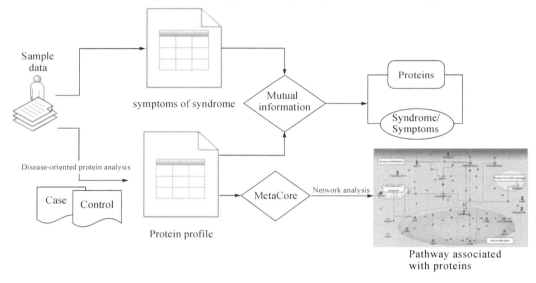

Figure 4　Bioinformatics workflow in the study of proteome-related TCM.

3.3　TCM meets metabolomics

Metabolites are the products that specific cellular processes leave behind. Metabolomics [36] is a novel discipline that studies the metabolic profiles, which contribute to the identification of metabolic features corresponding to medical treatment or drug therapies. As a systemic approach, metabolomics adopts a "top-down" strategy to reflect the function of organisms from the end products, and thus to understand the metabolic changes of a living system, usually through urine or plasma samples, which can further lead to the complete understanding of the body reaction.

The ability to understand the dynamic responses to the changes toward integrated living systems can make things easier in the study of complex systems such as TCM [37], with the observation of both endogenous and exogenous factors. Motivated by the intervention effects of Chinese formulas and herb medicine, the characters and changes of the metabolomics profiling can be analyzed with a range of statistical and machine-learning algorithms. The technologies of metabolomics have been successively applied to the key scientific issues in TCM by the international and domestic scholars with metabolomic technology, including syndrome, differential treatment of the individual, synthetic effect of Chinese herbs, molecular pharmacology [38] and quality control of Chinese medicine [39]. At the same time, metabolomics approaches may potentially benefit the combination between TCM and WM[40] by facilitating the evaluation of the therapeutic effects of TCM formula and understanding of the possible action mechanisms of herbal medicine.

1) Biomarker metabolites associated with certain Chinese herb

Chinese herbal medicine provides modern medicine with a collection of complementary remedies for disease treatment and health maintenance. Some of the natural herbs are known to have good effect on the diseases that are not fully understood regarding their molecular mechanisms. Metabolomics can study the biomarker metabolites and perturbed pathways associated with these herbs, providing insights for drug action mechanisms.

A famous Chinese herbal remedy, "*Suanzaoren decoction*", has been used in TCM to treat *insomnia* for a long time, yet the molecular mechanism and key metabolites underlying it are not fully clear. A research institute in China presented a method with regard to the natural product extracted from SuanZaoRen decoction, "*Jujuboside B (JuB)*" [41], which is considered to be the major pharmacological active compound responsible for insomnia treatment. Metabolic data of both control and case groups were analyzed to detect the enriched clusters. Multivariate projection approaches such as principal component analysis (PCA) and partial least-squares-discriminant analysis were applied to raw spectrometric data to identify various metabolites as potential biomarkers. Typically, the metabolic profiles of disease cases and controls are compared to identify spectral features and discriminatory variables. The supervised orthogonal projection to latent structures-discriminant analysis was implemented to separate significant metabolites from the two groups, which can be viewed as potential biomarkers, suggesting the metabolic profiles have significantly changed as a result of sleep deprivation. The intermediate data were subjected to computational systems analysis to further investigate the effects of JuB on the insomnia *Drosophila* metabolite profiles, the parallel PCA score trajectory plots, hierarchical clustering analysis and heatmap visualization was used to distinguish perturbed metabolomics models, which showed that JuB exhibits preventive efficacy by adjusting target metabolic pathways to their normal state. Once the influenced pathways are targeted and analyzed, new drugs can be designed for insomnia.

2) Metabolomics study on the toxicity on Chinese herbs

Although herbal remedies are available to treat various illnesses, little or no actual scientific basis of their toxicity and safety was presented. Under this circumstance, doctors cannot provide enough experimental evidence while guiding their patients regarding proper use or potential toxicity. Metabolites before or after herbal treatment provide measureable objects for studying the pharmacological activity and potential toxicity of herbs.

Aconite root (*Fuzi* in Chinese), a herb in TCM, has been popularly used in herbal medicine in Asia for thousands of years, commonly applied for various diseases, i.e. rheumatic fever, painful joints, etc. However, the original plant can be toxic and fatal and, to date, the toxicological risk of its usage is not clear. As a TCM herbal processing approach, *Paozhi* is supposed to reduce the toxicity of aconite root and exert maximal therapeutic efficacy. Studying the metabolomics profiling changes of processing can help define the scientific parameters for evaluating safety and toxicity of drugs [42].

To compare the metabolic profiles of crude herb and processed products, the resultant data matrices were processed for pattern recognition analysis of significant metabolic patterns. The data were imported to EZinfo 2.0 software for PCA, partial least-squares-discriminant analysis and orthogonal projection to latent structures analysis. To maximize cluster discrimination, the data were further analyzed using the orthogonal projection to latent structures-discriminant analysis method. Same as identifying targeting metabolites, variables in the computation results that contributed significantly to discrimination between groups were considered as potential biomarkers. The results indicated that NaK-ATP activity was increased and Lactate dehydrogenase (LDH) and Aspartate Transaminase (AST) values were decreased in the processed group compared with the crude group; this proved that herbal processing can actually achieve weak toxicity of toxic herbs.

Metabolomics approaches, as a strong link among genomics, proteomics and molecular biology, have shown increasing effect on providing biochemical evidence of the mechanisms of the metabolomics network in the study of TCM drug development and herbal medicine. Until now, using metabolomics in combination with TCM pharmacology is a convincing way for the discovery of novel biological active compounds as well as for proving herbal safety. No doubt that metabolomics will gradually promote Chinese medicine research, and bioinformatics methods such as pattern recognition algorithms will speed up the process.

4 TCM Herbal Medicine Meets Modern Pharmaceutics

In TCM, medical treatment is determined by a holistic characterization of the patient's health status (i.e. disease, syndrome), and is thus followed by a prescription that comprises a group of herbs specially tailored for the patient. Most of the Chinese medicinal prescriptions have relatively complex combination of herbs and complex targeting preparation, which usually lead to one or more pharmacological mechanisms [43]. The active components have been isolated from those TCM herbs for chemical compound analysis, and some findings are used in modern pharmaceutical drugs [44]. As multicomponent drug development is gaining rising interest among numerous drug companies, investigating the effective components of TCM herbal remedies and medicinal plants [45] become a novel trend to invent new drugs [46].

The core philosophy of modern drug development is the biochemical decomposing process of herbal medicine and tagging the targeting biomarkers. For instance, an herb that we mentioned before—*Fuzi*, the cardiotonic active substanceture related to catecholamines. The alternative way of studying the active components of the herbs is through targeted agents affected by herbs. The targeted agents refer to the drug carrier that selectively concentrates on the target site through local delivery or whole-body blood circulation, such as liposomes, nanoparticles and emulsion [47]. Research on targeted agents can help profoundly understand the structural characteristics and mechanism of drug carrier and achieve clinical targeting drug delivery system.

4. 1　TCM Herb databases

TCM database@ Taiwan [48] is claimed to be the world's largest 3D molecular structure database for TCM drug screening, download and search. The database contains >20000 pure compounds isolated from 453 TCM ingredients in the form of 2D and 3D structures. The database supports simple and advanced web-based query options that can specify search clauses, such as molecular properties, substructures, TCM ingredients and 2D/3D visualization of molecules.

An integrated knowledge portal TCMOnline (http://www. cintcm. com) [49] is developed and maintained by China Academy of Traditional Chinese Medicine. Currently, TCMOnline database system is the largest TCM data collection in the world, integrating 17 branches in China and >50 TCM-related databases, including chemical ingredients of Chinese herbal medicines constituting Chinese medicinal formula. A comprehensive e-Science architecture [50] was built above these databases to support large-scale database integration and knowledge-intensive applications.

4. 2　Exploring functional herbal network

Because of the common occurrence of compound therapies, studying functional herbal network of TCM herbs reflects the associations and the combinational patterns among various herbs, which can provide insights for studying the molecular mechanisms of herbs and improving drug design.

In the information science, mutual information (MI) of two variables refers to a quantity that measures the mutual dependence of the two variables, which, in this case, are two herbs. The MI between a pair of variables X and Y can be defined $I(X,Y) = H(X) + H(Y) - H(X,Y)$, where $H(X,Y) = -\sum\limits_{p(x,y)} \log p(x,y)$ is the joint entropy of X and Y.

A herb network can be constructed by studying the MI among herbs from the numerous herbal formulas. Li *et al*. [51] proposed a distance-based mutual information model to identify combination mechanisms among herbs. The formula data were collected from SIRC-TCM Herbal Formula database and transformed into a numeral matrix $A = (a_{ij})_{m \times n}$ ($a_{ij} = 0$ means herb j is absent in formula i) to indicate the relative position of the herbs in a formula. They provided an integrated scoring system combining the MI entropy characteristics and the "between-herb-distance" d between herbs: $score(x,y) = \dfrac{MI(x,y)}{d(x,y)}$, which describes the tendency of herbs x and y to form a herb pair. The efficacy of distance-based mutual information model method to uncover the combination rules of herbs has been successfully validated through a frequently used herbal formula Liu Wei Di Huang by co-module analysis.

Sometimes to remove the noisiness of the entropy data, random permutation test is used to set a sound threshold for MI process. Random permutation test estimates the approximate sampling distribution based on the large number of random permutation samples. The network construction of treatment cases based on this method applied in tumor diseases[52] indicated the complex entropy network is suitable for the analysis of interaction effects among multifactors through the analysis of examples. Similarly, the entropy network method can also be applied to construct subnetworks such as "herb-herb", "herb-syndrome", "herb-symptom" and " syndrome-symptom ", and assess the correlation of multifactors by the statistical information of networks. Network-based analysis can be useful in predicting therapeutic mechanisms of specific herb on specific disease, such as SAME and atherosclerosis [53].

Common biological networks shared by different diseases and various herbal formulas might have meaningful evidence corresponding to the commonly existing functional networks. For Rheumatoid Arthritis and CHD diseases that sometimes are treated with similar therapies, literature data were extracted from PubMed and SinoMed, and analyzed with data slicing algorithm [54] to generate commonly existing biological networks.

4.3　Identifying multicomponent targets

The multicomponent synergy in Chinese herbs is of great significance for understanding TCM herbal medicine, and most importantly, of great value nowadays for the novel drug discovery. Usually the action mechanism of the multiple components is studied separately; however, a novel concept, "*network target*" [55], has been proposed to consider simultaneously the disease mechanisms and drug actions on a network basis. A network target comes from the single target-based and multiple target-based drug studies, referring to a therapeutic target that is derived from systematic interventions of the biology network underlying a disease or pathological process. The mechanisms of herbal synergism [56] can be investigated by *in vivo* studies using drug combination analysis methods and network-based analysis of the molecular interaction profiles and pathways regulatory actions of active ingredients.

Li *et al*.[57] proposed a network target-based identification of multicomponent synergy (NIMS) method to access the synergistic strength of multicomponent therapeutics. They measured synergistic agent combinations by introducing and integrating two parameters, named topology score and agent score. Then, NIMS was applied to prioritize synergistic combinations from the agents including herbs or herb compounds. Two graph-based measures, betweenness and closeness, were used to capture the associations among variables, and the other measure, PageRank, to verify the node importance. Interestingly, when NIMS is applied to the angiogenesis network, two synergistic agent pairs, "Sinomenine and Matrine" and "Sinomenine and Honokiol", are found to be the main constituents of TCM herbal formulas Qing Luo Yin and Tou Gu Zhen Feng. The preliminary results demonstrated that NIMS, as a software tool, has the potential for screening synergistic combinations of Chinese herbal formulas, as well as modern drugs.

Wang *et al*.[58] developed a quantitative structure-activity relationship (QSAR) to study the multiobject optimization of component combination in drug design. The basic idea of optimal combination of drugs is to obtain best biological activities and minimal side effects. In QSAR, a multicomponent combination of different doses of n components $C_i(i=1,2,\cdots,n)$ was represented within a certain combination vector $[T_R^1, T_R^2,\cdots,T_R^n]$. They introduced a mathematical function $Y_R = f(X_R)$ to quantify the multicomponent combination of chemical composition and biological activities, where $X_R^i = C_i * T_R^i(i=1,2,\cdots,n)$ stands for the composition of R. This algorithm-based knowledge discovery method first quantitatively interprets the relationship between combinations and their activities into a model, and then uses the proposed model to simulate the real-life drug formula combinations. It was found to be valuable in providing potential association information for studying the design of Chinese formula Shenmai.

The biological activities of the Chinese herbal medicine are unclear because of their complex nature and the possible interaction among the combined therapies. With the DNA microarray data, gene expression profiles were analyzed to compare disease-altered genes and drug-altered genes, and transcriptomic analysis was used to perform pathway analysis and gene expression similarities in different formulas. This method [59] has been applied to study the top 15 most used Chinese herbal formulas and the comparison results indicated that the TCM formula treatments might be related to metabolic, cardiovascular, neuroskeletal and hepatic diseases.

Network-based computational technologies based on systems biology strategies have been widely used in modern drug discovery, mostly in herbal synergy study through mathematical modeling of specific biological processes or pathways to study global cellular effects of multitarget drugs or multicomponent therapies [60]. For example, recent work on CytoSolve [61], based on systems biology principles, aims to provide a broad-based platform, for whole cell modeling, which enables the integration of large-scale biological pathways to understand such cellular effects to discover multicomponent therapies [62]. As one part of the research, molecular networks provide potential target sets for constructing drug-or disease-associated networks, benefiting the development of TCM pharmacology [63].

4.4　Distinguishing the herbal properties

To improve the research of TCM pharmaceutics, studying the herb properties (HPs) of the herb recipes and keeping track of herb-related entities can be helpful in modulating the pharmacological and toxicological effects of the chemical ingredients of the constituent herbs. Here, HP refers to the fundamental parameters (such as characters, tastes, toxic states, meridians) in TCM herbs.

Ung *et al.*[64] divided the TCM-HPs into four classes: character (C), taste (T), meridian (M) and toxicity level (Tox). These classes can be further divided into 5, 5, 12 and 2 subclasses, respectively. Each herb can be represented with a vector $h = (C, T, M, Tox)$ of the TCM-HPs with 39 features. The value of HP is 1 if the herb possesses the corresponding property, and it is 0 if the herb does not possess the property. For an herb pair composed of herbs A and B, two separate vectors $h_{AB} = (h_A, h_B)$ and $h_{BA} = (h_B, h_A)$ of dimension 78 can be formed, both of which were used to represent the herb pair. Given TCM herb pairs and randomly generated non-TCM herb pairs, artificial intelligent methods were applied to attempt to distinguish TCM herb pairs from non-TCM herb pairs. Mainly, probabilistic neural network method is used to classify the HPs, and k nearest neighbor is used to predict the class of unclassified vector (new herb pair). Known TCM herb pairs and non-TCM herb pairs in a training set were adjusted by using a separate testing set of TCM herb pairs and non-TCM herb pairs. By projecting the feature vector of new multiherb pairs, support vector machine (SVM) method can be used to determine whether it is a valid TCM herb pair based on its location with respect to the hyperplane. The classification results suggested that TCM-HPs of TCM herb pairs contain distinguishable features that contribute to the synergistic combinations.

4.5　Novel drug discovery

Although the success of the antimalarial drug artemisinin was inspired by Chinese herbal therapies, the pharmacological effectiveness of Chinese material medica has not led to the successful development of new drugs. Systems biology technologies and bioinformatics approaches [65, 66] are making promising progress in opening up the opportunities of developing new drugs [67] from herb-drug interactions [68].

It is recognized that Chinese herbs are usually screened for compounds that may be active against certain targets. In modern biomedicine, enzymes and receptors represent the most common drug targets. Target-based drug discovery is an important strategy for developing new agents. Thus, a new concept of drug discovery is a reverse approach to find and separate the active compounds from TCM by using virtual screening, immobilized enzymes [69], polyclonal antibodies and molecularly imprinted polymers. Databases of Chinese herbal constituents are being created [70], providing the community with more detailed information of Chinese herbs.

Moreover, intelligent computing algorithms such as data mining approaches [71] can be applied in TCM-inspired drug discovery. Zhou *et al.* [72] proposed a structure-activity relationship method to identify potential active ingredients in natural products. An SVM model was trained to learn the structural activity relationship of bioactive NP ingredients. Decision tree algorithms and rule set algorithms were applied to pick out important descriptors in bioactive ingredient prediction. The method should find evidence about the therapeutic mechanisms and synergies of natural products, whose ingredients can potentially compose drugs.

There are so many active fields in the integration of TCM herbal medicine and modern pharmaceutics, and drug discovery based on effective Chinese herbs seems promising with the help of various computational analysis methods and emerging data resources. Except for manual curation, knowledge about herbal information can also be extracted from textual data [73], with the assistance of domain-specific ontology models. In addition, currently in the field of TCM herbal medicine, a novel concept "herbogenomics" is defined as the analysis of the biological effect of the target objects of aparticular herbal medicine through a profiling of the affected genomic and proteomic changes. Integrating genomic and proteomic profile changes into the research of the efficacy and toxicity of herbal medicine [74] will provide novel insights into all the mechanism and action studies of TCM herbal medicine.

5 TCM Meets Evidence-Based Medicine

In Chinese medicine, diagnosis is highly related to contextual information, including not only a detailed profile of the patient at the moment but also the external factors such as climate, emotional states, joint problems, types of pain, fever, etc. Practitioners collect these symptoms through four typical methods: inspection, auscultation-olfaction, inquiry and palpation. Doctors will deliver diagnosis and treatment based on a holistic understanding of the patient's condition. This diagnostic process in TCM is rather experience-based than science-based, so explicit evidence is missing in explaining the mechanisms, efficacy and safety of the diagnosis.

Recently, the novel discipline called "evidence-based medicine" [75] aims to deliver optimized health care by informing clinical decision making in diagnosis and systems biology-supported personalized health strategies [76] with the use of computation estimate of the benefits and the harm. It can potentially enable the researchers from both TCM and WM in assessing the strength of the evidence found in various data sets and analysis and benefit the integrated treatments. Until now, evidence-based approaches in TCM [77] have been focusing on major fields such as improvement of poor treatment, reduction of severe adverse effects, unwanted interactions of standard therapy with herbal medicines and efficacy and safety of TCM treatments. Moreover, there are a lot of successful case studies [78] that showed finding evidence in TCM helps improve new drug discovery and functional food therapies in modern drug development.

5. 1　Understanding TCM concepts

Here, the TCM concepts refer to the core entities in the basic theoretical systems of TCM that play an important role in mapping and shaping the universe, making treatment decisions and delivering personalized therapies. One of the understanding obstacles between WM and TCM is that they disagree with each other on the concept level. WM is based on modern mathematics and TCM is based on ancient understanding of the nature.

1）Understanding *Zheng*

"*Zheng*" (syndrome) differentiation is often used as a guideline in TCM disease diagnosis, and has been recently incorporated with biomedical diagnosis [79]. There is no equivalent concept in WM, although there could be a biomedical path that may explain the molecular and cellular mechanisms of the "*Zheng*" concept.

One of the explanations of the molecular basis of *Zheng* is the context of neuro-endocrine-immune (NEI) network system [80]. In modern medicine, NEI system acts as a pivot in modulating host homeostasis and adjusting health through complex communication among hormones, cytokines and neuro-transmitters. NEI network and *Zheng* network can be extracted from PubMed articles through text mining, and by topological comparison and the pathway analysis of networks of Hot *Zheng* and Cold *Zheng*, it was found that hormones are predominant in the Cold *Zheng* network, immune factor is predominant in the Hot *Zheng* network and these two networks are connected by neurotransmitters. Here, Hot *Zheng* and Cold *Zheng* are widely applied in the diagnosis and treatment of patients in TCM as two different patterns. The results demonstrated the distinguishable differences between Hot *Zheng* and Cold *Zheng* in TCM in terms of different targets and different receptors in a biological communication network.

Specifically, Ma *et al*. [81] focused on the implicit stratification of Cold Syndrome by surveying 4575 cases of Cold Syndrome patients and examining gene expression information of a typical Cold Syndrome pedigree by microarray. The symptom patterns of Cold Syndrome can be standardized using latent tree model. The Cold Syndrome was represented as quantitative scale that is composed of 20 factors, such as the 10 fixed cold body parts from head to feet. Each cold factor can have value 0, 1, 2 and 3, standing for none, mild, moderate and severe level, respectively. The latent variables derived from the latent tree model of Cold Syndrome are three categories of elements, namely, cold adaption, cold behaviors and cold areas. On combining the multifactor measurements with NEI network, results indicated that Cold Syndrome-related genes play an essential role in energy metabolism.

For more specific studies of syndromes, latent tree models have been applied in the validation of Kidney-Yin deficiency syndrome and Kidney-Yang deficiency syndrome [82] in elderly women with menopausal symptoms. In the study of multitarget molecular pharmacology of *Qi*-deficiency and Blood-stasis syndrome (QDBS), high-throughput gene microarrays before and after treatment with Fuzheng Huayu Capsule were analyzed [83]. Patients with QDBS suffer from energy deficiency and blood stasis. It is related with a bunch of diseases such as diabetes mellitus, dyslipidemia, hypertension, hepatitis and liver cirrhosis. Fuzheng Huayu Capsule is a recipe for treating liver fibrosis with QDBS. A pathway-based similarity comparison method was proposed based on a microarray database "Connectivity Map", which collects microarrays corresponding to treatment of different small molecules in different human cell lines. A gene set repository Sigpathway was referenced to sort out the meaningful gene sets and pathway information according to the microarray data. The expression pattern similarity between the microarrays and in the Connectivity Map Database in every selected pathway was calculated using KS-test, whose result will be either positive or negative.

2) Understanding Yin-Yang

It is a well-known concept that refers to contrary forces in the natural world, and how they give rise to each other. The basic theories of TCM fundamentally rely on the understanding of *Yin-Yang* balance in the diagnosis and treatment of diseases. However, the *Yin-Yang* balance has not been studied by modern scientific means. One of the convincing explanations of *Yin-Yang* balance is antioxidation-oxidation with Yin representing antioxidation and Yang oxidation [84]. In their article, they found the fact that the Yin-tonic traditional Chinese herbs have about six times more antioxidant activity and polyphenolic contents than the Yangtonic herbs on average.

5.2 Advanced medical diagnosis

Medical diagnosis in TCM is a complex reasoning process based on the identification and differentiation of symptoms, syndromes and diseases. Modern diseases can sometimes find corresponding description, symptoms and treatments in TCM, e.g. Parkinson's disease [85]. However, there are several challenging problems that need to be solved to transform the reasoning process to an interpretable model of diagnostic rules. First, no regularized architecture of these entities exists because of the relatively non-standardized naming in ancient descriptions. Second, although the diagnosis in TCM is based on individuals' experience, the clinical records of thousands of years of accumulation contain larger amount of information than well-structured data of prescriptions extracted manually from TCM literature. These data can be an important source for discovering useful patterns and regularities in TCM. Last, owing to different experience and background of TCM doctors, the same concept might be described in several different terms, which will cause inconsistency and duplicate issues.

Wang *et al*. [86] addressed the problem of automatic symptom name normalization by measuring the similarity between the clinical symptom name to be normalized and all possible standard forms. The background knowledge is that most of the symptoms listed in clinical records have >1 synonym. Based on the experiment evaluation, after all kinds of similarity distance calculation within the features of dynamic programming, vector space model, it was found that the symptoms can be normalized into reasonable and accurate standard ones among three similarity metrics—literal similarity metrics, remedy-based similarity metrics and hybrid similarity metrics. This automatic symptom name normalization method is important in advancing a unified system of medical theories and diagnosis. Apart from similarity metric normalization, MI among symptoms provides an alternative way to study the relations between symptoms based on clustering of associated symptoms with Bayesian network construction [87].

In the process of TCM diagnosis, not only the normalization of symptom names but also the differentiation of syndromes matters. Mapping into an abstract model, syndrome differentiation is basically a classifier that classifies patients into different classes based on their symptoms. For example, Kidney-Yang deficiency is a TCM syndrome concluded from the observation of manifestations, from symptoms such as "cold limbs". The relationships between symptoms and syndromes can be regarded as a model of latent trees [88, 89], in which syndrome is represented as a latent variable and symptoms as manifest variables. Abstractly speaking, the task of TCM diagnosis is to classify the input to latent variables that have been defined, based on the differentiation of manifest variables. Formally, a latent tree model can be represented as $M = (G, \theta)$, where G stands for the model structure plus cardinalities of variables, and θ stands for the vector of probability parameters. In a case study of a subdomain of TCM diagnosis—kidney deficiency, a bunch of symptom variables were selected in data collection phase and analyzed with the kidney data using learning algorithm, and consequently generate models of latent trees as natural clusters. The results showed that there exist natural clusters in data that correspond to TCM syndrome types.

More interesting attempts tried to associate the basic theories of TCM diagnosis and treatment principles with a multilateral system of mathematical representations and relationships [90], namely, two kinds of opposite relations and one kind of equivalence relation, to formalize the treatment principles in mathematical way, and the reasoning of the mathematical assertions proves that the principles are true.

In modern TCM research, it is possible to integrate syndrome differentiation [91] with orthodox medical diagnosis leading to new scientific findings in overall medical diagnosis and treatment. The key challenge in TCM syndrome differentiation research is how to standardize the diagnostic procedure for syndrome. Modern technologies are applied into the syndrome differentiation in diagnosis, clinical research, pharmacological research, new drug discovery and medical equipment development. The way toward to identify evidence of TCM syndrome differentiation in TCM practice requires multidisciplinary collaborations from biomedical, bioinformatics, medical, pharmaceutical and TCM disciplines. Pattern differentiation in TCM will help identify a subset of patients who are more likely to respond to combination biomedical therapy treatment [92]. In addition, specific diagnostic examples such as apoptosis pathways in cancer related with Chinese medicine [93] and the QSAR study of the bioactivity of the TCM compounds in stroke treatment [94] were studied to understand the mechanisms of diseases andthe novel therapeutics.

6　Next-Generation Platform for Biomedical Integration

6.1　The rise of Semantic Web technologies in biomedicine

A massive amount of biological data has been generated, which has led to the adoption of tools for automated analysis of the biological knowledge and the full integration of heterogeneous data. Because of the data diversity and semantic heterogeneity of biological data [95], it is essential for the whole biomedical community to share a standardized data and knowledge representation paradigm. In the past decade, the amount of biological ontologies [96] has been growing, within the definition that ontology is a technology in Semantic Web used to represent and share knowledge about a domain by modeling the things in that domain and the relationships between those things.

Specifically, ontology is becoming a technology advocated by computer scientists and bioinformaticians to overcome problems of heterogeneity and to form a linked web of structured knowledge instead of sparse data distributions. In Semantic Web, the basic idea of representing knowledge is resource description framework (RDF) [97] and Web Ontology Language [98], in which the resources (e. g. specific genes, gene-encoded proteins) are formatted and linked by binary associations. The resources form a directed knowledge graph with each node assigned with unique web identifiers, which can enable the contents to be stored, managed and queried within any persistent systems or web environment. Through the abstractions of biomedical semantics [99], the Semantic Web offers an ideal platform for representing and linking biomedical information among different researchers. Community efforts have already been made, including the growing repository Bio2RDF [100] that contains ~5 billion triples, including omics information [101] such as genes [102] and proteins [103] and other resources such as pathways [104], diseases [105] and drugs [106]. With the strong power of expressivity and connectivity of ontology resources, the knowledge-supported biomedical data should be able to import rules like "If Gene X is implicated in Disease D, and its Protein Product Y is a functional component of only Pathway P ⟶ Then Disease D directly perturbs Pathway P", and answer complex cross-discipline questions that are associated with customized requests such as drug discovery [107, 108].

In today's cyberinfrastructure of biological information processing [109], Semantic Web technologies are playing a more important role in greatly reducing the amount of coordination needed among participants, which will potentially accelerate the development of biomedical information communication.

6.2 Use case: modern biomedical integration

Standardized representation and computational analysis of biomedical data have become increasingly important, and this situation provides us with a speedy way of facilitating the communication of TCM and systems biology from accumulated high-throughput data. With the increasing amount of biomedical ontologies [110], we believe that the integration of biomedical data on the semantic level might bring hope to the research of TCM and modern medicine in two steps: (i) connect various kinds of information from published trustworthy data sources [111] and make the resources recognizable and linkable and (ii) introduce associated knowledge into the linked data and make the data available for association discovery and comprehensive knowledge inference. The basic idea of the connections is demonstrated in Figure 5.

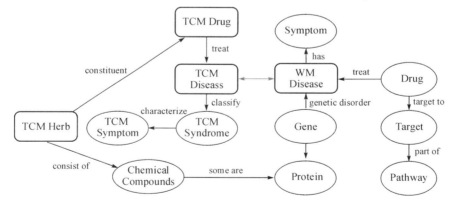

Figure 5 Future vision of the knowledge-based interconnections between modern biology and TCM.

By reconstructing the networks of biological entities such as gene, transcription factors, compounds and other regulatory molecules [112], and integrating significant findings in various facets of TCM mentioned in this article, a broader biomedical linked cloud can be built up and may be able to derive novel cross-discipline evidence based on logic-based reasoning, association discovery and network analysis. As an example, the idea of openly available RDF/Web Ontology Language data sets has been applied to integrate heterogeneous data of traditional medicine and modern pharmaceutical research [113], aiming to find evidence for pharmaceutical compounds from Chinese medicine that may treat expressive disorders or serve as leading compounds for the future pharmaceutical drug development. As a typical example of assessing the drug-target associations in semantically linked data [114], a wide range of databases that include compound-gene, drug-drug, protein-protein interactions, and side effects of drugs can be annotated with domain-specific semantic information, and the strength of association can be calculated based on the topology and semantics of the neighborhood in the drug linked data.

Cheung *et al.* [115] proposed a small specific example of the integration of WM and TCM on Alzheimer's disease based on semantic ontology representation and association discovery mechanisms. In this example, *Huperzia serrata* (HS) is a Chinese herb that strengths the kidney, mainly for curing aging disorders, whereas in some western biological experiments, it was found that a compound of the herb HS acts on the brain and can serve as a potential therapy for the Alzheimer's disease. This knowledge was represented as several linked graphs of resources, and after linking the knowledge with newly found statements, they could assert that HS targets the brain (WM) instead of the kidney (TCM). For more in-formation of drug discovery from Chinese medicine, researchers can refer to [116].

Another promising technology support for the biomedical domain is cloud computing of large-scale data [117], which is now becoming more important in the data-deluge era. It provides a group of hardware, software and computing frameworks to deal with the data effectively. Combining Semantic Web technologies and cloud computing together[118] can allow biomedical researchers to perform the integration of vast amount of data and knowledge in a comparably reasonable time.

7　Conclusion

With the development of integrative medicine, the integration of TCM and modern informatics technologies is increasing rapidly. Bioinformatics technologies, such as text mining, relational database construction, similarity calculation and latent clustering, have great potential in building and discovering the explicit and implicit associations between TCM and modern biomedicine. Currently, the major focus of research is divided into two directions, understanding the mechanisms of TCM from the systems biology perspective and facilitating novel drug design based on the analysis of TCM herbal medicine [119]. The applications are still limited and massive amounts of research data all over the world are private and isolated, which will restrict the communication of the community and weaken the power of integrative medicine. Advances in Semantic Web, especially the effort on linking open life science data together, open a gate for worldwide access and integration of the knowledge discipline. On the other hand, the capability of consuming large scale of data today will allow researchers focus more on the data itself.

There are two basic steps for us to enrich the life science data integration with Chinese medicine knowledge. First, as there exists a wide range of biomedical ontologies in WM but little in TCM, it is an urgent need to transform the knowledge of herbal medicine, basic theories and disease diagnosis in TCM into structured models of ontologies. Second, find the associations between the knowledge of genes, protein, drugs and the knowledge formatted, or import the existing associations into the big linked biomedical data, which can be further used to generate meaningful connections, especially implicit facts as novel discoveries.

Key Points

- Combining systems biology with modern bioinformatics technologies to probe the mystery of TCM will potentially help bridge the methodological gap between TCM and modern medicine, providing the scientific evidence to support simplification of the complexity of TCM, which can verify the value of TCM in modern medicine.

- Decomposing the biochemical components from TCM herbs and tagging the targeting biomarkers using MI and network-target identification, the active components of herbal medicine can be investigated to invent modern multicomponent drugs.

- The way toward to identify evidence of TCM syndrome differentiation in TCM practice requires multidisciplinary collaborations from biomedical, bioinformatics, medical, pharmaceutical and TCM disciplines, e.g. explaining the molecular basis of syndromes through NEI network and identifying the patterns during syndrome differentiation through latent tree models.

Funding

China's Natural Science Foundation Project (NSFC61070156/NSFC60525202); NSF of Zhejiang (LY13F020005); China National Cloud Initiative.

References

[1]Xu J, Yang Y. Traditional Chinese medicine in the Chinese health care system. Health Policy 2009,90:133-9, 2009.

[2]Cheung F. TCM: made in China. Nature 2011,480:S82-83.

[3]Ridley RG. Medical need, scientific opportunity and the drive for antimalarial drugs. Nature 2002,415:686-693.

[4]Tu Y. The discovery of artemisinin (qinghaosu) and gifts from Chinese medicine. Nat Med 2011,17:1217-1220.

[5]Normile D. The New Face of Traditional Chinese Medicine. Science 2003,299:188-190.

[6]Qiu J. China plans to modernize traditional medicine.Nature 2007;446:590-591.

[7]Stone R. Lifting the veil on traditional Chinese medicine.Science 2008;319:709-710.

[8]Jiang WY. Therapeutic wisdom in traditional Chinese medicine: a perspective from modern science. Trends Pharmacol Sci 2005,26:558-563.

[9]Bell IR, Caspi O, Schwartz GER, *et al*. Integrative medicine and systemic outcomes research: issues in the emergence of a new model for primary health care. Arch Intern Med 2002,162:133.

[10]Zhang A, Sun H, Wang P, *et al*. Future perspectives of personalized medicine in traditional Chinese medicine: a systems biology approach. Complement Ther Med 2012,20: 93-99.

[11]Hood L. Systems biology: integrating technology, biology, and computation. Mech Ageing Dev 2003,124:9-16.

[12]Hood L, Heath JR, Phelps ME, *et al*. Systems biology and new technologies enable predictive and preventative medicine. Sci Signal 2004,306:640.

[13]Cohen J. Bioinformatics—an introduction for computer scientists. ACM Comput Surveys 2004,36:122-158.

[14]Schäfer J, Strimmer K. An empirical Bayes approach to inferring large-scale gene association networks. Bioinformatics 2005,21:754-764.

[15]Baldi P, Brunak S. Bionformatics: The Machine Learning Approach. The MIT Press, 2001.

[16]Kitano H. Systems biology: a brief overview. Science 2002,295:1662-1664.

[17]Ralt D. Intercellular communication, NO and the biology of Chinese medicine. Cell Commun Signal 2005,3:8.

[18]Koo A, David N, Renato U, et al. In Silico Modeling of Shear-Stress-Induced Nitric Oxide Production in Endothelial Cells through Systems Biology. Biophys J 2013, 104:2295-2306.

[19]Buriani A, Garcia-Bermejo ML, Bosisio E, etal. Omic techniques in systems biology approaches to traditional Chinese medicine research: present and future. J Ethnopharmacol 2012,140:535-544.

[20]Mertz L. Creating Accurate Models of Life: merging biology and computer science. Pulse IEEE 2013,4:16-25.

[21]Lockhart DJ, Winzeler EA. Genomics, gene expression and DNA arrays. Nature 2000,405:827-836.

[22]Auffray C, Chen Z, Hood L. Systems medicine: the future of medical genomics and healthcare. Genome Med 2009,1:2.

[23]Fang YC, Huang HC, Chen HH, et al. TCMGeneDIT: a database for associated traditional Chinese medicine, gene and disease information using text mining. BMC Complement Alternative Med 2008,8:58.

[24]Wu Z, Zhou X, Liu B, et al. Text mining for finding functional community of related genes using TCM knowledge. In: Knowledge Discovery in Databases: PKDD 2004. Springer, 2004, 459-470.

[25]Zhou X, Liu B, Wu Z, et al. Integrative mining of traditional Chinese medicine literature and MEDLINE for functional gene networks. Artif Intell Med 2007,41:87-104.

[26]Zhao S, Li S. A co-module approach for elucidating drug-disease associations and revealing their molecular basis. Bioinformatics 2012,28:955-961.

[27]Jiang M, Xiao C, Chen G, et al. Correlation between cold and hot pattern in traditional Chinese medicine and gene expression profiles in rheumatoid arthritis. Front Med 2011,5: 219-228.

[28]Youns M, Hoheisel JD, Efferth T. Toxicogenomics for the prediction of toxicity related to herbs from traditional Chinese medicine. Planta Med 2010,76:2019.

[29]Joyce AR, Palsson BO. The model organism as a system: integrating "omics" data sets. Nat Rev Mol Cell Biol 2006,7: 198-210.

[30]Ayyadurai VAS. Service-Based Systems architecture for modeling the whole cell: a distributed collaborative engineering systems approach. FutVisions Biomed Bioinform 2011,1: 115-168.

[31]Cho WC. Application of proteomics in Chinese medicine research. AmJ Chin Med 2007,35:911-922.

[32]Guo P, Ma ZC, Li YF, et al. Effects of siwu tang on protein expression of bone marrow of blood deficiency mice induced by irradiation. China J Chin Material Med 2004,29: 893-896.

[33]Su SB, Lu A, Li S, et al. Evidence-based ZHENG: a traditional Chinese medicine syndrome. Evidence-Based Complementary and Alternative Medicine. 2012, 2012.

[34]Wang W, Zhao H, Chen J, et al. Bridge the gap between syndrome in Traditional Chinese Medicine and proteome in western medicine by unsupervised pattern discovery algorithm. In: IEEE International Conference on Networking, Sensing and Control, 2008 (ICNSC 2008). Hainan, China: IEEE. 2008, 745-750.

[35]Hung YC, Wang PW, Pan TL. Functional proteomics reveal the effect of Salvia miltiorrhiza aqueous extract against vascular atherosclerotic lesions. Biochim Biophys Acta 2010, 1804:1310-1321.

[36]Kaddurah-Daouk R, Kristal BS, Weinshilboum RM. Metabolomics: a global biochemical approach to drug response and disease. Annu Rev Pharmacol Toxicol 2008,48: 653-683.

[37]Zhang A, Sun H, Wang Z, et al. Metabolomics: towards understanding traditional Chinese medicine. Planta Med 2010,76:2026-2035.

[38]Wang M, Lamers RA, Korthout HA, et al. Metabolomics in the context of systems biology: bridging traditional Chinese medicine and molecular pharmacology. Phytotherapy Res 2005,19:173-182.

[39]Lao YM, Jiang JG, Yan L. Application of metabolomics analytical techniques in the modernization and toxicology research of traditional Chinese medicine. Br J Pharmacol 2009,157:1128-1141.

[40]Wang X, Sun H, Zhang A, et al. Potential role of metabolomics approaches in the area of traditional Chinese medicine: as pillars of the bridge between Chinese and Western medicine. J Pharmaceutical Biomed Anal 2011,55: 859-868.

[41] Wang X, Yang B, Sun H, et al. Pattern recognition approaches and computational systems tools for ultra performance liquid chromatography-mass spectrometry-based comprehensive metabolomics profiling and pathways analysis of biological data sets. Anal Chem 2011, 84:428-439.

[42]Wang X, Wang H, Wang A, et al. Metabolomics study on the toxicity of aconite root and its processed products using ultra performance liquid-chromatography/electrospray-ionization synapt high-definition mass spectrometry coupled with pattern recognition approach and ingenuity pathway analysis. J Proteome Res 2011,11: 1284-1301.

[43]Chan E, Tan M, Xin J, et al. Interactions between traditional Chinese medicines and Western Therapeutics. Curr Option Drug Discov Dev 2010,13:50-65.

[44]McEwen J, Cumming F. The quality and safety of traditional Chinese medicines. Aust Prescr 2003,26:130-131.

[45]Sharma V, Sarkar IN. Bionformatics opportunities for identification and study of medicinal plants. Brief Bioinform 2013, 14:238-250.

[46]Sanderson K. Databases aim to bridge the East-West divide of drug discovery. Nat Med 2011,17:1531.

[47]Li DC, Zhong XK, Zeng ZP, et al. Application of targeted drug delivery system in Chinese medicine. J Controlled Release 2009,138:103-112.

[48]Chen CY. TCM Database@Taiwan: the world's largest traditional Chinese medicine database for drug screening in silico. PLoS One 2011,6:e15939.

[49]Feng Y, Wu Z, Chen H, et al. Data quality in traditional Chinese Medicine. In: International Conference on BioMedical Engineering and Informatics 2008 (BMEI 2008), Vol. 1. Hainan, China: IEEE, 2008, 255-9.

[50] Chen H, Mao Y, Zheng X, et al. Towards Semantic e-Science for traditional Chinese medicine. BMC Bioinformatics 2007,8(Suppl 3):S6.

[51]Li S, Zhang B, Jiang D, et al. Herb network construction and co-module analysis for uncovering the combination rule of traditional Chinese herbal formulae. BMC Bioinformatics 2010,11(Suppl 11):S6.

[52]Ming Y, Lijing J, Peiqi C, et al. Complex systems entropy network and its application in data mining for Chinese Medicine Tumor Clinics. World Sci Technol 2012,14: 1376-1384.

[53]Chen G, Lu AP. Prediction of the mechanisms of salvia miltiorrhiza against atherosclerosis using text mining and network-based analysis. J Algorithms Computat Technol 2011, 5:139-144.

[54]Zheng G, Jiang M, He X, et al. Discrete derivative: a data slicing algorithm for exploration of sharing biological networks between rheumatoid arthritis and coronary heart disease. BioData Mining 2011,4:1-21.

[55]Li S. Network systems underlying traditional Chinese medicine syndrome and herb formula. Curr Bioinform 2009, 4: 188-196.

[56]Ma XH, Zheng CJ, Han LY, et al. Synergistic therapeutic actions of herbal ingredients and their mechanisms from molecular interaction and network perspectives. Drug DiscovToday 2009,14:579-588.

[57]Li S, Zhang B, Zhang N. Network target for screening synergistic drug combinations with application to traditional Chinese medicine. BMC Syst Biol 2011, 5(Suppl 1):S10.

[58]Wang Y, Yu L, Zhang L, et al. A novel methodology for multicomponent drug design and its application in optimizing the combination of active components from Chinese medicinal formula Shenmai. Chem Biol Drug Design

2010, 75:318-324.

[59] Cheng HM, Li CC, Chen CY, *et al*. Application of bio-activity database of Chinese herbal medicine on the therapeutic prediction, drug development, and safety evaluation. J Ethnopharmacol 2010,132:429-437.

[60] Leung EL, Cao ZW, Jiang ZH, *et al*. Network-based drug discovery by integrating systems biology and computational technologies. Brief Bioinform 2013,14:491-505.

[61] Ayyadurai VAS, Dewey CF,Jr. CytoSolve: a Scalable computational method for dynamic integration of multiple molecular pathway models. Cell Mol Bioeng 2011, 4:28-45.

[62] AI-Lazikani B, Banerji U, Workman P. Combinatorial drug therapy for cancer in the post-genomic era. Nat Biotechnol 2012,30:679-692.

[63] Zhao J, Jiang P, Zhang W. Molecular networks for the study of TCM pharmacology. Brief Bioinform 2010,11: 417-430.

[64] Ung CY, Li H, Cao ZW, *et al*. Are herb-pairs of traditional Chinese medicine distinguishable from others? Pattern analysis and artificial intelligence classification study of traditionally defined herbal properties. J Ethnopharmacol 2007, 111:371-377.

[65] Barlow DJ, Buriani A, Ehrman T, *et al*. In-silico studies in Chinese herbal medicines research: evaluation of in-silico methodologies and phytochemical data sources, and a review of research to data. J Ethnopharmacol 2012,140: 526-534.

[66] Jorgensen WL. The many roles of computation in drug discovery. Science 2004,303:1813-1818.

[67] Sucher NJ. The application of Chinese medicine to novel drug discovery. Expert Opinion Drug Discov 2013,8:21-34.

[68] Butterweck V, Derendorf H. Herb-Drug interactions. Planta Med 2012,78:1399-1399.

[69] Xu X. New concepts and approaches for drug discovery based on traditional Chinese medicine. Drug Discov Today Technol 2006,3:247-253.

[70] Ehrman TM, Barlow DJ, Hylands PJ. In silico search for multi-agent anti-inflammatories in Chinese herbs and formulas. Bioorg Med Chem 2010,18:2204-2218.

[71] Yang H, Chen J, Tang S, *et al*. New drug R&D of Traditional Chinese Medicine: role of data mining approaches. J Biol Syst 2009,17:329-347.

[72] Zhou X, Li Y, Chen X. Computational identification of bioactive natural products by structure activity relationship. J Mol Graph Model 2010,29:38-45.

[73] Cao C, Wang H, Sui Y. Knowledge modeling and acquisition of traditional Chinese herbal drugs and formulae from text. Artif Intell Med 2004,32:3-13.

[74] Kang YJ. Herbogeneomics: from traditional Chinese medicine to novel therapeutics. Exp Biol Med 2008,233: 1059-1065.

[75] Sackett DL. Evidence-based medicine. In: Seminars in Perinatology, Vol. 21. WB Saunders: Elsevier, 1997, 3-5.

[76] van der Greef J, van Wietmarschen H, Schroën J, *et al*. Systems biology-based diagnostic principles as pillars of the bridge between Chinese and Western medicine. Planta Med 2010,76:2036.

[77] Konkimalla VB, Efferth T. Evidence-based Chinese medicine for cancer therapy. J Ethnopharmacol 2008,116:207-210.

[78] Graziose R, Lila MA, Raskin I. Merging traditional Chinese medicine with modern drug discovery technologies to find novel drugs and functional foods. Curr Drug Discov Technol 2010,7:2.

[79] Lu A, Jiang M, Zhang C, *et al*. An integrative approach of linking traditional Chinese medicine pattern classification and biomedicine diagnosis. J Ethnopharmacol 2012,141: 549-556.

[80]Li S, Zhang ZQ, Wu LJ, et al. Understanding ZHENG in traditional Chinese medicine in the context of neuro-endocrine-immune network. Syst Biol, 2007,1:51-60.

[81]Ma T, Tan T, Zhang H, et al. Bridging the gap between traditional Chinese medicine and systems biology: the connection of Cold Syndrome and NEI network. Mol Biosyst 2010,6:613-619.

[82]Chen RQ, Wong CM, Cao KJ, et al. An evidence-based validation of traditional Chinese medicine syndromes. Complement Ther Med 2010,18:199-205.

[83]Yu S, Guo Z, Guan T, et al. Combining ZHENG Theory and High-Throughput Expression Data to Predict New Effects of Chinese Herbal Formulae. Evid Based Complement Alternat Med 2012,2012:986427.

[84]Ou B, Huang D, Hampsch-Woodill M, et al. When east meets west: the relationship between yin-yang and antioxidation-oxidation. FASEB J 2003,17:127-129.

[85]Li Q, Zhao D, Bezard E. Traditional Chinese medicine for Parkinson's disease: a review of Chinese literature. Behav Pharmacol 2006,17:403-410.

[86]Wang Y, Yu Z, Jiang Y, et al. Automatic symptom name normalization in clinical records of traditional Chinese medicine. BMC Bioinform 2010,11:40.

[87]Wang M, Geng Z, Wang M, et al. Combination of network construction and cluster analysis and its application to traditional Chinese medicine. In: Advances in Neural Networks-ISNN 2006. Chengdu, China: Springer, 2006,777-785.

[88]Zhang NL, Yuan S, Chen T, et al. Latent tree models and diagnosis in traditional Chinese medicine. Artif Intell Med 2008,42:229-246.

[89]Zhang NL, Yuan S, Chen T, et al. Statistical validation of traditional Chinese medicine theories. J Alternat Complement Med 2008,14:583-587.

[90]Zhang YS. Mathematical reasoning of treatment principle based on "Yin Yang Wu Xing" theory in Traditional Chinese Medicine. Chin Med 2011,2:6-15.

[91]Jiang M, Lu C, Zhang C, et al. Syndrome differentiation in modern research of traditional Chinese medicine. J Ethnopharmacol 2012,140:634-642.

[92]Lu C, Zha Q, Chang A, et al. Pattern differentiation in traditional Chinese medicine can help define specific indications for biomedical therapy in the treatment of rheumatoid arthritis. J Alternative Complement Med 2009, 15: 1021-1025.

[93]Li-Weber M. Targeting apoptosis pathways in cancer by Chinese medicine. Cancer Lett 2010.

[94]Chen KC, Chen CY. Stroke prevention by traditional Chinese medicine? A genetic algorithm, support vector machine and molecular dynamics approach. Soft Matter 2011,7:4001-4008.

[95]Li L, Singh RG, Zheng G, et al. A methodology for semantic integration of metadata in bioinformatics data sources. In: Proceedings of the 43rd Annual Southeast Regional Conference, Vol. 1. Kennesaw, GA, USA: ACM, 2005, 131-136.

[96]Antezana E, Kuiper M, Mironov V. Biological knowledge management: the emerging role of the Semantic Web technologies. Brief Bioinform 2009,10:392-407.

[97]Lassila O, Swick RR. Resource Description Framework (RDF) model and syntax specification. W3C, 1998.

[98]McGuinness DL, Van Harmelen F. OWL web ontology language overview. W3C 2012,10:1376-1384.

[99]Splendiani A, Burger A, Paschke A, et al. Biomedical semantics in the Semantic Web. J Biomed Semantics 2011, 2 (Suppl 1):S1.

[100]Belleau F, Nolin MA, Tourigny N, et al. Bio2RDF: towards a mashup to build bioinformatics knowledge systems.

J Biomed Inform 2008,41:706-716.

[101]Wang X, Gorlitsky R, Almeida JS. From XML to RDF: how semantic web technologies will change the design of "omic" standards. Nat Biotechnol 2005,23:1099-1103.

[102]Ashburner M, Ball CA, Blake JA, *et al*. Gene Ontology: tool for the unification of biology. Nat Genet 2000,25: 25-29.

[103]Bairoch A, Apweiler R, Wu CH, *et al*. The universal protein resource (Uniprot). Nucleic Acids Res 2005,33 (suppl 1): D154-159.

[104]Ye Y, Jiang Z, Diao X, *et al*. An ontology-based hierarchical semantic modeling approach to clinical pathway workflows. Comput Biol Med 2009,39:722-732.

[105]Schriml LM, Arze C, Nadendla S, *et al*. Disease Ontology: a backbone for disease semantic integration. Nucleic Acids Res 2012,40:D940-946.

[106]Wishart DS, Knox C, Guo AC, *et al*. DrugBank: a knowledge base for drugs, drug actions and drug targets. Nucleic Acids Res 2008,36(suppl 1):D901-906.

[107]Wild DJ, Ding Y, Sheth AP, *et al*. Systems chemical biology and the Semantic Web: what they mean for the future of drug discovery research. Drug Discov Today 2011, 17:469-474.

[108]Searls DB. Data integration: challenges for drug discovery. Nat Rev Drug Discov 2005,4:45-58.

[109]Stein LD. Towards a cyberinfrastructure for the biological sciences: progress, visions and challenges. Nat Rev Genet 2011,9:678-688.

[110]Rubin DL, Shah NH, Noy NF. Biomedical ontologies: a functional perspective. Brief Bioinform 2008,9:75-90.

[111]Bodenreider O, Stevens R. Bio-ontologies: current trends and future directions. Brief Bioinform 2006,7:256-274.

[112]Li S, Wu L, Zhang Z. Constructing biological networks through combined literature mining and microarray analysis: a LMMA approach. Bioinformatics 2006,22:2143-2150.

[113]Samwald N, Dumontier M, Zhao J, *et al*. Integrating findings of traditional medicine with modern pharmaceutical research: the potential role of linked open data. Chin Med 2010,5:43.

[114]Chen B, Ding Y, Wild DJ. Assessing drug target associations using semantic linked data. PLoS Computat Biol 2012, 8:21002574.

[115]Cheung K, Chen H. Semantic Web for data harmonization in Chinese medicine. Chin Med 2010,5:2.

[116]Ho YS, So KF, Chang RC. Drug discovery from Chinese medicine against neurodegeneration in Alzheimer's and vascular dementia. Chin Med 2011,6:15.

[117]Dudley JT, Butte AJ. In silico research in the era of cloud computing. Nat Biotechnol 2010,28:1181.

[118]Eberhart A, Hasse P, Oberle D, *et al*. Semantic technologies and cloud computing. In: Foundations for the Web of Information and Services. Berlin: Springer, 2011, 239-251.

[119]Parekh HS, Liu G, Wei MQ. A new dawn for the use of traditional Chinese medicine in cancer therapy. Mol Cancer 2009,8:21.

1.2 学位论文摘要

本节摘录了中医药科学数据库共建共享方向 2004—2014 年共 13 份硕士学位论文资料信息。

1.2.1 基于规则学习的中医药文献自动标引系统

周孟霞(指导教师:吴朝晖)

2004 年硕士学位论文

中医药学是中华民族具有几千年传统的医药学,中华民族繁衍生息到现在充分证明了中医顽强的生命力及其实用价值。近几年来,中医药科学问题的现代研究不仅是中医药本身的研究重点,也成为其他学科如化学、药物学研究的重点。随着信息化的深入,中医药信息越来越多,巨量数据有时也使一些特定的用户不知所措。

目前在中医药领域已经建立了文献数据库,几乎每年都会有几万篇文献。如何采用计算机技术来自动和半自动地完成文献的编辑如标引、关键字提取等任务,减少在文献编辑中人为的不确定性和错误,同时减少人力物力,从而提高文献分类、检索的效率和质量,变得异常突出和重要。

本文在以前工作的基础上,就中医药文献自动标引研究提出并开发了一个基于规则学习的主题自动标引系统。该系统从文献的题名中抽取并识别主题模式,相当有效地解决了医学科技文献的自动标引中涉及的主题词和副主题词的组配问题。开发完成的自动标引系统初期版本在大量中医药文献中进行了实验,标引结果远好于以前的系统。具体来讲,本文做了以下几个方面的工作。

(1)具体研究了信息抽取中的 WHISK 算法,并且针对中医药文献数据,对 WHISK 算法做了相应改动,作为自动标引的规则学习算法。

(2)开发了词库管理系统,由于自动标引系统中用到的主题词库和入口词库在不断更新和变化,这种词库的变化对于自动标引结果的准确性有很大的影响。开发的词库管理系统负责 Mesh 词更新与反插、主题词与入口词关联、主题词更新提示、更新词分析与统计等功能。

(3)提出了通过"规则学习"产生规则集的思想,并且利用由改进的 WHISK 算法产生的规则集,对 2001 年文献进行自动标引测试,标引结果表明系统具备了一定的实用性。

1.2.2 DartConsole:数据库网格管理平台的设计与实现

裘君(指导教师:吴朝晖)

2005 年硕士学位论文

网格是下一代 Internet 上的计算平台,其核心任务是管理分布在 Internet 广域环境中的各种类型的数据与服务资源,并为基于 Internet 的分布式应用提供一个统一的、虚拟的共享资源的计算平台。作为网格计算模型的一个重要组成部分,网格上的数据库管理问题一直以来是网格研究的一个热点。来自科学与商业领域的大量网格应用迫切需要数据库系统的支持,因此,如何管理数据库网格环境以及满足更广泛的网格应用的数据管理需求,已经成为一项亟待研究的新课题。

本文从动态开放的网格环境下数据的资源共享与协同管理的应用需求背景出发,综合了现有的 Internet 下的数据资源的信息共享与整合管理的解决方案,提出了 DartConsole 数据库网格管理平台。该平台提出了一套面向数据库资源的管理方案,解决了如下问题:统一的数据库资源访问、动态数据库网格环境的监控及性能管理、基于 VO 的数据库网格环境的安全管理等。在设计上,DartConsole 平台基于 OGSA 框架的网格服务体系进行设计,并充分利用 Eclipse 的插件机制进行开发,满足了网格管理软件严格的可靠性、稳定性、规范性和高性能等方面的各项要求,同时又具有很好的可重用性和可扩展性,便于根据用户需求进行裁剪和定制。它以采用基于语义的资源融合为主线,提出了资源在语义层次上的规则推理,不仅使用户可以高效地为计算任务寻找合适的资源,更重要的是能够对资源语义信息进行管理,以及进行更高层次的语义推理,并为故障监控、自修复等服务提供接口。本文阐述了数据库网格管理的基本思想,描述了管理服务模型架构的设计及实现。本文还介绍了 DartConsole 在传统中医药研究领域的一个应用测试床。最后,本文进行了总结并提出了进一步的工作展望。

1.2.3　基于语义本体的中医药科学数据共建工程

范宽(指导教师:吴朝晖、陈华钧)

2006 年硕士学位论文

如何建设保存海量的中医药科学数据,并使中医药科学数据能最大限度地发挥作用? 为了解决这些问题,中医药科学数据共建项目应运而生。数据库是绝大多数应用特别是 Web 应用不可或缺的后台组成部分,数据库的建设本身也成为一类工程和应用,专业领域的数据库建设慢慢从文本的电子存档或简单的结构化数据向语义知识库转变。浙江大学 CCNT 实验室与中国中医科学院合作,在中医药科学数据库建设方面,从摸索开发,发展到基于语义本体的中医药科学数据建设。本文主要做了以下几个方面的工作。

(1)整理维护遗留的中医药数据建设程序,主要包括使用 ASP 技术的 Web 应用和使用 VB 编写的本地局域网数据库工具集。从中找出中医药科学数据建设的特点并开发基于自定义元数据的通用数据共建平台 DartMani 1.0。

(2)学习语义网以及技术本体和 RDF,分析中医药科学数据共建对语义技术的需求,将相关技术应用到中医药科学数据共建工程中。将中医药本体视为中医药科学数据的科学元数据,将 RDF 数据模型视为透明化底层存储的中间数据。以此为基础,设计开发了基于本体的中医药科学数据共建平台 DartMani 2.0,并采用 AJAX 相关的技术,开发 RDF 数据处理的 Web 客户端。

(3)DartMani 2.0 的语义辅助模块应用中医药一体化语言系统,将其作为中医药的知识库,为中医药科学数据共建工程开拓新的发展空间。

总的来说,本文介绍了中医药科学数据共建项目的发展历程,并着重描述了中医药科学数据共建在采用了本体和 RDF 等语义网相关技术之后的设计和实现,提出了以后共建工程的发展方向。

1.2.4　基于语义的数据库全文检索系统

谢骋超(指导教师:吴朝晖、陈华钧)

2006 年硕士学位论文

在大规模科学数据共享以及大型企业应用中存在海量的数据库。由于系统的定制性和历史原因,这些数据库共享存在以下难题:封闭性、数据孤岛、缺乏规范和标准。中医药科技数据库群的共享正是大规模数据共享的一个例子。

为了解决异质异构数据的集成与共享难题,浙江大学网格实验室于 2002 年起开始用语义与网格技术,并于 2003 年底推出了 DartGrid V1,实现了用语义集成数据并投入应用。此后我们一直在改进、扩充 DartGrid V1 的功能与性能,提高它的稳定性,并于 2005 年推出了 DartGrid V3。

DartGrid V3 完全改造了已有 DartGrid 的内核,使它的稳定性、性能得到了本质提高,集成的数据也更全面。DartGrid V3 还扩充了新的功能,将语义集成的理念推广到了全文检索系统,使语义技术与当今最热门的搜索技术相结合,使数据的搜索比以前更加方便快速;同时它还提供了强大的 Web 应用支持,使整个查询构造、查询处理等功能都可以在 Web 浏览器上完成,从而使 DartGrid 系统更加贴近最终用户,更加实用。

笔者负责整个数据库全文检索引擎和基于 DartGrid V3 的 Web 查询处理系统的开发。将语义技术与全文检索引擎相结合来集成异质异构数据库的查询是一个不错的创意,而在全文检索系统中设计的全新的中文分词算法更是一个很好的创新。当然在开发过程中还有很多工程上的设计和思想,也是我在工程开发过程中的所得。以中医药数据库做切入点,全文检索系统已经在中国中医科学院成功运行。

本文介绍了整个 DartGrid V3 的基本设计理念和解决方案、基于 DartGrid V3 的 Web 查询平台的设计、基于语义的数据库全文检索系统的设计以及笔者自己设计的中文分词算法——树状词库法的思想和实现。

1.2.5 基于 SPARQL 的分布式语义查询处理

唐晶明(指导教师:吴朝晖、陈华钧)
2007 年硕士学位论文

在互联网飞速发展的背景下,海量数据是互联网发展的必然结果,而大规模数据的开放式共享则是网络时代的必然需求。由系统的定制性和历史原因造成的数据封闭性、数据孤岛等难题严重阻碍了科学数据的有效共享。

为了解决异质异构数据的集成与共享,浙江大学网格实验室致力于利用语义与网格技术来解决这个难题,并开发出 DartGrid V3 语义数据库网格系统。

DartGrid V3 利用基于语义视图的语义映射和查询重写的思想,解决传统数据资源语义化的关键问题,实现分布式数据库的语义集成。作为一个发展中的内核平台,DartGrid V3 仍有一些地方需要完善。首先是要提高分布式查询的效率,其次是要完善 DartGrid 内核对 SPARQL 语法的支持。

本文在分析原有 DartGrid V3 内核的基础上,借用传统分布式数据领域中半连接操作的思想,提出了基于 SPARQL 的分布式语义查询优化算法,并介绍了具体的实现过程。同时,对于部分新增 SPARQL 语法的设计和实现,本文也给予了具体的介绍。

DartGrid V3 内核是一个坚持面向实际应用的语义数据网格系统。基于 V3 内核,我们开发了数据库全文检索引擎和 Web 查询处理系统,有效解决了中医药领域科学数据库的集成与共享问题。

1.2.6　基于语义标注的中医药数据加工平台

吴振宇(指导教师:姜晓红、陈华钧)

2007 年硕士学位论文

中医药数据信息化建设是一项重要的课题,已经作为医药卫生事业基础信息建设的组成部分被列入国家"十一五"规划中。中医药信息数据库建设是中医药信息化的基础。浙江大学 CCNT 实验室与中国中医科学院中医药信息研究所合作开发了中医药科学数据加工大平台,目的就在于建设中医药信息数据库。在长期的合作中,CCNT 实验室已开发了多套针对中医药领域的专题数据库的应用平台。在这些中医药数据加工平台的基础上,本文主要做了以下两个方面的工作。

(1)从中医药科学数据加工的需求入手,分析了现有中医药在线数据加工平台的问题,提出了建立基于语义标注的离线数据加工平台 DartAnnotation。DartAnnotation 将中医药本体视为中医药科学数据的科学元数据,将 RDF 数据模型视为透明化底层存储的中间数据,以对加工文本标注的形式,为中医药数据加工人员提供便捷的加工数据方式,并能与在线数据加工平台形成互补。

(2)从整合现有加工平台管理的角度考虑,提出开发中医药虚拟研究院管理平台 TCM-Mannager。TCMMannager 为多个中医药数据加工平台提供了统一的账号管理,并提供了一站式登录到这些共建平台的功能。TCMMannager 还包括了项目管理模块,以提供诸如数据加工任务分配、数据加工质量考评等功能。TCMMannager 还向 DartAnnotation 提供了上传数据加工记录文件的功能。

总的来说,DartAnnotation 提供了基于中医药本体进行离线数据加工的方式,对在线加工方式是一种补充,通过 TCMMannager 的整合,中医药科学数据加工平台成为一个整体。

1.2.7　面向领域的关系数据库全文检索系统的优化设计

张慧敏(指导教师:陈华钧)

2008 年硕士学位论文

在互联网飞速发展的背景下,数据库应用体现出了不同以往的新特点,新的需求应运而生。海量数据及数据孤岛的产生,严重阻碍了科学数据的有效共享。

从这一背景出发,DartGrid 在传统的数据集成解决方案基础上引入了语义技术和网格技术,提出了基于语义的数据库网格的概念,作为异质异构数据库集成的一种解决方案。作为 DartGrid 内核的一个主要应用平台,DartSearch 全文搜索系统已经伴随着 DartGrid 发展到了第三个版本,本文主要介绍了 DartSearch V3 系统的设计和实现。

首先,本文简要介绍了 DartGrid 平台和搜索引擎技术的发展现状,然后介绍 Lucene 的实现机制。并通过分析 DartSearch V2 版本所存在的问题,提出了 DartSearch V3 所要解决的问题和系统的架构设计。

本文的重点是对 DartSearch V3 系统中中文分词方法、索引机制、Rank 机制这三个核心模块所采用的技术、架构、算法思想、核心模块、优化结果等多个方面进行了分析。此外,本文还介绍了 DartSearch V3 系统所开发的 VML 语义图工具包和相关图文聚合工具包。总之,探讨的重点始终围绕 DartSearch V3 面向数据库的全文搜索系统的功能性、实用性、易用性进行。

最后,本文还扼要地分析了 DartSearch V3 系统将来可能面临的问题,提出了 DartSearch 系统的发展方向。

1.2.8 中医药共享平台与 Mashup

王俊健(指导教师:陈华钧)
2010 年硕士学位论文

在海量数据、语义数据、数据服务的互联网发展背景下,数据网格的应用出现了诸多与以往不一样的新特征。DartGrid 是一种面向异质异构的数据语义集成解决方法,而中医药共享统一平台是 DartGrid 内核的一个典型示范用例。面对新的发展趋势,原来的各个独立共享系统暴露出开发零散、搜索结果缺乏语义关联、界面展示不够丰富等问题。因此本文着重介绍了新的中医药共享系统的设计和实现。

首先,本文简要介绍了语义网格技术、索引搜索技术、服务化和富客户端技术的发展现状,然后分析了当前共享搜索及可视化展示存在的问题,接着结合当前最新的计算机应用技术提出了针对这些问题的解决方法和新的面向中医药数据共享平台的架构设计。

本文的重点是对中医药共享平台的架构和各个模块所采用的技术、框架、算法等多方面的分析介绍。主要包括数据层、本体层、服务层、逻辑层和展现层。其中本文特别介绍了服务层共享服务的设计、发现和组合。总之,论述始终围绕着为中医药数据提供快速、准确、全面的搜索服务而展开。

此外本文还介绍了 Mashup 相关的内容,包括对 Mashup 社区用户行为模式的分析,参与研究实现的互联网信息聚合系统,在中医药共享服务与其他互联信息资源间进行 Mashup 等内容。

最后本文简要分析了中医药数据共享将来所要面对的问题,提出了整个中医药数据共享今后的发展方向。

1.2.9 基于隐语义的中医药文献搜索引擎

冯叶磊(指导教师:姜晓红、陈华钧)
2011 年硕士学位论文

随着计算机网络技术的日新月异,中医药信息化建设很快发展,中医药服务信息手段越来越先进、越来越方便,中医药信息化的巨大社会价值和经济潜力也日益显现。"十一五"期间,广大中医药工作者在中医药信息化建设方面做了大量基础性和开拓性的工作,取得了令人鼓舞的成绩。

但是,在中医文献信息化方面还面临许多挑战。大多医学文献搜索引擎都是针对英文文献开发的,而且国内中医文献搜索引擎起步较晚,信息资源有限,专业性不强。中医这个特定专业领域在信息检索、文献分类、文献导航、数据规模等方面都与国外著名医学搜索引擎有着一定差距。因此,针对中医文献的搜索引擎有着广泛的研究价值和应用场景。

本文提出的基于隐语义的中医文献搜索引擎的主要功能是为海量的文献数据(包括数据库中的文献和万维网上的文献)提供一个平台。该系统的功能特色如下。

(1)海量的数据通过机器学习的模型进行分析,挖掘出文献之间隐藏的语义关系,并利用挖掘出来的信息建立文献之间、概念词之间的关系,更好地为搜索引擎服务。

(2)针对中文搜索引擎,设计了一种基于广义后缀树的中文模糊自动补全方法,充分考虑了中文语境中以字为单位、基于拼音的音形相似度和基于感官上的字形相似度等不同于其他语言的特点,增强了中文自动补全的功能和适用性。

1.2.10　基于超链数据的中医药语义查询系统

盛浩(指导教师:陈华钧、姜晓红)
2011 年硕士学位论文

现代计算机信息技术的飞速发展,极大地推动了各科学研究领域的学术与科技进步,同时也积累了大量的科学数据,例如医学与生命科学数据库、国家地理信息科学数据库、大气基础科学数据库等。如何有效组织、共享和利用这些数据,将成为科学技术进一步发展的关键手段之一。另外,科学技术的创新与多学科研究领域的交叉融合,也越来越倚重科学数据的挖掘、集成以及将其转化为知识与信息的能力。

本文从中医药学科的海量信息出发,利用语义本体、语义查询等技术手段,设计并实现了一个面向中医药领域的语义查询系统。该系统将关系型数据库、超链数据等多种数据来源集成到一个统一的平台,并提供语义查询接口,根据用户的查询请求去查找语义相关的数据,最终把结果以一种集成的方式展示给用户。

本文的主要内容如下。

(1)介绍查询系统的应用背景和语义方面的相关技术。

(2)分析系统的整体结构设计,分别阐述数据模块、语义本体模块、语义逻辑查询模块、展示模块等子模块的具体功能。

(3)介绍基于中医药关系型数据库和中医药超链数据的语义查询的具体实现。首先提出一个关系型数据库到语义视图的映射,然后在语义视图的基础上,用查询重写算法将来自不同数据源的查询结果语义包装成 XML 格式后返回,并展示给用户。

(4)提出一种基于语义相似度的模糊查询技术。该技术以超链数据为基础,结合了知识体系分类和文献语料库统计等方法,实现了一个混合型的语义相似度模型。利用这个模型,计算出一组与输入关键词在语义上较为相近的词语集,然后将这一组词语作为查询系统的关键词,实现模糊查询。

1.2.11　基于语义的中医药数据采集工程及应用平台

陶金火(指导教师:陈华钧、姜晓红)
2011 年硕士学位论文

积累了两千多年的中医药数据文献是一个价值连城的知识宝库。将中医药数据结构化地收录到信息系统中,对中医药数据的分析、处理、利用有着至关重要的作用。十多年来,CCNT 实验室网格组与中国中医科学院合作,在中医药文献的结构化建模及数据采集方面做了大量工作,建立了一套中医药语义本体和多个中医药专题数据采集系统。尽管如此,中医药文献数据采集还有许多亟待改进的地方,比如数据采集系统数量太多,彼此之间相互孤立,无法相互连接访问,组件重用性较低,可维护性差,数据采集智能化程度偏低等。

　　针对这些问题,本文提出了一种采用语义本体配置元数据对中医药数据模型和存储逻辑进行配置的方法。该方法实现了对数据模型的语义描述,并且描述了如何将数据存储到存储逻辑中。另外本文还提出了一种语义关系图标注算法,用以辅助数据采集。该算法以语义本体知识库为基础,对中医药文献进行关键词抽取、高频关键词计算以及关键词之间语义关系的识别和预测,得到语义关系图,实现数据采集的半自动化。最后本文设计实现了一体化中医药数据采集平台,以语义配置信息为系统配置元数据,将不同专题的数据集成到一个统一的平台中采集。

　　一体化中医药数据采集平台以语义本体对中医药数据模型的描述为基础,实现数据采集的高度可配置性,解决了中医药文献数据模型繁多的问题。一体化中医药数据采集平台支持基于语义关系图标注的半自动化的文献加工。一体化中医药数据采集平台是一个坚持面向实际应用的语义数据网格系统。目前平台已经投入实际使用,提高了数据采集的效率,大幅降低了运维成本。

1.2.12　对等结构的 NoSQL 存储在图数据库上的应用研究

郭健(指导教师:姜晓红)
2013 年硕士学位论文

　　随着互联网的发展,传统关系型数据库(RDBMS)已不能满足大数据时代系统水平扩展的需要。NoSQL 存储提供了一个具有巨大的可扩展性、容错性、可用性、可靠性的下一代数据库方案,同时避免了传统关系数据库复杂的连结操作造成的效率低下和难于扩展。

　　图数据关系在描述和表达互联网时代大数据如社交网络、推荐系统等大规模图关系数据上,有着天然的优势。所以,我们可以把具有高水平扩展性的 NoSQL 存储和图数据库分析结合起来,构建分布式云处理的在线事物处理系统(OLTP)。本文主要研究非关系型数据库(NoSQL)作为图数据库存储后端的解决方案,主要贡献如下。

　　(1)梳理了以 CAP 定理为代表的分布式系统的基本理论,为实践中对可用性、一致性、分区容忍性进行权衡以选取合适的分布式系统奠定理论基础。

　　(2)介绍了以 Dynamo、Cassandra 和 Riak 为代表的对等结构的 NoSQL 大规模数据存储系统的系统方案,为适应互联网时代大数据的挑战和系统水平扩展的需要提供实际的技术方案。

　　(3)讨论了对以 TinkerPop 图数据库技术栈为基础的分布式图数据库 Titan 进行存储后端扩展的技术路线,将其扩展的各种非关系型数据库(NoSQL)作为存储后端。同时,通过将扩展 Riak 作为分布式图数据库的存储后端的实践以及遇到的挑战,总结了部分 NoSQL 牺牲 RDBMS 特性所带来的新的局限性。

1.2.13　基于图论的空间大数据仓库的实现

陈云路(指导教师:陈华钧)
2014 年硕士学位论文

　　撰写本文是为了能够针对空间信息下大数据的特征,提出一套关于大数据仓库的实现理论和具体实现方法。根据空间信息的概念定义和特点,将空间信息数据整体分类为两类,包括遥感影像数据和传统文件数据。然后作者在文中介绍了宏观的大数据仓库架构及其包含的各个模块的理论和实现细节,包括基于图论的大数据存储架构、I/O 加速缓存优化层、多维度空间信息数据发布模块、基于空间信息和网络协议的数据监控等一系列模块设计。最后介绍了大数据仓库的代码实现情况、测试结果、传统关系型数据库 MySQL 以及其他非关系型数据库的性能比较结果,得出该文提到和设计的大数据仓库系统在其特殊领域的优势性。

1.3　学术论文摘要

本节摘录了中医药科学数据库共建共享方向 2001—2016 年共 23 篇主要学术论文(分别发表在《中国中医药信息杂志》、《中国数字医学》、《计算机科学》、*BEMI*、*ICTAI*、*APWeb*、*KES*、*IRI* 等国内外期刊和会议论文集上)。

1.3.1　TCMMDB: A Distributed MultiDatabase Query System and Its Key Technique Implement

Xuezhong Zhou, Zhaohui Wu, Wei Lu
首发于 *SMC*,2001:1095-1100

With information exploding, the number of databases and information stored in the database increases very quickly. Those databases are more likely to be heterogeneous. There are many distributed databases systems to resolve this problem, but the main drawback is that they don't do well in database cooperation. In this paper, we provide a general architecture of a Distributed MultiDatabase Query system: TCMMDB (Traditional Chinese Medicine MultiDatabase). We will discuss some key techniques, such as distributed query plan generation, distributed query synchronization and distributed error handling in TCMMDB related to Distributed Database.

1.3.2　Dart Database Grid: A Dynamic, Adaptive, RDF-Mediated, Transparent Approach to Database Integration for Semantic Web

Zhaohui Wu, Huajun Chen, Yuxing Mao, Guozhou Zheng
首发于 *APWeb*,2005,*LNCS* 3399:1053-1057

This paper demonstrated the Dart Database Grid system developed by Grid Research Center of Zhejiang University. Dart Database Grid is built upon several Semantic Web standards and the Globus grid toolkits. It is mainly intended to provide a Dynamic, Adaptive, RDF-mediated and Transparent (DART) approach to database integration for semantic web. This work has been applied to integrate data resources from the application domain of Traditional Chinese Medicine.

1.3.3　基于 SOAP 的 Web Databases 实现

周雪忠,陆伟,吴朝晖
首发于《计算机科学》,2002,29(8):151-153

We describe an architecture called WWDB-Ferry that is an Internet databases infrastructure. It can dynamically couple all the Web accessible databases and provide various kinds of applications such as Internet Database Search Engine, Web information retrieval and other Web intelligent applications. XML is the universal data-exchanging standard on Internet, and also HTTP is the basic protocol of WWW. We use SOAP (Simple Object Access Protocol)—a protocol combined of HTTP and XML to make an Internet databases implementation. Also we discuss the SOAP middleware technology infrastructure.

1.3.4 RDF-Based Ontology View for Relational Schema Mediation in Semantic Web

Huajun Chen, Zhaohui Wu, Yuxin Mao
首发于 *KES*, 2005, *LNAI* 3682:873-879

One fundamental issue for semantic web applications is how to define the mapping between the relational model and the RDF model, so that the legacy data in relational databases can be integrated into the semantic web. In this paper, we propose an view-based approach to mediate relational schema using RDF-based ontology. We formally define the Ontology View, and precisely define the semantics of answering queries using ontology view. With our approach, we highlight the important role played by RDF Blank Node in defining semantic mappings and representing the incomplete part of relational schema.

1.3.5 基于 XML 的 Web 数据库全文搜索引擎

陆伟,周雪忠,吴朝晖
首发于《中医药网络与数据库》,2003:129-132

随着计算技术的发展,信息共享及信息利用有了更大需求,同时 Internet 的发展使得通信范围日益扩大。如何利用 Internet 将分布在各地的数据库连接融合并且统一访问是信息产业急需解决的问题之一。我国的中医药领域有着大量宝贵的中医药文献资料和医药信息,但这些资源分门别类地分布在全国各地的不同研究所及院校和医疗单位,这无疑给这些信息的再利用带来很大困难。我们的目的就是利用 Internet 将这些分布在各地的各种异质异构并且自治性很强的数据库融合成为统一的访问平台,并在此基础上建立全文数据库搜索引擎以帮助用户使用。本文将讨论由浙江大学和中国中医研究院中医药信息研究所联合开发的 Web 数据库全文搜索引擎 FTSS_TCM。FTSS_TCM 采用 XML 和 Web 技术相结合的方法成功地解决了 Internet 环境下数据通信受防火墙等网络安全设备影响的问题。

1.3.6 数据库中知识发现在中医药领域的若干探索

吴朝晖,封毅
首发于《中国中医药信息杂志》,2005,12(10):93-95;12(11):92-95

数据库中知识发现(KDD)技术是从海量数据中获取有效、新颖、有潜在应用价值和最终可理解的模式的信息技术。中医药学是中华民族的文化瑰宝,几千年来积累了海量的数据。采用 KDD 技术从数据的汪洋大海中发现有意义的知识,对于中医药的信息化来讲既是必要的,也是可行的。近几年来,我们在中医药海量数据数字化的基础上进行了中医药领域的 KDD 探索,取得了一系列成果。实践表明,利用 KDD 技术进行中医药知识发现是有效的、有前景的,并能推动中医药的信息化进程。

1.3.7　Interactive Semantic-Based Visualization Environment for Traditional Chinese Medicine Information

Yuxin Mao, Zhaohui Wu, Zhao Xu, Huajun Chen, Yumeng Ye

首发于 *APWeb*,2005,*LNCS* 3399:950-959

Vast amount of Traditional Chinese Medicine（TCM）information has been generated across the Web nowadays. Semantic Web opens a promising opportunity for us to share Web TCM information by standardizing the protocols for metadata exchange. To fulfill its long-term goal, we need to build universal and intelligent clients for end-users to retrieve and manage useful information based on semantics and services. In this paper, we propose a set of design principles for such an intelligent information client and describe a novel semantics-based information browser, Semantic Browser, to resolve the problem of sharing and managing large-scale information towards data-intensive fields like TCM.

1.3.8　Rewriting Queries Using Views for RDF-Based Relational Data Integration

Huajun Chen, Zhaohui Wu, Yuxin Mao

首发于 *ICTAI*,2005:260-264

We study the problem of answering queries through a target RDF ontology, given a set of view-based mappings between one or more source relational schemas and this target ontology. We design a novel query rewriting algorithm that can efficiently rewrites a RDF query into relational queries using a set of RDF views. With our approach, we highlight the important role played by RDF Blank Node in representing incomplete semantics of relational data when integrating them using RDF.

1.3.9　基于 OWL 本体论映射的数据库网格语义模式集成研究

裘君,吴朝晖,徐昭

首发于《计算机科学》,2005,32(5):4-7

本文提出了数据库网格中基于 OWL 本体论映射的数据库网格语义模式。首先把关系模式转化为 RDF/OWL 语义描述以完成局部映射,再对局部数据语义与全局共享本体建立联系以完成全局映射。本质是把异构数据库模式的语义通过本体显性地表达出来,并在语义 Web 层完成模式的集成。特点是实现了在统一的语义层次上进行共享与查询,同时采用了局部映射与全局映射松耦合的构架,其特有的分层结构使得在跨库/单库环境中进行语义查询变得更加灵活。

1.3.10　Query Optimization in Database Grid

Xiaoqing Zheng, Huajun Chen, Zhaohui Wu, Yuxin Mao

首发于 *GCC*,2005,*LNCS* 3795:486-497

DartGrid Ⅱ is an implemented database gird system whose goal is to provide a semantic solution for integrating database resources on the web. Although many algorithms have been proposed for optimizing query-processing in order to minimize costs and/or response time, associated with obtaining the answer to query in a distributed database system, database grid query optimization problem is fundamentally different from distributed query optimization. These differences are shown to be the consequences of autonomy and heterogeneity of databases in database grid. Therefore, more challenges have arisen for query optimization in database grid than traditional distributed database. Following this observation, we present the design of a query optimizer in DartGrid Ⅱ, and a heuristic, dynamic, and parallel query optimization approach for processing query in database grid is proposed.

1.3.11　DartGrid: A Semantic Infrastructure for Building Database Grid Applications

Huajun Chen, Zhaohui Wu, Yuxin Mao, Guozhou Zheng

首发于 *Concurrency and Computatation: Practice and Experience*, 2006, 18(14): 1811-1828

In the presence of a Database Grid where a huge number of highly diverse, widely distributed, autonomously managed databases can be involved in a sharing cycle, database tools and middleware should be well suited for schema mediation and query processing in a semantically meaningful way. In this paper, an implemented system called DartGrid is presented. DartGrid is intended to provide a semantic infrastructure for building database grid applications. We explore the essential and fundamental roles played by Resource Description Framework (RDF) semantics for database grids and implement a set of semantically enabled tools and grid services such as semantic browser, semantic mapping tools, ontology service, semantic query service and semantic registration service. We propose an RDF-View-based approach for relational schema mediation and describe the view-based semantic query rewriting algorithm implemented in DartGrid. DartGrid has been used to build a real database grid application for Traditional Chinese Medicine in China.

1.3.12　基于本体的网络数据工作平台 NetData

范宽, 吴朝晖, 陈华钧

首发于《计算机科学》, 2006, 33(9): 85-88

近年来, 网格、语义网络等新技术迅速发展并日臻成熟。互联网发展焦点开始从信息的发布和互联转向知识的交互框架。随着语义网络的迅速发展, 世界各地各个领域的研究爱好者组成虚拟社区, 对同一领域的知识信息一起协作研究。其中, 对数据的整理、保存、检索、分析是实现语义网络远景的基础工作。本文为了带动研究社区的研究人员更有效方便地加入社区的研究, 利用长期帮助中国中医科学院建设专业结构化数据库群的项目中所取得的经验, 结合了语义网络和数据库网格的研究, 设计并初步实现了基于本体的网络数据工作平台。

1.3.13　DartGrid: A Semantic Grid and Application for Traditional Chinese Medicine

Zhaohui Wu

首发于 *PRIMA*, 2006, *LNAI* 4088: 7-9

The rapid growth of web along with the increasing decentralization of organizational structures has led to the creation of a vast interconnected network of distributed electronic information in many fields such as medical science, bioinformatics, highenergy physics etc. The data produced and the knowledge derived from it will lose value in the future if the mechanisms for sharing, integration, cataloging, searching, viewing, and retrieving are not quickly improved. Building upon techniques from both Semantic Web and Grid research areas, we propose the DartGrid which exhibits a Dynamic, Adaptive, RDF-mediated and Transparent (DART) approach for building semantic grid applications.

1.3.14　Dynamic Query Optimization Approach for Semantic Database Grid

Xiaoqing Zheng, Huajun Chen, Zhaohui Wu, Yuxin Mao

首发于 *Journal of Computer Science and Technology*, 2006, 21(4): 597-608

Fundamentally, semantic grid database is about bringing globally distributed databases together in order to coordinate resource sharing and problem solving in which information is given well-defined meaning, and DartGrid Ⅱ is the implemented database gird system whose goal is to provide a semantic solution for integrating database resources on the Web. Although many algorithms have been proposed for optimizing query-processing in order to minimize costs and/or response time, associated with obtaining the answer to query in a distributed database system, database grid query optimization problem is fundamentally different from traditional distributed query optimization. These differences are shown to be the consequences of autonomy and heterogeneity of database nodes in database grid. Therefore, more challenges have arisen for query optimization in database grid than traditional distributed database. Following this observation, the design of a query optimizer in DartGrid Ⅱ is presented, and a heuristic, dynamic and parallel query optimization approach to processing query in database grid is proposed. A set of semantic tools supporting relational database integration and semantic-based information browsing has also been implemented to realize the above vision.

1.3.15　Data Quality in Traditional Chinese Medicine

Yi Feng, Zhaohui Wu, Huajun Chen, Tong Yu, Yuxin Mao, Xiaohong Jiang

首发于 *BMEI*, 2008, 1: 255-259

Data quality is a key issue in medical informatics and bioinformatics. Although many researches could be found that discuss data quality in the area of health care and medicine, few literature exist that particularly focuses on data quality in the field of traditional Chinese medicine (TCM). Due to the high domain-specificity of data quality, it is of essential necessity to identify key dimensions of data quality in TCM. In this paper, based on TCM practice in past years, three data quality aspects are highlighted as key dimensions, including representation granularity, representation consistency, and completeness. Moreover, practical methods and techniques to handle data quality problems in these dimensions are also provided, showing how to enhance data quality in TCM field.

1.3.16　A Chinese Fuzzy Autocompletion Approach

Yelei Feng, Huajun Chen, Hao Sheng

首发于 *IRI*, 2010: 355-358

Autocompeltion is a feature for predicting a word or phrase that the user wants to type in without actually typing it completely. Fuzzy autocompletion technologies have been presented recently to deal with the typing error. However, they do not perform well in Chinese circumstances. In the paper, it extends autocompletion by (1) supporting Chinese character fuzzy match, (2) considering phonetic similarity and shape similarity of Chinese characters, and (3) allowing infix match as well as prefix match. When typing a Chinese character string, minor mistakes are tolerated and expected autocompletion strings are presented to the user. Our empirical evaluation demonstrates that our autocompletion algorithm has high-real-time performance to meet the demand of user interaction. We have developed a autocompletion framework using this algorithm and has been used in a Traditional Chinese medicine (TCM) application.

1.3.17　基于域驱动的链接数据的社区发现研究与实现

曹凌,陈华钧
首发于《计算机应用与软件》,2011,28(5):78-81

在语义网上不断出现的链接数据能够为社会网络分析提供大规模的数据资源,尤其是能够用于对特定的域结构进行社会社区结构的探索。使用基于本体的知识结构,通过从域中的链接数据来发现特定的属性,并结合提出的距离计算方法和聚类方法,能够改进域中人之间的相关性和聚类的定制,从而从链接数据中发现域中包含的社会社区结构。在真实的域中的链接数据上进行测试,结果证明该方法能够在各个不同的域中(如音乐、电影)发现可靠的、有价值的社会社区。

1.3.18　Knowledge-Driven Diagnostic System for Transitional Chinese Medicine

Peiqin Gu, Huajun Chen
首发于 JIST,2012,LNCS 7185:258-267

Recognizing diseases from theoretical perspectives can help ordinary people have a general understanding of medicine. The usual process of identifying syndromes or diseases in Traditional Chinese Medicine (TCM) is by confirming the frequently symptom patterns. The Semantic Web and ontologies introduce well-structured controlled vocabularies for biomedical science. The direct correspondence between symptoms and syndromes can be formatted to semantic inference rules as an additional knowledge upon a medical ontology.

In this paper, we present a simplified rule-based diagnostic system for febrile disease theory in TCM, which makes use of the capability of semantic inference based on medical ontology. Actually the method is rather general for logic-based medical diagnosis, and we show that without interpreting clinical data, the medical knowledge itself can be applied to do basic clinical diagnosis.

1.3.19　一种基于 Hadoop 的语义大数据分布式推理框架

陈曦,陈华钧,顾珮嵌,张宁豫,陈娇彦,于彤
首发于《计算机研究与发展》,2013,50(Suppl.):103-113

随着语义万维网(Semantic Web)和关联数据集项目(linked data project)的不断发展,各领域的语义数据正在大规模扩增。同时,这些大规模语义数据之间存在着复杂的语义关联性,挖掘这些关联信息对研究者来说有着重要的意义。为解决传统推理引擎在进行大规模语义数据推理时存在的计算性能和可扩展性不足等问题,本文提出了一种基于 Hadoop 的语义大数据分布式推理框架,并且设计了相应的基于属性链(property chain)的原型推理系统来高效地发现海量语义数据中潜在的

有价值的信息。实验主要关注医疗和生命科学领域各本体之间的语义关联发现。实验结果表明,该推理系统取得了良好的扩展性和准确性。

1.3.20 面向特定领域的语义搜索结果排序算法

杨克特,陈华钧

首发于《计算机应用与软件》,2011,28(12):172-174

为了提高面向特定领域的语义搜索的准确性,在分析现有本体排序算法的基础上,对现有的中医药领域本体的重要性进行了评估。同时在计算检索关键词与结果的匹配度之后,给出综合评估后的排序结果。实验结果表明,该算法给出较合理的排序结果,能较好地满足用户的需求。

1.3.21 中医药三维虚拟世界构建研究

于彤,陈华钧,王超,姜晓红,顾珮嵚,张竹绿

首发于《中国数字医学》,2013,8(10):73-75

三维虚拟世界是一种新型的虚拟社区系统,它为中医药领域知识的获取、保护和共享提供了有效手段,为该领域的学术交流和医患互动提供了理想的平台。本文提出了一个面向中医药领域的三维虚拟世界原型系统,对其中的名医古镇、中医名家、名家医馆和中医学堂等核心组件进行了介绍。

1.3.22 语义维基技术在中医药领域的应用研究

于彤,贾李蓉,刘丽红,朱玲,高博,董燕,朱彦,刘静

首发于《第一届中国中医药信息大会论文集》,2014:130-132

近年来,随着信息革命的兴起,中医药信息化建设取得迅猛发展,中医药信息学作为一门独立学科应运而生。中医药知识工程是其中的一项核心内容。近年来,中医药工作者使用知识工程方法,建成了大量富含中医药科学知识的数据库和本体,从而实现了中医药经验性知识的结构化,为中医药知识创新提供了宝贵的资源。

1.3.23 中医养生知识管理的现状和发展思路

于彤,崔蒙,高宏杰,李敬华,于琦,张竹绿,毛郁欣

首发于《中国数字医学》,2016,11(4):73-75

目的:完善和发展中医养生知识管理体系,促进中医养生知识的系统梳理和广泛传播。方法:通过文献检索、互联网浏览等方式,对中医养生领域的知识资源进行调研,分析知识管理的现状并提出未来的发展思路。结果:中医养生学已成为一个独立的学科,形成了相对完整的知识体系。该领域的知识资源众多、内容丰富,主要包括古籍、期刊文献、教材、网页等多种形式。结论:该领域已积累了海量的知识资源,但大多是基于自由文本的,其内容难于被计算机直接处理。可采用本体、语义网等新兴技术逐步实现术语标准化、知识结构化及系统智能化,从而改进知识管理的效果。

1.4 学术著作

本节主要介绍了中医药科学数据库共建共享方向于 2012 年由 Elsevier 和浙江大学出版社联合出版的一部著作 *Modern Computational Approaches to Traditional Chinese Medicine*，摘录了著作前言和一级目录信息。

1.4.1 Modern Computational Approaches to Traditional Chinese Medicine

Zhaohui Wu, Huajun Chen, Xiaohong Jiang

首发于 Elsevier 和 Zhejiang University Press, 2012

Preface

Traditional Chinese medicine (TCM) is both an ancient and a living medical system using fully developed theoretical and practical ideas. In China, traditional medicine accounts for around 40% of all health care delivered. TCM is recognized as an essential component of Chinese culture, and the preservation and modernization of this Chinese cultural heritage is prioritized in the Chinese government's planning program.

TCM has an independently evolving knowledge system, which is expressed mainly in the Chinese language. TCM knowledge discovery and knowledge management have emerged as innovative approaches for the preservation and utilization of this knowledge system. It aims at the computerization of TCM information and knowledge to provide intelligent resources and supporting evidence for clinical decision making, drug discovery, and education.

Specifically, the expansion of TCM practice results in the ongoing accumulation of more and more research documents and clinical data. The major concern in TCM is how to consolidate and integrate the data, and enable efficient retrieval and discovery of novel knowledge from the massive data. Typically, this requires an interdisciplinary approach involving Chinese culture, modern health care, and life sciences. For example, in order to map a global network of herb-drug interactions revealing drug communities, explicit knowledge should be integrated from a plurality of heterogeneous data resources in health care and the life science domain, including electronic health records, literature databases, and domain knowledge databases.

Additionally, TCM knowledge is commonly available in the form of ancient classics and confidential family records, which are disparate among people and organizations across geographical areas. Novel knowledge integration and discovery approaches are thus required to link data across database and organizational boundaries so as to enable more intuitive queries, search, and navigation without the awareness of these boundaries.

The goal of exploring effective methods for knowledge discovery and management in TCM in this book is to provide a systematic interface which can bridge the linguistic gap, cultural gap, and methodological gap between TCM and Western science, by extracting intelligent resources from physicians' theoretical and practical knowledge and applying computational approaches to promote the automatic progress of clinical decision making, drug discovery, and education.

This book compiles a number of recent research results from the Traditional Chinese Medicine Informatics Group of Zhejiang University. This book reports systematic approaches for developing knowledge discovery and knowledge management applications in TCM. These approaches feature in the utilization of the modern Semantic Web and data mining methods for more advanced data integration, data analysis, and integrative knowledge discovery. Driven by the heterogeneous distribution and obscure literature of TCM data, these methods and techniques mentioned in this book aim to analyze and understand such huge amounts of data in a controllable style and turn this into integrated knowledge. The digested knowledge could thus be used to promote systemized knowledge discovery and mining, so that TCM experts, physicians, even ordinary people, can gain excellent experience of effective knowledge acquisition. For example, a large-scale TCM domain ontology is utilized to improve the quality of search and query, and to interpret statistically important patterns in those reported approaches. Semantic graph mining methodology is developed for discovering interesting patterns from a large and complex network of medical concepts. The platform and underlying methodology has proved effective in cases such as personalized health care with TCM characteristics, TCM drug discovery, and safety analysis. This book can be a reference book for researchers in TCM informatics. Generally, the topics in this book cover major fundamental research issues, track current challenges, and present core applications. Specifically, we mainly make important contributions to TCM knowledge discovery and management from the following aspects.

1) TCM Data Mining

TCM is a completely dependent discipline, and is a complementary knowledge system to modern biomedical science. Due to diverse and increasing biomedical data, it is difficult to obtain effective information for applications from such massive data. Different forms of TCM data also hinder integration of information sources from different disciplines. Data mining techniques provide flexible approaches to uncovering implicit relationships in these data sources.

Chapter 2 assumes that related genes of the same syndrome will have some biological functional relationships, and thus constitute a functional gene network. We generated syndrome-based gene networks from 200,000 syndrome-gene relations, in order to analyze the functional knowledge of genes from the syndrome perspective. The primary results suggest that it is worthy of further investigation. In Chapter 3, a path-finding algorithm in the context of complex networks was designed to detect network motifs. Performance evaluation is made to learn about the data block size, node number, and network bandwidth in considering the MapReduce-based path-finding performance. In addition to the architectural level of data mining methods, Chapter 5 presents a unified Domain-driven Data Mining platform, which carries out data mining applications by resource orchestration through web services from a variety of heterogeneous intelligence resources and data. The effectiveness of this platform has been proved by a series of in-use applications in the TCM domain. Semantic associations are complex relationships between resource entities, which is a topic studied in Chapter 10 to explore and interpret the knowledge assets of TCM. A case study is demonstrated that discovers and integrates relationships and interactions on TCM herbs from distributed data sources. Chapter 13 presents a novel approach, which utilizes node and link types together with the topology of a semantic graph to derive a similarity graph from linked datasets. Semantic similarity is calculated through semantic similarity transition during the process of generating a similarity graph.

2) TCM Knowledge Discovery and Retrieval

Confronted with the increasing popularity of TCM and the huge volume of TCM data, there is an urgent need to explore these sources effectively so as to generate useful knowledge, by the techniques of knowledge discovery and retrieval. Knowledge discovery is one proper methodology for analyzing such heterogeneous data.

Chapter 1 provides readers with a perfect overview of knowledge discovery in TCM, including knowledge discovery in a database (KDD) for the research of Chinese medical formula, Chinese herbal medicine, TCM syndrome research, and TCM clinical diagnosis. Chapter 4 attempts to investigate data-quality issues particularly in the field of TCM. Three data-quality aspects are highlighted as key dimensions, including representation granularity, representation consistency, and completeness, and practical methods and techniques are proposed to handle data-quality problems. In order to achieve seamless and interoperable e-Science for TCM, Chapter 6 presents a comprehensive approach to building dynamic and extendable e-Science applications for information integration and service coordination of TCM. The semantic e-Science infrastructure uses domain ontologies to integrate TCM database resources and services, and delivers a semantic experience with browsing, searching, querying, and knowledge discovery for users. Chapter 11 introduces an in-use application deployed at the China Academy of Traditional Chinese Medicine (CATCM), in which over 70 legacy relational databases are semantically interconnected by a shared ontology, providing semantic query, search, and navigation services to the TCM communities. Chapter 12 proposes a probability-based semantic relationship discovery method, which combines a TCM domain ontology and more than 40, 000 relative publications so as to uncover hidden semantic relationships between resources. A probabilistic RDF model is defined and used to store semantic relations identified as uncertain and assigned with a probability.

3) TCM Knowledge Modeling

Knowledge representation is a primary step in understanding the nature of diverse domains and conducting useful applications, especially in scientific fields such as biology, economics, and medicine. A lot of knowledge modeling techniques are proposed to solve different levels of knowledge representation obstacles so as to construct an applicable infrastructure.

As a complete knowledge system, TCM researches into human health care via a different approach compared to orthodox medicine. In Chapter 7, a unified traditional Chinese medical language system (UTCMLS) is developed through an ontology approach, which will support TCM language knowledge storage, concept-based information retrieval, and information integration. It is a huge project which was collaborated on by 16 distributed groups. Moreover, unlike Western Medicine, knowledge in TCM is based on inherent rules or patterns, which can be considered as causal links. Chapter 8 presents a semantic approach to building a TCM knowledge model with the capability of rule reasoning using OWL 2, a kind of web ontology language defined by the W3C consortium. The knowledge model especially focuses on causal relations among syndromes and symptoms and changes between syndromes. The evaluation results suggest that the approach clearly displayed the causal relations in TCM and shows great potential in TCM knowledge mining. The on-demand and scalability requirement ontology-based systems should go beyond the use of static ontology and be able to self-evolve and specialize in the domain knowledge. Chapter 9 refers to the context-specific portions from large-scale ontologies like TCM ontology as sub-ontologies. A sub-ontology evolution approach is proposed based on a genetic algorithm for reusing large-scale ontologies.

For a short overview, the book is specifically organized as follows: Chapter 1 gives an overview of the progress of knowledge discovery in TCM; Chapter 2 introduces a specific text mining application that integrates TCM literature and MEDLINE for functional gene networks analysis; Chapter 3 introduces a novel approach that utilizes a MapReduce framework to improve mining performance with an application of network motif detection for TCM; Chapter 4 discusses the data-quality issue for knowledge discovery in TCM; Chapter 5 reports on a service-oriented mining engine and several case studies from TCM; Chapter 6 elaborates on a systematic approach to TCM knowledge management based on Semantic Web technology; Chapter 7 introduces a large-scale ontology effort for TCM and describes the unified traditional Chinese medical language system; Chapter 8 reports an approach to modeling causal knowledge for TCM using OWL 2; Chapter 9 discusses the ontology evolution issue as related to TCM web ontology; Chapter 10 proposes an ontology-based technical framework for hypothesis-driven Semantic Association Mining, which allows a knowledge network to emerge through the communication of Semantic Associations by a multitude of agents in terms of hypotheses and evidence; Chapter 11 describes a Semantic Web approach to knowledge integration for TCM; Chapter 12 introduces a probabilistic approach to discovering semantic relations from large-scale traditional Chinese medical literature; Chapter 13 presents methods of analyzing semantic linked data for TCM.

This book is the result of years of study, research, and development of the faculties, Ph. D. candidates, and many others affiliated to the CCNT Lab of Zhejiang University. We would like to give particular thanks to Xuezhong Zhou, Peiqin Gu, Xiangyu Zhang, Yuxin Mao, Xiaoqing Zheng, Yi Feng, Yu Zhang, Chunyin Zhou, Tong Yu, Jinhua Mi, Yang Liu, Junjian Jian, Sen Liu, Mingkui Liu, Hao Shen, Jinhuo Tao, and many others who have devoted their energy and enthusiasm to this book and relevant projects.

We would also like to give particular thanks to our long-term collaborator: the China Academy of Chinese Medical Science (CACMS). We would like to thank Hongxin Cao, director of CACMS, and Baoyan Liu, vice director of CACMS, who gave us ongoing strong support over the past 10 years. Also, we are grateful to Meng Cui, the director of the Institute of TCM informatics of CACMS, and all of his kind colleagues. Without their strong support, this book could not have been finished.

In addition, the work in this book was mainly sponsored by the "973" Program (National Basic Research Program of China) of the Semantic Grid initiative (No. 2003CB317006); the National Science Fund for the Distinguished Young Scholars of China NSF Program (No. NSFC60533040); and the Program for New Century Excellent Talents in University of the Ministry of Education of China (No. NCET-04-0545). The work was also partially supported by the National Program for Modern Service Industry (No. 2006BAH 02401); "863" Program (National HighTech Research and Development Program of China) (No. 2006AA01 A122, 2009AA011903, 2008AA01Z141); the Program for Changjiang Scholar (IRT0652); the NSFC Programs under Grant No. NSFC61070156, NSFC60873224, Important Programs of Zhejiang Sci-Tech Plan (No. 2008C03007).

Contents

3　MapReduce-Based Network Motif Detection for Traditional Chinese Medicine

4　Data Quality for Knowledge Discovery in Traditional Chinese Medicine

5　Service-Oriented Data Mining in Traditional Chinese Medicine

6　Semantic E-Science for Traditional Chinese Medicine

7　Ontology Development for Unified Traditional Chinese Medical Language System

8　Causal Knowledge Modeling for Traditional Chinese Medicine Using OWL 2

9　Dynamic Subontology Evolution Traditional Chinese Medicine Web Ontology

10　Semantic Association Mining for Traditional Chinese Medicine

11　Semantic-Based Database Integration for Traditional Chinese Medicine

12　Probabilistic Semantic Relationship Discovery from Traditional Chinese Medical Literature

13　Deriving Similarity Graphs from Traditional Chinese Medicine Linked Data on the Semantic Web

1.5　发明专利

本节摘录了中医药科学数据库共建共享方向 2 项相关发明专利(分别于 2010 年和 2013 年得到授权)。

1.5.1　本体模式与关系数据库模式之间语义映射信息的编辑方法

吴朝晖,周春英,王恒,陈华钧

专利号:ZL200710156361.5;授权公告号:CN100590621C;授权公告日:2010-02-17

本发明公开了一种本体模式与关系数据库模式之间语义映射信息的编辑方法。通过对本体模式与关系数据库模式的分析,定义从异质异构的关系数据库模式到本体模式的语义映射。本发明有效地实现了自动化配置本体模式与关系数据库模式之间的语义映射,从而使用户可以简便地使用图形化工具进行语义映射信息的定义,而且还第一次实现了复杂关系数据库模式,提供了自动化的配置。

1.5.2　基于广义后缀树的中文搜索引擎模糊自动补全方法

陈华钧,冯叶磊,姜晓红,吴朝晖

专利号:ZL201110003711.0;授权公告号:CN102063508B;授权公告日:2013-06-05

本发明公开了一种基于广义后缀树的中文搜索引擎模糊自动补全方法。步骤一,建立词的广义后缀树索引,利用现有的建立后缀树的方法,对中文词库中的所有词建立广义后缀树索引;步骤二,计算字的相似度;步骤三,计算相似度接近的词的权重值;步骤四,模糊自动补全。本发明依据中文语境中以字为单位的特点,利用广义后缀树,能够高效地保存词库中所有词的后缀,根据相似度权重,在计算机上实现了中文搜索引擎的模糊自动补全,从而增强了计算机中文自动补全的功能和适用性。本方法中的模糊自动补全,不仅可以支持传统的中文前缀补全,而且能够支持中文的任意中缀补全。

第2章　中医药与语义网络知识图谱

知识工程是符号主义人工智能的典型代表,知识图谱就是新一代的知识工程技术。一般认为,人工智能分为计算智能、感知智能和认知智能三个层次。计算智能即快速计算、记忆和储存能力;感知智能即视觉、听觉、触觉等感知能力;认知智能则为理解、解释的能力。目前,计算智能已经基本实现,近几年在深度学习推动下,感知智能也取得不错的成果。然而,相比于前两者,认知智能实现难度较大。认知智能本是人独有的能力。人工智能的研究目标之一,就是希望机器具备认知智能,能够像人一样"思考",拥有理解和解释的认知能力。知识图谱和以知识图谱为代表的知识工程系列技术是认知智能的核心。

美国计算机科学家、专家系统之父、知识工程奠基人爱德华·费根鲍姆(Edward Albert Feigenbaum)指出,传统的人工智能忽略了具体的知识,人工智能必须引进知识。在他的带领下,专家系统诞生了。专家系统作为早期人工智能的重要分支,是一种在特定领域内具有专家水平解决问题能力的程序系统,一般由两部分组成:知识库与推理引擎。它根据一个或者多个专家提供的知识和经验,通过模拟专家的思维过程,主动推理和判断,从而解决问题。1977年费根鲍姆在第五届国际人工智能会议上提出知识工程的新概念。知识工程主要包括知识获取、知识表示和知识应用。

20世纪70年代到90年代,知识工程蓬勃发展,使得人工智能逐步开始商业应用。随后,万维网的出现为知识的获取提供了极大方便。1998年,万维网之父蒂姆·伯纳斯·李(Tim Berners-Lee)再次提出语义网。语义网可以直接向机器提供能用于程序处理的知识,通过将万维网上的文档转化为计算机所能理解的语义,使互联网成为信息交换媒介。但是,语义网是一个比较宏观的设想,需要"自顶向下"的设计,很难落地。由此学界提出了连接数据的概念,希望数据不仅仅发布于语义网中,更需要建立起自身数据之间的链接,从而形成一张巨大的链接数据网。这一类结构化知识的知识库就是知识图谱的雏形。

知识工程在知识图谱技术引领下进入了全新阶段。知识图谱使机器语言认知成为可能。机器想要认知语言、理解语言,需要背景知识的支持。而知识图谱富含大量实体和概念间的关系,可以作为背景知识来支撑机器理解自然语言。知识图谱使可解释的人工智能成为可能。在人工智能发展的任何阶段,我们都需要事物的可解释性,现在的深度学习也常因为缺少可解释性而受人诟病。知识图谱中包含的概念、属性、关系是天然可拿来做解释的。知识将显著增强机器学习能力。传统的机器学习通过大量的样本习得知识,在大数据红利渐渐消失的情况下,逐渐遇到发展瓶颈。而通过知识图谱等先验的知识去赋能机器学习,降低机器学习对于样本的依赖,增强机器学习的能力,或许是连接主义和符号主义在新时代下的共生发展。

在中医药与语义网络知识图谱研究中,我们着重从以下几个方面进行了研究。

(1)中医药本体的构建和大规模重用

对中医药知识工程项目进行了总体性和原理性的讨论及系统的总结,针对本体构建提出了语言系统的应用以及 TCMSearch 信息基础建设,见文献[1-6]。针对大规模本体重用提出了一个支持中医药领域的大规模本体重用的子本体原型系统 DartOnto,建立了面向本体的诊断系统,提出了基于子本体的领域知识资源管理方法,开发了基于语义维基技术构建了中医药知识共享网站,见文献[7-13]。提出了一种半自动图像标准框架,提高了图像标注能力,提出了一种基于统计决策理论和贝叶斯分析的语义网格知识融合与集成方法,提出了一种通过使用半监督学习方法学习语义贝叶斯网络来构建 Web 混搭网络的方法,介绍了 sGRAPH-a 领域本体驱动的语义图自动提取系统等,见文献[14-17]。

[1] 于彤,陈华钧,姜晓红.中医药知识工程[M].北京:科学出版社,2017.

主要对如何实施关于中医药学知识工程项目进行了总体性和原理性的讨论,对相关知识工程领域中所积累的实践经验进行了系统的总结,从中提炼出基本原理、指导原则和最佳实践方法,阐述中医药知识系统的架构和实现过程。

[2] 方青.基于本体论的中医药一体化语言系统[D].杭州:浙江大学,2004.

主要针对中医药数字资源缺乏知识层次的表达和统一的术语定义标准,提出了建立基于本体论的一体化语言系统的方案,目的是将现有的数字资源有效利用起来,以开放、简便的方式供用户使用。

[3] Zhou X,Wu Z,Yin A,*et al*.Ontology development for unified traditional Chinese medical language system[J].Artificial Intelligence in Medicine,2004,32(1):15-27.

主要研究了中医专业领域的本体建模与开发,提出了基于本体构建方法的传统中医语言系统(UTCMLS),解决了中医语言领域内的知识存储、基于概念的信息检索以及信息整合等应用难题。

[4] 汤萌芽.中医药本体工程及相关应用[D].杭州:浙江大学,2007.

主要研究了中医药领域的本体构建工程,提出了语言系统在中医药共享和共建两大平台上的应用,同时介绍了语言系统在中医药领域的中文分词中的贡献。这些应用是对中医药本体的科学利用的大胆尝试,解决了中医药本体构建的应用难题。

[5] Yu T,Cui M,Li H,*et al*.TCMSearch:An in-use semantic web infrastructure for traditional Chinese medicine[J].International Journal of Functional Informatics & Personalised Medicine,2013,4(2):103-125.

主要研究了统一中医药语言系统,提出了一个名为 TCMSearch 的信息基础设施。它集成了中医药领域的多个数据库,并通过 Web 门户提供了中医药知识资源的统一视图。TCMSearch 可以为中医从业人员提供涵盖基础理论、诊断学、疾病学、治疗学、针灸学、药物治疗学等多个领域的知识资源。

[6] 于彤,刘静,贾李蓉,等.大型中医药知识图谱构建研究[J].中国数字医学,2015(3):80-82.

主要研究了如何构建中医药知识图谱,从数据来源、研究内容、图形化展示几方面探讨如何构建中医药知识图谱,实现中医药知识资源的有效整合,最后提出中医药知识图谱的应用前景。

[7] 毛郁欣. 面向大规模本体重用的子本体模型研究[D]. 杭州:浙江大学,2008.

主要研究了面向大规模本体重用的子本体模型,提出了一个支持中医药领域的大规模本体重用的子本体原型系统 DartOnto,解决了大规模领域本体的重用问题。

[8] 宓金华. 中医药知识工程应用[D]. 杭州:浙江大学,2010.

主要研究了中医药知识工程应用,介绍了 DartOnto 平台,包括中医基础本体、五行本体模型、温病本体模型、OntoTool 工具、DartWiki 语义维基,解决了中医药知识工程中需要专家知识才能解决的应用难题。

[9] Gu P,Chen H,Yu T. Ontology-oriented diagnostic system for Traditional Chinese Medicine based on relation refinement[J]. Computational & Mathematical Methods in Medicine,2013:317803.

针对复杂的中医知识难以应用于计算机辅助诊断的问题,提出将中医诊断定义为发现症状与证候之间的模糊关系,建立了一个面向本体的诊断系统,以解决基于知识的诊断问题。

[10] 毛郁欣,陈华钧,姜晓红. 基于子本体的领域知识资源管理[J]. 计算机集成制造系统,2008,14(7):1434-1440.

主要提出了一种基于子本体的知识资源管理方法,以子本体为基本单位,通过建立语义映射动态地集成知识资源,利用遗传算法实现基于子本体演化的知识缓存,支持动态的、自适应的知识资源管理,提高了知识系统的效率。

[11] Mao Y,Wu Z,Tian W,et al. Dynamic sub-ontology evolution for traditional Chinese medicine web ontology[J]. Journal of Biomedical Informatics,2008,41(5):790-805.

主要提出了在本体缓存中发展子本体,以优化子本体的知识结构。提出了基于遗传算法的子本体进化方法,用于重用大规模本体。

[12] Wu Z,Mao Y,Chen H. Subontology-based resource management for web-based e-Learning[J]. IEEE Transactions on Knowledge & Data Engineering,2009,21(6):867-880.

主要研究了用于 Web 按需电子学习的基于子本体的资源管理,提出了静态地使用领域本体,并提出一种语义映射机制及一种基于子本体的资源重用方法,解决了电子资源学习的共同管理和重用相关资源困难的问题。

[13] 于彤,陈华钧,李敬华. 中医药语义维基系统研发[J]. 中国医学创新,2013(34):143-145.

主要研究了中医药领域的语义维基,基于中医药领域本体来整合知识与作品,向网络用户提供百科全书式的知识服务,提出了通过语义维基技术构建的中医药知识共享网站——中医百科,以期为中医药信息化领域的研究和开发人员提供参考。

[14] 丁艳春. 基于图像语义和内容的半自动标注系统[D]. 杭州:浙江大学,2008.

主要提出一种新的半自动图像标注框架,通过一个搜索-反馈的循环过程,数据库中图像标注的覆盖率和准确率都将会逐步地得到提高。这样的一个算法,与基于语义的搜索相比效率更高,与基于内容的搜索相比精度更高。

[15] Zheng X,Wu Z,Chen H. Knowledge fusion in semantic grid[C]//5th International

Conference on Grid and Cooperative Computing（GCC'2006），IEEE，2006：424-431.

如何处理不同的信息源，尤其是如何组合各种知识源以帮助用户进行有效的推理或协作解决问题，是实现愿景的一大障碍。在此背景下，我们提出了一种基于统计决策理论和贝叶斯分析的语义网格知识融合与集成方法。

［16］Zhou C，Chen H，Peng Z，et al. A semantic Bayesian network for web mashup network construction［C］//2010 IEEE/ACM Interational Conference on Green Computing and Communications & International Conference on Cyber，Physical and Social Computing. IEEE，2010：645-652.

主要提出了一种通过使用半监督学习方法学习语义贝叶斯网络来构建 Web 混搭网络的方法。定义了 RDF 模型来描述应用程序的属性和活动。为了处理语义网上的所有信息源，提出了一种语义贝叶斯网络，其中使用 SPARQL 查询定义的语义子图模板用于描述有关图结构的信息。

［17］Zhou C，Chen H，Tao J. Graph：A domain ontology-driven semantic graph auto extraction system［J］. Applied Mathematics & Information Sciences，2011，5（2）：9S-16S.

主要介绍了 sGRAPH-a 领域本体驱动的语义图自动提取系统，该系统用于从中医药的文本出版物中发现知识。由本体架构和包含 153692 个单词和 304114 个关系的知识库组成的中医语言系统（TCML）被用作领域本体。

（2）面向中医药的知识建模和语义搜索查询

针对面向中医药的知识建模和语义搜索查询问题，提出了一种领域本体和领域文献的语义关系抽取和验证方法，以及语义关系发现和验证方法，见文献［18-19］。提出了基于中医药集成知识库的智能搜索，开发了分布式语义搜索系统、多元语义搜索引擎、面向中药新药研发的语义搜索系统，提出了基于 Linked Open Data 的语义关联发现方法，面向异构生物医学数据的集成和查询方法，见文献［20-25］。提出了基于语义 Web 技术对中医临床知识建模，基于 OWL 的中医理论语义模型及应用，基于 Spark 大规模知识图谱语义查询方法，以及基于 Deepdive 的领域文本知识抽取方法，见文献［26-32］。设计开发了基于语义的移动 Mashup 应用生成系统，中医药数据挖掘平台，以及基于知识图谱的医疗问答系统，见文献［33-36］。

［18］Zhang X，Chen H，Ma J，et al. Ontology Based Semantic Relation Verification for TCM Semantic Grid［C］//4th ChinaGrid Annual Conference（ChinaGrid'2009），2009：185-191.

主要介绍了中医药语义网 DartGrid 中的本体工程的相关工作。为解决领域本体手工建设效率低下的问题，提出了一种基于领域本体和领域文献的语义关系抽取与验证方法。利用改进的向量空间模型从领域文献中抽取语义关系，并用关联规则过滤方法找出重要的语义关系，向用户推荐语义关系并显示其可能概率，由用户确认是否采纳该语义关系。

［19］张小刚. 基于中医药本体的语义关系发现及验证方法［D］. 杭州：浙江大学，2010.

主要研究了基于中医药本体的语义关系发现及验证，提出了一种基于中医药领域本体和领域文献的语义关系发现与验证方法，并在此基础上进一步提出了基于概率的语义关系发现方法，解决了利用现有的领域知识推动中医药本体建设和发展的问题。

［20］付志宏，陈华钧，于彤. 基于中医药集成知识库的智能搜索［J］. 东南大学学报（英文版），

2009，25（4）：460-463.

设计实现了中医药智能搜索引擎 TCMSearch。该搜索引擎的核心为一个集成语义知识库，知识库利用领域本体来表示中医药领域的实例及其之间的关系。该系统对异质异构数据资源进行语义集成并提供了统一的智能访问接口，支持智能搜索等功能。

[21] 付志宏．面向中医药的分布式语义搜索系统[D]．杭州：浙江大学，2010.

主要研究了中医药领域中分布式语义搜索系统。通过分析中医药领域数据集成及搜索的新需求以及原 DartSearch V3 存在的缺陷，提出了新的分布式语义搜索系统的解决方案，介绍了该系统的具体设计以及详细实现方法，解决了不同背景的数据之间的共享与集成以及对数据资源进行有效利用的难题。

[22] 杨克特．面向中医药的多元语义搜索引擎[D]．杭州：浙江大学，2010.

主要研究了中医药领域的多元语义搜索引擎系统的解决方案，提出了多元语义数据索引方法，该方法能够集成中医药领域多种来源的异构异质数据，并且具有足够的灵活性来兼容以后新添加的数据类型。提出了基于本体的搜索结果排序算法，该算法在考虑本体重要性的基础上，综合用户查询与结果的匹配度，对结果进行排序。最终，文献提出的方法解决了特定领域进行高效搜索的难题。

[23] 于彤，陈华钧，李敬华．面向中药新药研发的语义搜索系统[J]．中国医学创新，2013（33）：158-160.

主要研究了本体驱动下基于概念的内容检索问题，提出了以语义视图来定义关系型数据库与领域本体之间的模式映射，设计并实现了语义搜索系统 TCMSearch，实现了分布式异构数据库的语义集成和一致性访问，解决了中药新药研发中的信息集成和检索应用难题。

[24] 郑清照．基于 Linked Open Data 的语义关联发现及其应用[D]．杭州：浙江大学，2010.

主要研究了分布式场景下数据语义关联的发现问题，提出并设计实现了一个多代理协作的分布式语义关联发现框架。提出了一种新的知识表示模型、一种新的多代理协作式语义关联发现机制；设计并实现了两类代理以及语义关联发现的核心算法，研究分析了算法可以采用的不同策略。通过对该语义关联发现框架进行模拟实验，证明了多代理之间协作进行语义关联发现的可行性。

[25] Chen X，Chen H，Bi X，*et al*．BioTCM-SE：A semantic search engine for the information retrieval of modern biology and traditional Chinese medicine[J]．Computational and Mathematical Methods in Medicine，2014：1-13.

传统的搜索引擎只支持基于关键字的搜索，无法为语义相关知识提供准确、全面的搜索结果。针对异构生物医学数据难以集成和查询的难点，提出并实现了一个现代生物学和中医学信息检索的语义搜索引擎 BioTCM-SE，为生物学家提供了一个全面、准确的关联知识查询平台，极大地促进了中西医之间的隐性知识发现。

[26] Wu Z，Yu T，Chen H，*et al*．Semantic web development for traditional Chinese medicine[C]//23rd AAAI Conference on Artificial Intelligence，and 20th Innovative Applications of Artificial Intelligence Conference（AAAI-08/IAAI-08），vol.3，2008：1757-1762.

主要研究了传统中医里的语义 Web，首次提出采用最先进的语义 Web 技术用于中医信息及知识资源的编码、管理和利用，有效弥合了异构的中医数据库间的语义差距，提供了各种创新的信息检索和知识发现服务。

［27］Mao Y，Wu Z，Chen H．Semantic browser：An intelligent client for Dart-Grid［J］．Lecture Notes in Computer Science,2004,3036:470-473.

主要研究了语义浏览器的应用,提出了一种用于 DartGrid 的语义浏览器的通用体系结构(一个智能的 Grid 客户端),可为用户提供一系列语义功能。

［28］梁欣颖．基于 OWL 的中医理论语义模型及应用［D］．杭州:浙江大学,2012.

主要介绍了温病知识模型、中医基础理论模型及其应用。对疾病和治疗的本体表达进行了深入探索,并在该模型的基础上开发相应的应用系统,用以指导温病的防治。中医基础理论针对阴阳学说和五行学说,描述了其基础理论,并对其开发应用系统,实现中医领域内的文献检索、模型展示和养生指导。

［29］于彤,陈华钧,吴朝晖,等．中医"象思维"的 OWL 语义建模［J］．中国数字医学,2013,8(4):29-33.

主要研究了中医"象思维"的语义建模和计算模拟,提出了基于语义 Web 技术的"象思维"语义建模,这对建设面向中医药领域的语义 Web 以及构建辅助中医临床实践的"智能体"起到了基础性作用。

［30］于彤,崔蒙,吴朝晖,等．基于语义 Web 的中医临床知识建模［J］．中国数字医学,2013,8(11):81-85.

以"郁怒"的中医药临床诊断为例,主要研究了中医辨证论治的思维过程,探讨了基于语义 Web 技术对中医临床知识建模的方法,为致力于将中医药与语义 Web 结合起来进行研究的中医药信息学家提供了参考。

［31］陈华钧,陈曦,张宁豫,等．一种基于 Spark 的大规模知识图谱语义查询方法:201710326554.4［P］.2019-09-06.

公开了一种基于 Spark 大规模知识图谱语义查询方法。该方法支持海量语义数据的高效查询,具有很强的扩展性,对基于大规模语义数据的查询应用具有很高的实用价值。

［32］陈华钧,陈曦,张宁豫,等．一种基于 Deepdive 的领域文本知识抽取方法:201710326192.9［P］.2019-09-20.

公开了一种基于 Deepdive 的领域文本知识抽取方法。该方法能够用于完成领域知识库的构建工作,具有很强的扩展性,对非结构化数据的利用和提取工作具有很高的实用价值。

［33］彭志鹏．基于语义的移动 Mashup 技术及应用［D］．杭州:浙江大学,2012.

主要提出基于语义的移动 Mashup 应用生成系统——MMAI(Mashup-based Mobile App Inventor)系统,该系统不仅使移动 Mashup 应用的开发不再局限于专业的编程人员,而且让不懂技术但富有想法的普通用户能够将自己的 Mashup 想法转化为一个可安装执行的移动 Mashup 应用程序。

［34］毛宇．中医药症状的中文分词与句子相似度研究［D］．杭州:浙江大学,2017.

主要研究了中医药信息化过程中的中医药症状,重点研究了中医药症状分词和中医药症状句子相似度的计算,设计并实现了一个完整的、易用的、可扩展的中医药数据挖掘平台。

[35] 杨笑然. 基于知识图谱的医疗问答系统[D]. 杭州：浙江大学，2018.

设计并开发了一种基于知识图谱的医疗问答系统。设计并实现了针对非结构化数据的医疗知识图谱构建系统，设计并实现了基于知识图谱的医疗语义搜索模型。

[36] 陈广. 基于关键语义信息的中医肾病病情文本分类问题研究[D]. 杭州：浙江大学，2019.

主要提出了基于关键词的中医病情文本关键语义信息提取方法，构建了中医药智能服务平台。深入分析了中医病情文本的特点，提出了一种基于病位的中医病情文本关键词提取算法（TF-IDF-DP），一种基于关键词的中医病情文本关键语义信息提取方法（DKSIEK），以及一种融合病情文本关键语义信息的分类方法。考虑到中医辨证的特点，进一步提出了基于 two stage 的分类方法。

（3）基于知识图谱的推理和知识表示应用

针对知识图谱中的推理和知识表示应用问题，研究了面向海量数据的语义推理，Web 语义查询与推理，基于 MapReduce 的分布式语义推理，语义图推理，基于 Spark 的语义推理引擎，以及面向大规模知识图谱的弹性语义推理，见文献[37-42]。研究了语义 Web 在中医药领域中的应用，基于实例的知识共享和管理方法，基于语义的专家综合决策系统，以及语义万维网的不确定知识表示与信任计算方法，见文献[43-48]。建立了统一的中医药语言系统，并提出生物学领域大量孤立的数据资源建模、集成和分析的方法，以及关系数据库的集成方法，见文献[49]。提出了基于 3D 技术的中医五行模型在线展示的实现方法，基于浏览器的本体 3D 可视化和在线编辑系统及方法，基于组合特征的网页主题块识别算法，以及基于表示学习的知识图谱融合算法与系统实现；提出了一个面向语义 Web 的知识网格服务体系和一种基于贝叶斯决策理论的计算信任模型，见文献[50-54]。

[37] 陈华钧. Web 语义查询与推理研究[D]. 杭州：浙江大学，2004.

主要研究了 Web 语义查询与推理，提出了一个面向语义 Web 的知识网格服务体系，建立了一个基于语义的数据库网格原型系统 DartGrid，介绍了三种最基本的知识服务在数据库资源的模式集成和协同共享中所起的作用。

[38] 郑耀文. DartReasoner 面向海量数据的语义推理[D]. 杭州：浙江大学，2012.

主要研究了基于查询翻译的推理算法，设计并实现了基于该算法的推理引擎 DartReasoner，将元数据映射关系转换为语义映射图，结合翻译算法将 SPARQL 查询转换为多个 SQL 查询，利用成熟的关系型数据库技术提升性能。同时针对海量数据推理问题，设计并实现了属性链的分布式推理算法。

[39] 顾珮嵚. 语义图推理及中医药应用研究[D]. 杭州：浙江大学，2013.

以语义图推理的三大实用性科学问题为研究内容，重点解决了面向因果循环的因果语义图建模及推理，面向不精确主观描述的模糊语义图建模及推理以及面向大规模语义图整合需求的弹性语义推理等问题。

[40] 顾珮嵚，吴朝晖，陈华钧，等. 基于 Open Linked Data 的中西医关联发现云平台[J]. 中国数字医学，2014，9(5)：88-92.

主要研究了海量链接数据下基于 MapReduce 框架的分布式语义推理，提出了一个用于中西医关联发现的云平台——BioTCM Cloud。该平台基于跨领域知识整合的需要，在大量的开放链接数据（Linked Data）的基础上，解决基于领域规则的知识推理问题。

［41］黄崛.一种基于 Spark 的语义推理引擎实现及应用［D］.杭州:浙江大学,2017.

主要研究了基于 Spark 的语义推理引擎技术。设计了一个模块化分层的且推理规则可配置的完整分布式推理引擎架构;实现了推理引擎中 RDFS 推理、OWL Horst 推理、通用规则推理的分布式推理算法。实验验证了相应推理算法的效率要高于基于 MapReduce 的推理实现,同时具有高可扩展性。

［42］陈曦.面向大规模知识图谱的弹性语义推理方法研究及应用［D］.杭州:浙江大学,2017.

主要研究了面向大规模知识图谱弹性语义推理的若干实用性科学问题,包括基于 OWL 属性链的弹性语义关联推理方法、基于分布式内存的弹性语义查询推理方法、基于规则的弹性语义流推理方法。设计实施了两个实用的面向大规模知识图谱弹性语义推理系统:基于 Spark 的大规模知识图谱规则推理系统和领域相关的大规模中西医知识图谱关联发现系统。

［43］高琦,陈华钧.互联网 Ontology 语言和推理的比较和分析［J］.计算机应用与软件,2004(10):73-76.

从描述逻辑和语义互联网两个角度比较和分析了几种 Web 本体描述语言(RDF/RDFS、DAML＋OIL 和 OWL)的表达力和相关的推理以及现有的推理工具,总结了推理的分类,说明了推理在本体建设、维护和应用中的作用。

［44］于彤.知识服务:语义 Web 在中医药领域的应用研究［D］.杭州:浙江大学,2011.

主要研究了语义 Web 在中医药领域中的应用,阐述了语义 Web 在中医药领域的应用现状和发展前景,为语义 Web 技术在中医领域的推广应用提供参考。

［45］Chen H,Yu T,Chen J Y. Semantic Web meets Integrative Biology:A survey［J］. Briefings in Bioinformatics,2012,14(1):109-125.

主要研究了集成生物学领域中跨学科整合所带来的一系列生物信息学问题,指出集成生物学可以从语义 Web 技术支持的集成解决方案中受益。在系统生物学、综合神经科学、生物药剂学和转化医学方面提供了丰富的案例研究,以突出软件在集成生物学中应用的技术特点和优势。

［46］Chen H,Wu Z. On case-based knowledge sharing in semantic web［C］// IEEE International Conference on Tools with Artificial Intelligence. IEEE,2003.

主要研究了语义网设定方面基于实例的知识共享和管理方法,在开放分布式环境中以整合实例知识和网络本体为重点,为基于案例的推理开发了一种通用体系结构,解决了语义 Web 中的知识共享对语义一致性要求较高的问题。

［47］景鲲.基于语义的中医药专家综合决策系统 DartSurvey［D］.杭州:浙江大学.2006.

主要研究了中医药领域的专家综合决策系统 DartSurvey,提出了采用语义技术解决中医药领域知识分散、无统一标准的问题,并且对系统中的数据进行元信息描述,使得 DartSurvey 中所引用的基础数据、平台数据和讨论数据均有很好的重用性,最终实现了协助领域专家进行决策,进而找到最优解决方案的应用。

［48］郑骁庆.语义万维网的不确定知识表示与信任计算［D］.杭州:浙江大学,2007.

主要研究了语义万维网技术的逻辑层、证明层和信任层,提出了描述逻辑 ALCNR、霍恩规则和事实集合相结合的推理算法,解决了结合两种或两种以上知识表示方法的混合知识表示应用难题。

[49] Chen X，Chen H，Zhang N，*et al*. OWL reasoning over big biomedical data[C]//2013 IEEE International Conference on Big Data. IEEE，2013：29-36.

主要研究了生物学领域大量孤立的数据资源建模、集成和分析的方法，提出了一个通用的 OWL 推理框架来研究生物实体之间的隐含关系。利用中西医结合的生物本体论，建立了生物网络的概念模型。然后将相应的生物数据作为数据模型集成到生物知识网络中。在概念模型和数据模型的基础上，利用一种可扩展的 OWL 推理方法从生物网络中推断出生物实体之间的潜在关联。

[50] 陈华钧，吴朝晖，王超，等. 一种基于 3D 技术的中医五行模型在线展示的实现方法：201110053929.7[P].2013-07-31.

公开了一种基于 3D 技术的中医五行模型在线展示的实现方法.首次实现了五行理论中平面五行生克模式与中土模式在三维空间中的结合，将二者合为同一个空间体系。

[51] 陈华钧，王超，顾珮嵚，等. 基于浏览器的本体 3D 可视化和编辑的系统及方法：201110048281.4[P].2013-07-31.

公开了一种基于浏览器的本体 3D 可视化和在线编辑系统及方法。能支持多用户通过浏览器随时随地进行 OWL、RDF 本体文件的结构可视化和可视化结果保存，并可通过可视化操作对本体文件进行再加工。

[52] 张思. 基于组合特征的网页主题块识别算法[D]. 杭州：浙江大学，2017.

针对仅利用视觉特征或文本特征来识别 Web 页面主题信息算法的不足，提出了一种基于组合特征的主题块识别算法。提出了计算网页块内容与主题相关性的算法模型 BBM25，以及基于组合特征的主题块识别算法。

[53] 罗丹. 一种基于表示学习的知识图谱融合算法与系统实现[D]. 杭州：浙江大学，2018.

主要提出了一个基于知识表示学习的双向监督迭代融合算法，将实体和属性映射到同一个低维的向量空间。实现了一个基于 Web 的实体融合工具，提供了良好的交互界面以及详细的操作指南，实现了高效的在线融合计算与数据传输。

[54]Zheng X，Chen H，Wu Z，*et al*. A computational trust model for semantic web based on bayesian decision theory[C]//Asia-Pacific Web Conference（APWeb'2006），2006：745-750.

主要提出了一种基于贝叶斯决策理论的计算信任模型。信任模型结合了多种信息来源，可帮助用户根据先验信息和实用功能所表达的偏好来选择合适的提供商，从而做出正确的决定，并将三种成本(运营、机会和服务费用)纳入考虑范围。

2.1 代表性学术论文全文

本节选取了中医药与语义网络知识图谱方向的 2 篇代表性学术论文"Ontology Development for Unified Traditional Chinese Medical Language System"和"Semantic Web Development for Traditional Chinese Medicine"全文(分别于 2004 年、2008 年发表于国际期刊 *Artificial Intelligence Medicine* 及国际会议论文集 *AAAI/IAAI* 2008)。

Ontology Development for Unified Traditional Chinese Medical Language System

Xuezhong Zhou, Zhaohui Wu, Aining Yin, Lancheng Wu, Weiyu Fan, Ruen Zhang

首发于 *Artificial Intelligence Medicine*, 2004, 32(1):15-27

Summary

Traditional Chinese medicine (TCM) as a complete knowledge system researches into human health conditions via a different approach compared to orthodox medicine. We are developing a unified traditional Chinese medical language system (UTCMLS) through an ontology approach that will support TCM language knowledge storage, concept-based information retrieval and information integration. UTCMLS is a huge knowledge project, which is a broad collaboration of 16 distributed groups, most of them with no prior experience of formal ontology development. Therefore, the cooperative and comprehensive ontology engineering is crucial. We use Protégé 2000 for ontology development of concepts and relationships that represent the domain and that will permit storage of TCM knowledge. This paper focuses on the methodology, design and development of ontology for UTCMLS.

Keywords

traditional Chinese medicine; ontology development; medical language system

1 Introduction

Traditional Chinese medicine (TCM) is a complete system of medicine encompassing the entire range of human experience. Thousands of scientific studies that support traditional Chinese medical treatments are published yearly in journals around the world. However, even patients who benefit from treatments such as acupuncture or Chinese herbal therapy may not understand all the components of the TCM system. That may be, in part, because TCM is based on a dynamic understanding of energy and flow that has more to do with Western physics than Western medicine. TCM embodies rich dialectical thoughts, such as the holistic connections and the unity of *yin* and *yang*. The ideas of integration and *bianzhenglunzhi* are the fundamental infrastructure of TCM [1].

With the development of information technology and wide use of the Internet, immense amount of disparate isolated medical databases, electronic patient record (EPR), hospital information systems (HIS) and knowledge sources were developed. In 2000, we developed a unified web accessible to multi-databases query system of TCM bibliographic databases and specific medical databases to address the distributed, heterogeneous information sources retrieval in TCM. It has been available on the website for registered user online for 5 years [2]. As a complete system with complex disciplines and concepts, TCM has a main obstacle that large amount of ambiguous and polysemous terminologies existed during the information processing procedure. We have initiated the unified traditional Chinese medical language system (UTCMLS) project since 2001, which is funded by China Ministry of Science and Technology to study the terminology standardization, knowledge acquisition and integration in TCM. We recognized that there are three main challenges in UTCMLS project.

- To design a reusable and refinable ontology that integrates and accommodates all the complex TCM knowledge.

- To harness a broad collaboration of different domain experts in distributed sites in ontology development.

- To develop a knowledge infrastructure for semantic web.

This article mainly addresses the former two challenges, which are relevant to the design and development of TCM ontology. Ontology building is a non-trivial and valuable work for domain data, information and knowledge integration, especially for the complicated and comprehensive domain like TCM. Using Protégé 2000, we try to facilitate the development of TCM ontology and alleviate the labor through methodology and structure design of ontology. The rest of this paper is arranged as follows. To illuminate TCM as a complete system and to clarify the methodology of ontology design, Section 2 gives a detailed overview of the knowledge system of TCM from the disciplines perspective. An ontology overview is proposed in Sections 3 and 4 to introduce Protégé 2000, the ontology tool we use to build the UTCMLS. Section 5 discusses the methodology, knowledge acquisition and information integration for ontology development. Section 6 gives current main results of ontology development. Finally, the concluding remarks and future work are proposed.

2   The principle and knowledge system of TCM

TCM is a medical science that embodies Chinese culture and philosophical principle, which are the basis and essence of the simple and naive materialism in China. Because the understanding of TCM concept, theory and philosophy is vital to this ontology's development, we give a brief overview of TCM knowledge system.

Traditional Chinese medicine embodies rich dialectical thought, such as that of the holistic connections and the unity of yin and yang. It deals with many facets of human anatomy and physiology: *zang-fu* (organs), meridians (main and collateral channels), *qi* (vital energy), blood, *jing* (essence of life), body fluid, the inside and outside of the body, as well as the connections between the whole and the parts. It also examines the effect of the social and natural environment—the universe, the sun and the moon, weather, seasons and geography on the interrelations and conditioning of *yin* and *yang*. The result has been the formation of a system of thought about the interrelations behind spirit and organism, zang and fu, and the inside and outside of the body. Traditional Chinese medicine puts the human body into a large system for observation and explores the interrelationship among formations, factors and variables, both within and outside the body; it regards and deals with these interrelations with reference to data that are correspondingly interrelated; it uses the principle of stabilization to "harmonize *yin* and *yang* to reach a state of equilibrium" and adjust their relationship so that they remain in a healthy state. The detailed discussions and remarks about the methodology of TCM can be found in [1,3].

Given the difficulties to TCM concept (i. e. complex, vast, variable and non-standard), and the importance given to that enormous amount of ancient literatures, which have been a general and core knowledge source in TCM, it is a great challenge and central role to develop an ontology of formally specified concepts and relationships for UTCMLS. The design, implement and use will be described in detail in the next several sections.

3 What is an ontology

Ontology is a branch of philosophy concerned with the study of what exists. "Ontology" is often used by philosophers as a synonym for "metaphysics" [4]. Philosophical ontology is a descriptive enterprise. It is distinguished from the special sciences not only in its radical generality but also in its primary goal or focus: it seeks, not predication or explanation, but rather taxonomy. Formal ontologies have been proposed since the 18th century, including recent ones such as those by Carnap [5] and Bunge [6].

It was McCarthy [7] who first recognized the overlap between the work done in philosophical ontology and the activity of building the logical theories of AI systems. McCarthy affirmed already in 1980 that builders of logic-based intelligent systems must first "list everything that exists, building an ontology of our world". According to Gruber [8] an ontology is a "specification of a conceptualization". While Guarino [9] argued that "an ontology is a logical theory accounting for the *intended meaning* of a formal vocabulary". Ontologies are essential for developing and using knowledge-based systems. Every knowledge model has an ontological commitment [10], that is, a partial semantic account of the intended conceptualization of a logical theory. Ontologies form the foundation for major projects in knowledge representation such as CYC [11], TOVE [12], KACTUS [13] and SENSUS [14]. Medicine has been the active ontology research and construction area for large knowledge bases. There are several distinguished efforts in medical terminology systems like SNOMED-RT [15] and "Canon group" [16]. The semantic network in unified medical language system (UMLS) [17] is also considered a distinguished terminological ontology [18]. GALEN [19] is a project developing medical terminology servers and data entry systems based on ontology, the common reference model, which is formulated in a specialized description logic, GRAIL [20]. Also reusable medical ontologies were strongly recommended by Schreiber and Musen [21,22] in intelligent systems; furthermore, Van Heijst *et al.* [23,24] had a case study in construction of library of reusable ontologies and proposed several important and useful principles to address the corresponding hugeness problem and the interaction problem. TCM is a specific domain with large amount of knowledge. The goal of TCM ontology development is to facilitate the development of TCM terminological KBS by providing a reusable core generic ontology and relevant skeleton sub-ontologies.

4 Protégé 2000: the tool we use

We use Protégé 2000 [25] as an ontology editor (also as knowledge acquisition tool) with RDFS as the underlying representation language. Protégé 2000 is a frame-based knowledge base development and management system that offers classes, slots, facets and instances as the building blocks for representing knowledge. The Classes Tab is an ontology editor, which designs classes in flexible style and organizes classes as hierarchy. Classes have slots whose value may or may not be inherited. Facets specify the cardinality and data type of the slot value. The Instances Tab can help the user acquire the knowledge of domain. The ontology plus instances can be viewed as a domain knowledge base. We choose Protégé 2000 because:

- it integrates ontology editors and knowledge acquisition tools in a single application to facilitate the knowledge engineering process;

- it has the extensible component architecture; and

- it defines a flexible metaclass architecture and supports many formats such as OKBC, RDF/RDFS and database storage [26], and the DAML + OIL is also supported by the additional plug-ins in the current version.

There is huge amount of knowledge and data that are required to put into knowledge base. Protégé 2000 user interfaces are intuitive for domain experts to work with for knowledge acquisition. Figure 1 is an interface screen shot for ontology development in Protégé 2000. As it can be seen on the left frame of Protégé interface, we defined six core top level classes, namely semantic type, semantic relationship, concept name, concept definition, concept interpretation and concept relationship in TCM ontology. The right frame contains the specific definitions of a class (i. e. name, documentation, constraints, role, template slots). Section 5 gives the detailed description of the six core top-level classes definitions.

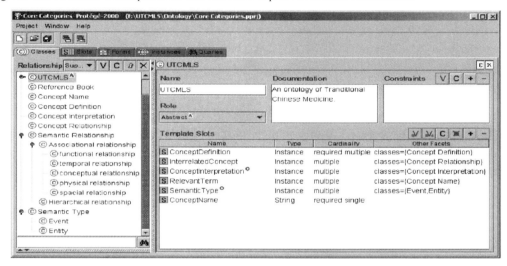

Figure 1   Protégé 2000 user interface and the overview of TCM ontology in editing.

5   Ontology design and development for UTCMLS

The development of ontologies is a modeling activity that needs the ontological engineers (also called ontologists) that have sufficient understanding of the domain of concern and are familiar with knowledge representation languages. Problems like ontology and conceptual modeling need to be studied under a highly interdisciplinary perspective [27]. Ontology construction is a complex and labor-intensive activity. There have existed several controlled vocabularies and many special terminology lexicons in TCM, but combining and synchronizing individual versions of existing medical terminology vocabularies into a unified terminological system is still a problem, because of the heterogeneity and indistinctness in the terminology used to describe the terminological systems [28]. It is accelerated by the various and non-standard using of words in the clinical practice. The ontology development for UTCMLS is still in the preliminary stage. Only small part of sub-ontologies (e. g. the basic theory of TCM, formula of herbal medicine, Chinese materia medica and acupuncture) has been developed. About 8000 class concepts and 50,000 instance concepts are

中医药智能计算

defined in the current TCM ontology. Whereas we estimate the number of concepts of TCM will up to several hundreds of thousand, maybe even reach several millions. Furthermore, because the terminology knowledge is mastered and used in practice by different groups of experts, there should be a broad co-operation in knowledge acquisition procedure. A methodology of loosely coupled development and quality assurance is needed to build a formal final ontology. Although agreement on a high level schema is a prerequisite for effective co-operation between different groups of modelers, it is not practically possible to build a philosophically perfect model. We would rather aim to assure the ontology to fit closely enough with most usage requirements, to be refinable and to be reusable. We give a summary discussion of the methodology, knowledge acquisition, design and development of ontology in TCM in the successive sections.

5.1 Methodology of ontology development

The use and importance of ontologies is widespread, however, building ontologies is largely a black art. All the methodologies, such as TOVE [12], SENSUS [15], etc. are task-specific. Uschold [18] emphasized that no unified methodology is suitable to all the jobs, but different approaches are required for different circumstances. Jones *et al*. [30] had an overview of ontology methodologies and proposed guidelines for ontology development. It shows that ontological engineering is still a craft rather than a science at present. There are two main tasks involved in content development for the TCM ontology: (1) knowledge acquisition and conceptualization from disparate TCM information sources; and (2) formulization and implementation of ontology schema. The building of TCM domain ontology conforms to several principles.

- Refinement is needed. The methodology, which based on the prototype ontology, is preferred in TCM ontology building for the vast, complex and dynamic knowledge system in TCM.

- Development should be based on informal ontologies. There are many terminology lexicons and a number of controlled vocabularies. These knowledge sources can be viewed as the informal ontologies at the start point.

- Evaluation is essential and important. Ambiguity and polysemia is the characteristic phenomenon of TCM concepts. No standard has been agreed on the concept structure and relationship in the TCM discipline. The ontology development of TCM is a continuous procedure of evaluation and development.

- The methodology of distributed loosely coupled development is required. The task of building TCM ontology is distributed across 16 sites in China, and each site is responsible for corresponding sub-domain terminology work of TCM.

Rector *et al*. [31] had the practice of distributed cooperative ontology development in medical domain, in which an intermediate representation at the knowledge level has been used to control the quality of ontology development. We also adopt the intermediate representation mechanism based on tabular and graph notations. The knowledge acquisition, conceptualization, integration, implementation, evaluation and documentation activities are involved in the ontology development. The evaluation mainly focuses on the quality control of the intermediate representation from the distributed domain experts. We also make guidelines and the criteria of Gruber [8] for domain experts to control process of knowledge acquisition and conceptualization. According to the above principles, we applied development criterion to both whole TCM ontology and individual sub-ontologies as shown in Figure 2. The current practice showed that this criterion

82

assured the quality control of ontology, interaction, communication between domain experts and central knowledge engineering team.

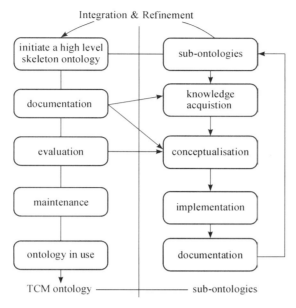

Figure 2　The cooperative loosely coupled development of TCM ontology.

A core generic framework of TCM ontology is designed at the start point of ontology development. About 14 sub-ontologies and six core top level classes (Figure 4 depicts the definitions of each class) are defined as the initial skeleton ontology. The sub-ontologies are defined according to the disciplines of TCM based on the most domain experts' viewpoints as shown in Table 1.

Table 1　The initial indispensable sub-ontologies defined corresponding to the disciplines of TCM

Sub-ontologies	Characterization of content
The basic theory of traditional Chinese medicine	Defines TCM basic theoretical notions such as *yin yang*, five elements, symptoms, etiology, pathogenesis, physiology and psychology, etc.
The doctrines of traditional Chinese medicine and relevant science	Defines basic notions about the doctrines of TCM, which based on Chinese ancient philosophy and TCM clinical practice. The concept knowledge of TCM relevant science is also defined
Chinese materia medica (herbal medicine)	Contains the natural medicinal materials used in TCM practice such as plants, animals and minerals
Chemistry of Chinese herbal medicine	Contains basic notions of chemical ingredients such as rhein, Arteannuin and Ginsenoside Rb2, which are distilled, separated, identified from herbal medicine and their structures are also measured
Formula of herbal medicine	Defines basic notions such as benzoin tincture compound, rhubarb compound and Cinnabar compound, etc. which are based on the theory of prescription of formula
Acupuncture	Defines basic notions of the modern acupuncture discipline, which are on the basis of thoughts of ancient acupuncture and uses traditional and modern techniques to study the issues of meridians, point, rules of therapy and mechanism, etc.

Table 1(**continued**)

Sub-ontologies	Characterization of content
Pharmaceutics and agriculture	Defines basic concepts of medical techniques in the manufacture and process of medicinal materials and ontological categories of agriculture issues relevant to medicine planting
Humanities	Defines basic notions about terminology interpretation and relevant knowledge of TCM ancient culture and TCM theories
Informatics and philology	Contains basic notions of TCM relevant informatics and philology
Medicinal plants and other resources	Defines the medicinal plants and other resources, which are used to health care and disease prevention/cure
Other natural sciences	Defines basic notions of TCM relevant disciplines, which study on the natural and physical phenomenon
Prevention	Defines basic notions of the science of preventing the occurrence and development of disease
Administration	Defines basic notions of medical research organizations and relevant administration
Geography	Contains the basic notions (e. g. toponym, climate and soil) that are relevant to TCM

Each subclass of sub-ontologies is mainly defined by the different experts of institutions we have also established a nomenclature committee to evaluate the definitions.

5. 2　Knowledge acquisition

In 2001, China Academy of Traditional Chinese Medicine and College of Computer Science, Zhejiang University initiated and organized the project of UTCMLS as the basis of all the TCM information related work. We aim to implement a unified TCM language system, which stimulates the knowledge and concept integration in TCM information processing. The National Library of Medicine in the United States has assembled a large multidisciplinary, multi-site team to work on the unified medical language system [17], aimed at reducing fundamental barriers to the application of computers to medicine [29].

UMLS is a successful task in medical terminology research, which inspired our research of TCM knowledge and terminology problem. Much good experience has been learned from UMLS. The structure of TCM ontology is heavily influenced by the semantic network of UMLS. However, the work of TCM as a complete discipline system and complex giant system is much more complicated. Some principles should be adhered to during the knowledge acquisition procedure.

- Deep analysis of specialized lexicons as the knowledge source. The scientific control of the conceptual glossary of a discipline is the most import issue in natural and artificial language processing. We combine the pre-controlled vocabulary and post-controlled vocabulary as the whole and have a multi-level description of conceptual glossary such as morphologic, lexics, semantics and pragmatics, etc.

- A good construction of the TCM oriented concept framework. TCM involves the complete discipline system including medicine, nature, agriculture and humanities, etc. The knowledge system of TCM has complex semantic concept structures, types and relationships, which refers to multi-disciplines content. Therefore, comprehensive analysis and research of the terminology of TCM is needed before the ontology design. A TCM oriented concept framework should be constructed to address all the knowledge engineering problems of related disciplines.

- Efficient combination of controlled vocabularies and specialized lexicons. As TCM has various concept taxonomical frameworks, a unified concept infrastructure should be established on the basis of controlled vocabularies and specialized lexicons. The controlled vocabulary can be viewed as an ontology, which has no instances. The specialist lexicon can be viewed as the instances of ontology. Both of them constitute a knowledge base.

- On basis of the TCM science and referring to the other relevant disciplines. We develop the UTCMLS not only for the information integration and processing in TCM field, but also for those in the agriculture, pharmaceutical technology and western scientific medicine, etc. This is coordinated along with the characteristics of TCM discipline system.

From the perspective of TCM discipline, considering the medical concept and its relationship, we define the TCM knowledge system by two components: (1) concept system; and (2) semantic system. The concept system initially contains about 14 subontologies according to the division of TCM discipline and four basic top-level classes to define each concept. The semantic system concerns the semantic type and semantic relationship of concept (Figure 3).

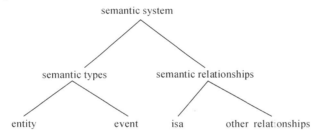

Figure 3　The semantic system framework. The detailed class definitions and instances of semantic types and semantic relationships are provided in Section 6.

According to the time, function, space, entity and concept attributes of TCM knowledge, we have defined 59 kinds of semantic relationships between concepts and about one hundred and four kinds of TCM semantic types plus all the semantic types of UMLS. In Section 6, we will introduce the current version of TCM ontology.

5.3　Integrating and merging of TCM ontology

Information integration is a major application area for ontologies. Ontology integration is possible only if the intended models of the original conceptualizations that the two ontologies associated with overlap [9]. In the procedure of TCM ontology development, we must let ontology be built by different experts in distributed environment for the very complex knowledge acquisition work of TCM. We use the top-down approach to develop the 14 sub-ontologies and other six core top-level classes and distribute the 14 sub-ontologies to the domain experts of about 16 TCM research organizations in China. The bottom-up approach is used during the development of each sub-ontology. Therefore, ontology merging (information integration) is a must. We use IMPORT to merge the subontologies from different sources to a unified TCM ontology. IMPORT is a plug-in of the Protégé 2000, which is the latest version of SMART [32]. It is showed from the TCM ontology practice that IMPORT is an effective tool to merge ontologies.

6 Results

The development of UTCMLS is a process of building a systematized general knowledge oriented TCM terminological system through an ontology approach. We have a nomenclature committee consisting of seven TCM linguistic and terminological experts to evaluate the nomenclature standard and fix the final definitions with the other participant linguistic and domain experts. More than 30 experts in the fields of traditional Chinese medicine, medical informatics, knowledge engineering, and medical administration were consulted about the development of TCM ontology. The categories of the structure of the TCM ontology are formed according to the structures of the controlled vocabularies and the standard textbooks. More than one hundred controlled vocabularies and terminologies have been chosen as the sources for TCM ontology, which are stored in a simple ontology named reference book ((8) in Figure 4). Some of the reference books as main knowledge sources are *Chinese Traditional Medicine and Materia Medical Subject Headings* [33], *Traditional Chinese Medical Subject Headings* [34], *Chinese Library Classification* (4th ed.) [35], *National Standard* [36-38] and *Pharmacopoeia of the People's Republic of China* [39], etc.

Based on these existing controlled vocabularies and terminologies, manual knowledge distilling and knowledge extraction are the approaches taken to concept definition and organization. A basic principle we conform to is that the three controlled vocabularies, namely *Chinese Traditional Medicine and Materia Medica Subject Headings*, *Traditional Chinese Medical Subject Headings* and *Chinese Library Classification* (4th ed.) are considered as the main knowledge sources of ontology, but we prefer to use *National Standard* and *Clinical Diagnosis and Treatment Terms* (e.g. *Classification and codes of diseases and ZHENG of traditional Chinese medicine/GB/T* 15657-1995, *Clinic terminology of traditional Chinese medical diagnosis and treatment — diseases, syndromes, therapeutic methods/GB/T* 16751.11997, *GB/T* 16751.2-1997, *GB/T* 16751.3-1997) when the terminology definitions of the above three controlled vocabularies are conflicts with those of the two terminological systems, and then the final definitions are defined by the participant domain experts and nomenclature committee. The translation is done from those sources to the TCM ontology by building the relations between terms. 16 medical information institutes or medical libraries joined the research group to establish the principles and rules for TCM ontology development, as well as to build the ontology. The translation from the sources to the TCM ontology was done according to the following principles. The relationships between terms were built based on the concepts. Different terms from various sources with the same concepts were connected by this way. The synonyms in different forms were translated by the system into the corresponding subject headings. All the terms with same concepts were selected from the sources first, and then the relationships between terms were built. The nomenclature committee and experts defined the subclasses of each category in TCM ontology. There were some intensive debates. For example, there were 12 subclasses under the category of the basic theory of traditional Chinese medicine on the first draft of the structure, but some of experts did not agree to this classification. After the discussion, a new structure with six subclasses was developed. The UTCMLS project is still in progress. The core top-level categories such as the concept relevant categories, semantic type and semantic relationship, and the first level sub-class definitions of 14 essential sub-ontologies are currently finished. Furthermore, the complete ontology

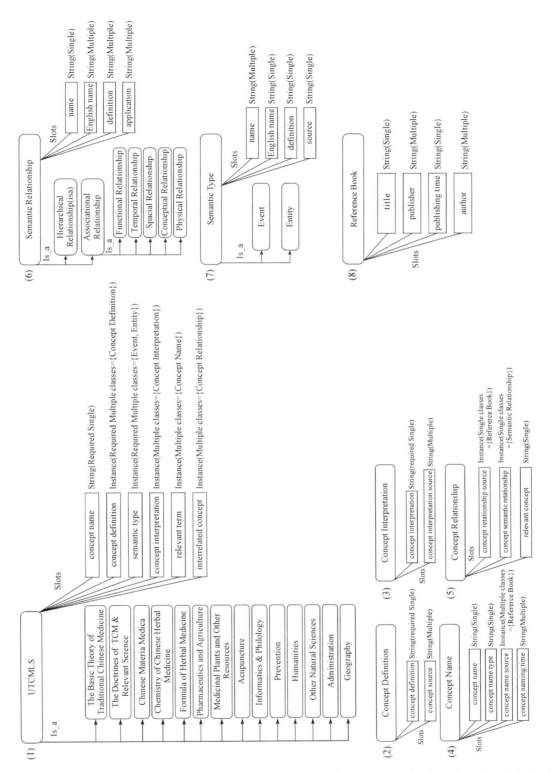

Figure 4　The core top-level categories of TCM ontology. In which：（1）is the highest-level ontology has six basic slots and 14 sub-ontologies；（2），（3），（4），（5）constitute the concept system；（6），（7）form the semantic system；and（8）is a simple ontology of reference book.

definitions and knowledge acquisition of some sub-ontologies (e.g. the basic theory of TCM, acupuncture and formula of herbal medicine) also have been completed. This section provides the current main results and experience of the ontology development by introducing the whole framework of the skeleton top-level categories of TCM ontology and the semantic types. Figure 4 shows the whole framework of the skeleton top-level class definitions of TCM ontology in Protégé 2000 (RDFS is the underlying knowledge representation language and storage format).

6.1 The core top-level categories

To unify, and initiate the whole ontology development and knowledge acquisition, we have defined the core top-level categories of TCM ontology with essential instances (e.g. 104 TCM semantic types and 59 semantic relationships). The semantic types and relationships are depicted in detail in Section 6.2. We provide six core top-level categories, which are treated as the instances of the metaclass: STANDARD-CLASS in Protégé 2000, and on the basis of them define all the intentional and extensional content of concepts in UTCMLS. Meanwhile, 14 subontologies with first level sub-classes are defined, but the second or deeper level sub-class definitions are mainly determined by the corresponding groups of domain experts who take change of the knowledge acquisition work, because the bottom-up method is used to facilitate the knowledge acquisition and to decrease the labor efforts. As is shown in Figure 4, three basic components constitute the core top-level TCM ontology.

1) Sub-ontologies and the hierarchical structure

The sub-ontologies and their hierarchical structure reflect the organization and content of TCM knowledge. The initial 14 sub-ontologies (Table 1 illustrates the definitions of sub-ontologies and their contents) and the six basic slots have been defined ((1) of Figure 4). The six basic slots are concept name, concept definition, concept interpretation, relevant term, interrelated concept and semantic type. Concept name slot gives the standard name of a concept, and the concept definition slot and interpretation slot give the descriptive content about the meaning of a concept. The relevant term slot defines the different terms of a concept used in the other relevant vocabulary sources, by which we can construct the relations between UTCMLS and other terminological sources. The interrelated concept slot defines the concepts, which has some kinds of semantic relationships with a concept. The semantic type slot gives the semantic type definition of a concept. More slots can be defined for an individual sub-ontology if necessary. The complete sub-ontologies with concept instances will become a medical language knowledge base system. Now there are 8000 concepts (e.g. herbal medicine, chemistry of herbal medicine and disease, etc.) and 50,000 concept instances (e.g. Rhubarb, Rhein and diabetes, etc.) in UTCMLS.

2) Concept structure

Using Protégé 2000, we provide a knowledge representation method to define the concept in a unified mode. We consider that every TCM concept consists of three basic intentional attributes, namely definition, interpretation and name, hence three classes, namely concept definition, concept name and concept interpretation ((2), (3), (4) in Figure 4) are defined to construct a terminological concept. The class of concept definition involves the definitions of essential meanings of a concept. The class of concept interpretation gives the explanation of a concept. The class of concept name defines the synonyms, abbreviations and lexical variants of a concept, that is to say, the concept name gives the relevant terminological names of a concept from different controlled vocabularies. Together with the concept name slot of each sub-ontology, these three classes give the lexicon level knowledge of a concept. However, the semantic structure aims at the semantic level knowledge of a concept.

3) Semantic structure

The semantic type and relationship classes ((6), (7) in Figure 4) form the foundation of semantic level knowledge of a concept. The semantic types provide a consistent categorization of all concepts represented in UTCMLS, and the semantic relationships defining the relations may hold between the semantic types. Classification and inference are supported by these definitions of semantic type and relationship of a concept. As Figure 4 shows, we define semantic relationship as a slot of concept relationship class and semantic type as an essential slot of TCM ontology to assign the semantic content to concept. Each concept of UTCMLS is assigned at least one semantic type. In all cases, the most specific semantic type available in the hierarchy is assigned to the concept. The semantic structure enables to construct an abstract semantic network of all the concepts in UTCMLS, so is vital to TCM ontology. This paper will list all the TCM oriented semantic types in Section 6.2.

6.2　Semantic types and semantic relationships

The semantic network of UMLS [17] is a high-level representation of the biomedical domain based on semantic types under which all the Metathesaurus concepts are categorized. The semantic network makes UMLS a unified medical language system, which is different from other classification and terminological system. We define the semantic structure in UTCMLS to construct the semantic level knowledge framework of TCM concept from the idea of semantic network of UMLS. We define the semantic type and semantic relationship as one of the two top-level categories of TCM ontology. The structures of semantic type and semantic relationship are defined as Figure 4 shows. Most of semantic relationships in TCM ontology are same as UMLS, but there are five more semantic relationships in TCM ontology than UMLS, namely *being exterior-interiorly related*, *produces*, *transform to*, *restricts*, and *cooperates with*. Those are special ones used in the unique system of traditional Chinese medicine. For example, *being exterior-interiorly related* is the relationship between the concepts with zang-fu semantic type, which is a special semantic category in TCM. We have defined 104 semantic types (including 40 entity definitions and 64 event definitions) to describe the high-level concept categories in TCM. The 40 TCM oriented entity semantic types and the hierarchical structure are depicted in Figure 5, and the 64 TCM event semantic types are listed in Figure 6. All the definitions of semantic system are finally fixed by intensive debates and rigorous evaluation. However, incompleteness and imperfection is practically allowed for. The detailed definitions of semantic types and relationships, and the rules of their applications to concepts are given in the technical report [40] and also are contained in the core top-level ontology of TCM. The whole ontology will be published and shared on the Internet when finished, so this article does not give further descriptions of them.

7　Concluding remarks and future work

In the current literature on knowledge management, it is often observed that the main challenges are in

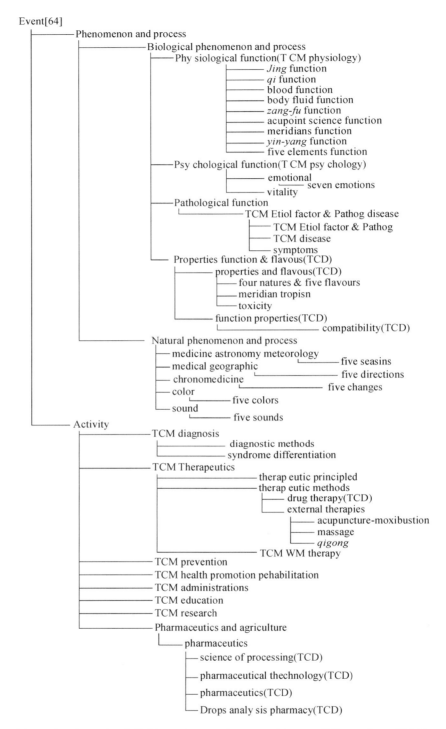

Figure 5   The entity definitions of semantic type, which are different from UMLS.

the realm of human organizational culture and practices. The key to providing useful support for knowledge management lies in how meaning is embedded in information models as defined in ontologies. In China, various kinds of TCM terminology systems with differing purposes have been developed during the past two

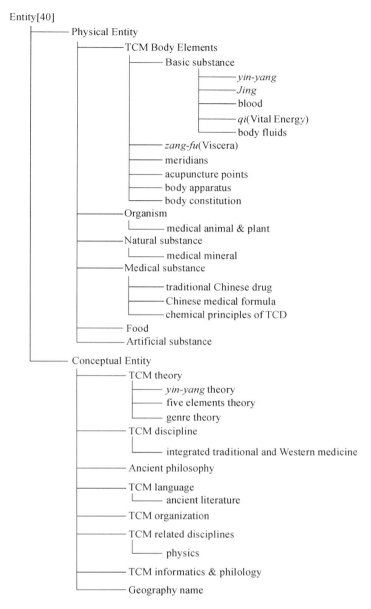

```
Entity[40]
├── Physical Entity
│   ├── TCM Body Elements
│   │   ├── Basic substance
│   │   │   ├── yin-yang
│   │   │   ├── Jing
│   │   │   ├── blood
│   │   │   ├── qi(Vital Energy)
│   │   │   └── body fluids
│   │   ├── zang-fu(Viscera)
│   │   ├── meridians
│   │   ├── acupuncture points
│   │   ├── body apparatus
│   │   └── body constitution
│   ├── Organism
│   │   └── medical animal & plant
│   ├── Natural substance
│   │   └── medical mineral
│   ├── Medical substance
│   │   ├── traditional Chinese drug
│   │   ├── Chinese medical formula
│   │   └── chemical principles of TCD
│   ├── Food
│   └── Artificial substance
└── Conceptual Entity
    ├── TCM theory
    │   ├── yin-yang theory
    │   ├── five elements theory
    │   └── genre theory
    ├── TCM discipline
    │   └── integrated traditional and Western medicine
    ├── Ancient philosophy
    ├── TCM language
    │   └── ancient literature
    ├── TCM organization
    ├── TCM related disciplines
    │   └── physics
    ├── TCM informatics & philology
    └── Geography name
```

Figure 6　The 64 TCM special event definitions of semantic type. The definitions such as *yin-yang* function, *zang-fu* function and seven emotions fully reflect the characteristics of TCM terminological knowledge.

decades. Unfortunately, most of them are paper-based that cannot satisfy anymore the desiderata of healthcare information systems, such as the demand for re-use and sharing of patient data. The unambiguous communication of complex and detailed medical concepts is now a crucial feature of medical information systems. An ontological approach to the description of terminology systems will allow a better integration and reuse of these systems. Ontology development for the UTCMLS is a systematic and comprehensive procedure of knowledge acquisition and knowledge integration in TCM. TCM embodies knowledge of systematics, cybernetics and informatics, and involves a wide range of multi-discipline terminologies. It is tempting to build a unified knowledge oriented terminological system with consistent, formal and extensible structure to integrate the existing terminology systems, but it will be a huge, labor and intelligence intensive work, like the UMLS project. 16 TCM institutes and colleges with several hundred researchers have been involved in this project to build the ontology and to acquire the knowledge. To satisfy the requirement of distributed development, scalable and extensible methodology is focused on in TCM ontology development. The process of ontology development for UTCMLS is also a course of medical concept standardization and unification. Due to the vast knowledge storage and very much complex knowledge system involved in TCM research, the UTCMLS and ontology development is a continuous refinement procedure.

More precisely, this article presents a preliminary ontology development experience of TCM medical language system. The main efforts of this article are to provide an ontology approach to standardize TCM medical terminology. Furthermore, the TCM oriented methodology of ontology development and an ontology structure are defined to facilitate the development of UTCMLS KBS. According to the knowledge system of TCM, two sub-systems (e.g. concept system and semantic system) are defined to describe and construct the terminological system. The structure of the semantic system is inherited from the semantic network of UMLS, but many more semantic types (about 104 additional semantic types) are defined to reflect the essential of TCM science. Four core top-level categories, namely concept definition, concept name, concept interpretation and concept relationship constitute the concept system, which build a unified approach to define the TCM concept. We aim to build a unified ontology framework to effectively organize and integrate the terminological knowledge of TCM. Although the core top-level categories and essential ontology structures are defined, much more work (e.g. terminology standardization, problem-solving methods and knowledge acquisition) should be done to construct a final version of TCM ontology and medical terminology system, which will support various medical applications.

Now the applications of UTCMLS such as concept-based medical information retrieval and TCM specific semantic browser (exploring the information and structure of UTCMLS online) are in progress. Future work on UTCMLS includes: (1) completion of TCM ontology and expansion of the sub-ontologies; (2) completion of knowledge acquisition to build a final medical language system; (3) interrelating to the existing medical database sources; (4) development of a TCM semantic web terminology server; and (5) development of healthcare information systems based on UTCMLS terminology server.

Acknowledgements

Our special thanks go to Dr. Yongsheng Gao (Salford Health Informatics Research Environment, School of Health Care Professions, The University of Salford, Great Manchester, UK) who has read the whole draft and provided valuable comments. We are also appreciative of comments by the three anonymous reviewers, which prompt a considerable revision and improvement to the final article. We gratefully acknowledge all the domain experts for their collaboration and hard work. We are also grateful to all the members of the UTCMLS project for the valuable suggestions and innovative discussions. This research is partly supported by National Basic Research Priorities Programme of China Ministry of Science and Technology under grant number 2001DEA30039.

References

[1] Yin HH, Zhang BN. The basic theory of traditional Chinese medicine. Shanghai: Shanghai Science and Technology, 1984 (in Chinese).

[2] http://www.cintcm.com.

[3] Huang JP. Methodology of traditional Chinese medicine. Beijing: New World Press, 1995.

[4] Mealy GH. Another look at data. In: Proceedings of the AFIPS Fall Joint Computers Conference. Washington, DC: Thompson Book Co., 1967, p. 525-534.

[5] Carnap R. The logical structure of the world: pseudoproblems in philosophy. California: University of California Press, 1967.

[6] Bunge M. Treatise on basic philosophy: ontology. I. The furniture of the world. New York: Reidel, 1977.

[7] Smith B, Welty C. Ontology: towards a new synthesis. In: Welty C, Smith B, editors. Formal ontology in information systems. New York: ACM Press, 2001, p.3-9.

[8] Gruber TR. Toward principles for the design of ontologies used for knowledge sharing. Hum-Comput Stud 1995,43: 907-928.

[9] Guarino N. Formal ontology and information systems. In: Guarino N, editor. Formal ontology in information systems. Amsterdam: IOS Press, 1998, p. 3-15.

[10] Noy N, Hafner C. The state of the art in ontology design: a survey and comparative review. AI Mag 1997,18:53-74.

[11] Lenat DB. CYC: a large-scale investment in knowledge infrastructure. Commun ACM 1995,38:33-38.

[12] Uschold M, Gru¨ninger M. Ontologies: principles, methods and applications. Knowledge Eng Rev 1996,11:93-155.

[13] Schreiber G, Wielinga B, Jansweijer W. The kactus view on the "o" word. In: Proceedings of the Workshop on Basic Ontological Issues in Knowledge Sharing/International Joint Conference on Artificial Intelligence. Menlo Park, CA: AAAI Press, 1995.

[14] Swartout B, Patil R, Knight K, Russ T. Toward distributed use of large-scale ontologies. In: Proceedings of the AAAI97 Spring Symposium on Ontological Engineering, March 1997, Stanford, CA.

[15] Spackman KA, Campbell KE, Cote RA. SNOMED RT: a reference terminology for health care. In: Proceedings of the AMIA Fall Symposium, 1997.

[16] Evans DA, Cimino J, Hersh WR, Huff SM, Bell DS, The Canon Group. Position statement: towards a medical concept representation language. Am Med Inform Assoc 1994, 1:207-214.

[17] Lindberg DAB, Humphreys BL, McCray AT. The unified medical language system. Methods Inform Med 1993,32: 281-291.

[18] Uschold M. Building ontologies: towards a unified methodology. In: Proceedings of the 16th Annual Conference of the British Computer Society Specialist Group on Expert Systems, Cambridge, UK, 1996.

[19] Rector AL, Nowlan WA, GALEN Consortium. The GALEN project. Comput Methods Programs Biomed 1993,45: 75-78.

[20] Rector AL, Bechhofer S, Goble C, Horrocks I, Nowlan W, Solomon W. The GRAIL concept modelling language for medical terminology. Artif Intelligence Med 1997,9: 139-171.

[21] Musen M. Modern architectures for intelligent systems: reusable ontologies and problem-solving methods. Am Med Inform Assoc Symp Suppl 1998,46-54.

[22] Musen M, Schreiber G. Architectures for intelligent systems based on reusable components. Artif Intelligence Med 1995,7:189-199.

[23] Van Heijst G, Falasconi S, Abu-Hanna A, Schreiber AT, Stefanelli M. A case study in ontology library construction. Artif Intelligence Med 1995,7:227-255.

[24] Van Heijst G, Schreiber AT, Wielinga BJ. Using explicit ontologies for KBS development. Hum-Comput Stud 1997,42:183-292.

[25] http://protege.stanford.edu.

[26] Eriksson H, Fergerson R, Shahar Y, Musen MA. Automatic generation of ontology editors. In: Proceedings of the 12th Banff Knowledge Acquisition Workshop, Banff, Alta., Canada, October 1999.

[27] Guarino N. Formal ontology, conceptual analysis and knowledge representation. Hum-Comput Stud 1995,43: 625-640.

[28] De Keizer NF, Abu-Hanna A, Zwetsloot-Schonk JHM. Understanding terminological systems. I. Terminology and typology. Methods Inform Med 2000,39:16-21.

[29] Humphreys BL, Lindberg DA. The unified medical language system: an informatics research collaboration. Am Med Inform Assoc 1998,5:1-11.

[30] Jones D, *et al*. Methodologies for ontology development. In: Proceedings of the IT&KNOWS Conference, XV IFIP World Computer Congress, Budapest, August 1998.

[31] Rector AL, *et al*. Untangling taxonomies and relationships: personal and practical problems in loosely coupled development of large ontologies. In: Gil Y, Musen M, Shavlik J, editors. K-CAP'01. p. 139-146.

[32] Fridman Noy N, Musen MA. SMART: automated support for ontology merging and alignment. In: Proceedings of the 12th Workshop on Knowledge Acquisition, Modelling and Management (KAW'99), Banff, Canada, October 1999.

[33] Wu LC (chief editor). Chinese traditional medicine and materia medical subject headings. Beijing: Chinese Medical Ancient Books Publishing, 1996.

[34] Beijing College of Traditional Chinese Medicine, Zhongyiyao Zhuti Cibiao. Traditional Chinese Medical Subject Headings. Beijing: Beijing Science & Technology Press, 1987.

[35] Editing Committee of Chinese Library Classification, Chinese Library Classification. 4th ed. Beijing: Beijing Library Press, 1999.

[36] General administration of technology supervision of the People's Republic of China, national standard: clinic terminology of traditional Chinese medical diagnosis and treatment—diseases, Beijing, 4 March 1997.

[37] General administration of technology supervision of the People's Republic of China, national standard: clinic terminology of traditional Chinese medical diagnosis and treatment—syndromes, Beijing, 4 March 1997.

[38] General administration of technology supervision of the People's Republic of China, national standard: clinic terminology of traditional Chinese medical diagnosis and treatment—therapeutic methods, Beijing, 4 March 1997.

[39] The pharmacopoeia commission of PRC, pharmacopoeia of the People's Republic of China. Beijing: Chemical Industry Press, 1997.

[40] Yin AN, Zhang RE. The blue print of unified traditional Chinese medical language system. Technical report, 2001 (in Chinese).

Semantic Web Development for Traditional Chinese Medicine

Zhaohui Wu, Tong Yu, Huajun Chen, Xiaohong Jiang, Chunying Zhou, Yu Zhang, Yuxin Mao, Yi Feng, Meng Cui, Aining Yin

首发于 *AAAI/IAAI*, 2008:1757-1762

Abstract

Despite its centrality to Chinese culture and wide adoption in Chinese communities, Traditional Chinese Medicine (TCM) has rarely been the application domain of computational analysis in previous academic works. Here we present the first systematic adoption of the state-of-the-art Semantic Web technologies in the codification, management, and utilization of TCM information and knowledge resources. These technologies are proved effective in bridging the semantic gaps between a plurality of legacy and heterogeneous relational databases, enabling ontology-based query and search across database boundaries. A global herb-drug interaction network is constructed and represented in Semantic Web language, on which the semantic graph mining methodology is applied for discovering and interpreting interesting patterns. This deployed Semantic Web platform provides various innovative information retrieval and knowledge discovery services to the TCM domain experts with positive feedbacks. This project demonstrates Semantic Web's advantages in connecting data across domain and community boundaries to facilitate interdisciplinary and cross-cultural studies.

1 Introduction

Traditional Chinese Medicine (TCM) is an ancient medical system that accounts for around 40% of all health care delivered in China (WHO 2002). However, the applications of computational analysis in TCM domain, if exist, have rarely been documented in previous academic works. Our joint group of the Zhejiang University and the China Academy of Chinese Medical Sciences (CACMS), has taken the first systematic approach to leverage the progress of biomedical informatics to address the preservation and modernization of this Chinese cultural heritage (Chen *et al*. 2006, Feng *et al*. 2006). We have constructed over 70 relational databases and various Web applications that provide knowledge and information services for TCM practitioners. However, the rapid accumulation of TCM data resources makes data integration across institutions a difficult and time-consuming task. Implicit or even lost data semantics hinders the efforts to link the data from disparate databases. Autonomous and arbitrary designs of database schemas make the data exclusively understood by originators and processed by ad hoc applications. The situation of database management and integration hinders the sharing and utilization of TCM information and knowledge resources.

The Semantic Web (http://www.w3.org/2001/sw/) technologies, by providing a common framework that allows data to be shared and reused across application, enterprise, and community boundaries, can potentially address the challenges of TCM informatics. The health care and life sciences communities have already taken efforts in the adoption of Semantic Web technologies. Most notably, the World Wide Web Consortium (W3C) established a Semantic Web interest group to focus on Health Care and Life Sciences (http://www.w3.org/2001/sw/hcls/). This community conducted a series of projects including ontology engineering (Smith *et al*. 2007) and Semantic Web applications (Sougata 2005, Cheung *et al*. 2005, Stephens *et al*. 2006), demonstrating that the Semantic Web is a feasible technical framework for knowledge representation, integration, and discovery in biomedical domain (Neumann *et al*. 2004). However, these successful projects focus exclusively on orthodoxy medicine, and never on TCM domain.

We have conducted the first project to adopt the Semantic Web solution in the integration, management, and utilization of TCM information and knowledge resources. As the result, a set of semantic-based tools and systems is developed and deployed to facilitate TCM practitioners in achieving collective intelligence. We have engineered the Unified TCM Language System (UTCMLS), the largest TCM Semantic Web ontology including 5,000 concepts and 20,000 instances. This ontology provides a common knowledge representation scheme to improve the quality of semantic search and query, and to infer semantic suggestions such as synonyms and associated concepts. We have also deployed at CACMS the ontology-based query and search engine (Figure 3), which maps legacy relational databases to the Semantic Web layer for query and search across database boundaries. Based on this semantic integration capability, we have mapped a global herb-drug interaction network (Figure 6), and developed the Spora system (Figure 4) based on *Semantic Graph Mining* methodology for discovering interesting patterns from complex networks in TCM domain. TCM domain experts evaluate the platform's major technical features as original and productive in TCM drug usage, discovery, and safety analysis.

2 Approach

Our approach put a special emphasis on making connections between TCM and biomedicine in purpose of facilitating interdisciplinary and cross-cultural information retrieval and data analysis. The major concern of TCM informatics is how to consolidate and utilize its own data, and how to connect its data with the data of other domains, especially the biomedicine. Figure 1 reveals that the two independent medical systems have potential in connecting points, such as: (1) the *patient* that represents electronic medical records and clinical trials that record the methods and results of integrative clinical practices, and (2) the *chemical* that refers to bioactive compounds from Chinese herbal medicine serving for drug discovery and safety analysis. We first engineer the TCM domain ontology based on this conceptual map, and then use the ontology to glue more and more databases. The resulting Semantic Web Platform provides a set of applications for end users, enabling searching, querying, navigating around an extensible set of databases. Semantic graph mining capabilities are also implemented on the Semantic Web layer for discovering interesting patterns from various large biomedical networks.

2.1 Mapping from Relational Data to Ontologies

The semantic mediator maps relational schemas into a shared domain ontology, and defines each relational table as a *Semantic View* over classes defined in the ontology (Chen *et al*. 2006). A visualized mapping tool has been developed and deployed to facilitate the TCM database administrators to define such Semantic Views in a graphical view (Figure 2). The database administrators can specify table-to-class mappings in a drag-and-drop fashion aided by the intelligent schema reasoner. This paradigm can improve efficiency and reduce errors compared with editing configuration files. Given table-to-class mappings, the

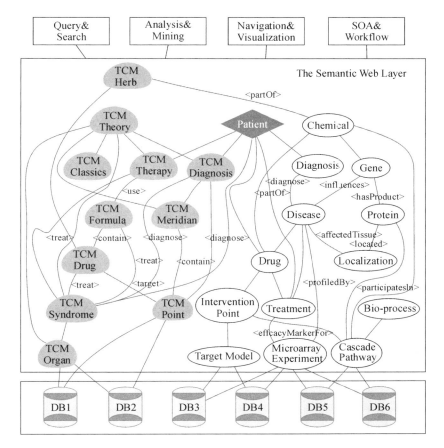

Figure 1 **The Semantic Web layer integrates heterogeneous relational databases from both TCM and Western Medicine, supporting various Web-based applications.**

engine infers potential table joins based on semantic associations inferred in the ontology. If two tables have foreign key relationships in relational schema, the engine is able to define the semantics of this join automatically. Class-level matching can also be inferred based on instance-level similarities. The generated semantic views can be deployed via invoking a semantic registration service and then take effect in query-rewriting mechanism. A query-rewriting engine translates a Sparql (Prud'hommeaux and Seaborne 2007) query into a series of SQL queries against underlying relational schemas, based on mapping rules derived from semantic views.

2.2　Ontology-based Query and Search

The Semantic Web portal (Figure 3) supports interactive discovery of TCM information and knowledge across database boundaries. In response to a keyword search, the portal displays content entries in the middle, and a recommended list of synonyms and associated concepts on the right. Using the classes and concepts in the searching results, the user can start to specify an accurate semantic query. Based on the semantic associations defined at the ontological level, the user can keep searching and navigating information and knowledge unaware of database boundaries.

In the paradigm of *Semantic Search*, the system accepts one or more keywords, performs a thorough

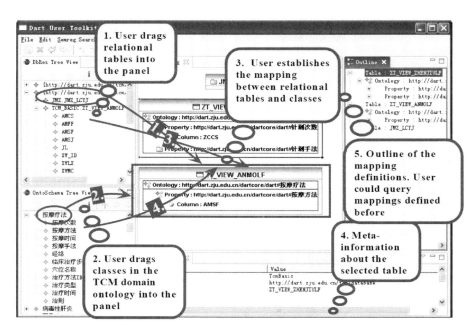

Figure 2   The relational-database-to-ontology mapping tool.

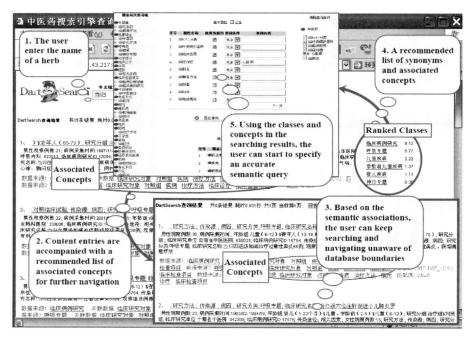

Figure 3   The ontology-based query and search portal.

content search on the Semantic Web, and presents searching results as a logical chain of evidences. The TCM knowledge is not organized as explicitly-linked Web resources, which makes link-based analysis not applicable for searching of the TCM knowledge, so we utilize the TCM domain ontology to improve the quality of search. The multimedia content, such as textual documents, images, and reporting tables, are annotated and indexed in terms of the ontology. The semantic associations of concepts are analyzed to determine the relevance and importance scores of concepts and content entries.

Semantic Query facilitates interactive and dynamic generation of the Sparql query, which is informally a graph pattern involving a set of variables, the class and property constraints for these variables, and the relationships between these variables. The system guides users through specifying and refining a query in an intuitive way. First, users can specify interesting classes by navigating on a graphical view of domain ontology. Second, a query form corresponding to property definitions of each selected class will be automatically generated and displayed. Third, users can check and select interesting properties and input query constraints into the text boxes. Finally, the constructed semantic query is translated into SQL queries based on the mapping rules derived from semantic views.

Semantic Navigation enables users to navigate TCM information and knowledge on the semantic level. The association between a patient's disease and a therapy that cures the disease can be critical for a clinical decision-making. However, the patient's EMR and the document for the therapy may not have explicit links or shared keywords. In our approach, semantic associations of concepts are inferred and ranked based on the ontology together with other knowledge resources, and are used to enhance the connectivity of the knowledge base. Among the results of a semantic query or search, in addition to multimedia content, there is a recommended list of associated concepts serving for users to pursue the navigation.

2. 3 Semantic Graph Mining

We developed the Spora system (Figure 4) that implements the semantic graph mining algorithms as generic operators that work on top of the Semantic Web layer and query semantic graph models in Sparql. The *Spora* system facilitates TCM domain experts to perform knowledge discovery experiments in an intuitive manner. Users can create an *experiment* by specifying a knowledge discovery process as a tree of operators with customizable properties, and then execute the process and review the visualized results. The user interface contains four units: (1) *Login, Introduction, and Navigation panels*; (2) *Explorer panel* that manages Semantic Web resources(including experiments and operators) that are visible and controllable by users; (3) *Operator and Operator Parameter panels* that display operators and their customizable parameters; (4) *Result panel* that visualizes data mining results through interactive tables, histograms, etc. Based on the above semantic integration capability, a global network of herb-drug interactions (Figure 6) can be mapped. Here we present our approach of semantic graph mining in analyzing this herb-drug interaction network.

The Semantic Web can be modeled as a directed graph that represents a statement with (1) a node for the subject, (2) a node for the object, and (3) an arc for the predicate, directed from the subject node to the object node. The merging of two semantic graphs is essentially the union of the two underlining sets of statements. Within a multiple semantic graph, a member graph can obtain a URI as its name for its provenance to be traced. This model gives an elegant solution to connect data from different sources and domains.

Definition 1 (Semantic Graph). We define a semantic graph as $SG = \{C, P, NCP, ST\}$ in which $C = \{c_1, c_2, \cdots, c_m\}$ is a set of classes, $P = \{p_1, p_2, \cdots, p_n\}$ is a set of properties, $NCP = \{r_1, r_2, \cdots, r_o\}$ is a set of normal resources that are neither classes nor properties, and $ST = \{st_1, st_2, \cdots, st_l\}$ is the set of statements. Let $R = C \cup P \cup NCP$ be the set of resources. Let $st \in ST$ be a statement in the form of subject-predicate-

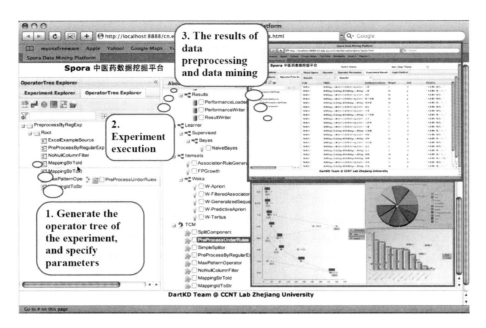

Figure 4   The *Spora* system for TCM knowledge discovery.

object triplet: $\langle s, p, o \rangle$ in which $s \in R$, and $p \in P$. We call s, p, and o the subject, the predicate, and the object of st, respectively.

Domain knowledge and/or personal preference can be used to assign various types of weights to resources and statements.

Definition 2(Weighted Semantic Graph). A weighted semantic graph $WSG = \{R, ST, W\}$ has a function $W: R \cup ST \rightarrow D$, which relates a resource or a statement to a value of set D. By default these weights are 1.0. Assigning a weight of type W and value v to a resource r is achieved by inserting a statement $\langle r, W, v \rangle$. Assigning a weight of type W and value v to a statement $st = \langle s, p, o \rangle$ is achieved by inserting the following statements: $\langle st, rdf: type, rdf: Statement \rangle$, $\langle st, W, v \rangle$, $\langle st, rdf: subject, s \rangle$, $\langle st, rdf: predicate, p \rangle$, and $\langle st, rdf: object, o \rangle$.

Given a weighted semantic graph $WSG = \{R, ST, W\}$, the *in-degree centrality* C_I of a resource is measured by the weighted sum of statements with the resource as object, the *out-degree centrality* C_O is measured by the weighted sum of statements with the resource as subject.

The *Closeness Centrality* (Brandes 2001) C_C of a resource r is defined as the inverse of the sum of the distance d_G from r to all other resources.

$$C_C(i) = \frac{1}{\sum_{j \in R} d_G(i,j)} \tag{1}$$

The *Betweenness Centrality* (Brandes 2001) C_B of a resource r is defined as the ratio of shortest paths across the resource in the graph. Let $\sigma_{st} = \sigma_{ts}$ denote the number of shortest paths from $s \in R$ to $t \in R$. Let $\sigma_{st}(r)$ denote the number of shortest paths from s to t that some $r \in R$ lies on.

$$C_B(r) = \sum_{s \neq r \neq t \in R} \frac{\sigma_{st}(r)}{\sigma_{st}} \tag{2}$$

Similarly, the *Betweenness Centrality* C_B of a statement is defined as the ratio of shortest paths across the statement in the graph.

Frequent patterns are item-sets, subsequences, or substructures that appear in a data set with frequency no less than a user-specified threshold (Han *et al.* 2007). In the traditional frequent pattern mining problem setting, a transaction is abstracted as a set of items, and frequent item-sets are extracted from a set of transactions. In medical domain, documents (EMRs or clinical trials) are better abstracted as a semantic graph of interrelated terms rather than a set of terms, and a knowledge base can be abstracted as a set of named semantic graphs. The problem of mining frequent semantic subgraph is therefore defined as follows.

Definition 3 (**Frequent Semantic Subgraph**). In a knowledge base KB, every transaction can be represented as a named semantic graph of statements. One graph α occurs in another graph β *iff*. $\alpha \subseteq \beta$. $ST = \{s_1, s_2, \cdots, s_n\}$ is the set of all statements in KB. A semantic graph α, which contains k statements from ST, is frequent if α occurs in graphs of knowledge base KB no lower than $\theta|KB|$ times, where θ is a user-specified minimum support threshold (called *min_sup* in our text), and $|KB|$ is the total number of graphs in KB.

The frequent semantic subgraph discovery (FSSD) process first construct a set of named semantic graphs using semantic queries, and then feed the resultset to an existing frequent pattern mining operator which treats each statement as an item. For example, the analyst retrieves a set of "Kidney Yang Deficiency (KYD)" (an instance of Syndrome) related EHRs to discover interesting patterns related to drug efficacy:

(1) These EHR transactions are represented as semantic graphs of statements.

(2) Merge EHR graphs with domain knowledge, and add annotations to every EHR transaction utilizing Sparql construction queries.

(3) Specify restrictions in Sparql, and run the Sparql to get a resultset of named graphs.

(4) Run frequent semantic subgraph discovery algorithm against the resultset, and again add annotations to every discovered pattern using semantic search.

(5) Visualize patterns for user interpretation.

Many complex networks have the property of community structure, in which network nodes are joined together in tightly knit groups, between which there are only looser connections (Girvan and Newman 2002). The problem of Semantic Graph Clustering is defined as follows.

Definition 4 (**Semantic Graph Clustering**). In a knowledge base KB, given a problem-solving context PC, grouping individuals of a given class D into communities, such that there is a higher density of interactions within communities than between them.

Suppose our problem is to discover significant patterns from the global network of herb-drug interactions. The inputs are an integrated knowledge base KB in TCM domain, a problem-solving context PC specifying the user's preference, and targeted class of population D (e.g. the set of herb-drugs); and the output is a set of frequent patterns and community structures extracted from KB that meet the criteria of PC. Our generic approach is defined in Algorithm 1. The first step is to ask the PC to find all interesting semantic associations between individuals of D from KB (by generating and executing a set of Sparql queries), and to merge the resulting semantic associations into a set SGs of named semantic graphs. The second step is to ask the PC to extract frequent patterns from SGs w.r.t. KB, and these frequent patterns are then merged together into a concise, weighted graph WSG. The third step is to add all components (a graph component refers to a connected subgraph) of WSG into the set CS.

Algorithm 1 Semantic Graph Mining

```
1: SGs ← PC.getAssociations(KB,D);
2: WSG = PC.frequentPattern(KB,SGs);
3: CS.add(getComponents(WSG));
4: for all (c ← CS) do
5:     if isCommunity(c) then
6:         move(c,CS,RS);
7:         continue;
8:     end if
9:     removeCentralityResources(c);
10:    while notDivided(c) do
11:        removeCentralityStatement(c);
12:    end while
13:    addCentralityVertices(getComponents(c));
14:    CS.add(getComponents(c));
15:    CS.remove(c);
16: end for
17: for all (c ← RS) do
18:    c.merge(PC.getAssociations(KB,c));
19: end for
20: return WSG,RS;
```

In the fourth step, we recursively pick a component c in CS to test if c satisfies the criteria for a community. We move c from CS to the result set RS if c is a community, and split c into smaller components otherwise. The splitting of c takes three major sub-steps: (1) remove centrality resources (whose closeness centrality ratio exceed a user-defined value) from c; (2) recursively remove the statement with max betweenness centrality ratio until the c ceases to be connected. (3) add centrality resources into every components of c. After c is divided into a set of components, we add these components into CS, and remove c from CS.

The final step is to generate semantic annotations for discovered communities with context analysis. For every community c in RS, ask the PC to find all interesting semantic associations between individuals of c from KB (by generating and executing a set of Sparql queries), and to merge the resulting semantic associations to c.

3   TCM Use Cases

TCM pharmacists primarily compound prescriptions as mixtures of multiple herbs, and establish a system of *TCM Herbal Formulae* as significant patterns of herb community structure. For example, *Four-Gentleman decoction*(FGD) is an ancient herbal formula with medical actions " to nurture the *qi* (the vital substance of human body as is stated in TCM)". It consists the following four herbs: (1) *Ginseng*, the king herb (FGD-K for short), (2) *Atractylodis*, the minister herb (FGD-M for short), (3) *Sclerotium*, the assistant herb (FGD-A for short), and (4) *Glycyrrhizae uralensis*, the carrier herb (FGD-C for short). A deeper understanding of TCM formulae system with its herb-drug interactions, can contribute to the drug discovery and safety analysis.

Based on the combination of TCM EMR warehouse and database of Chinese Medical Formula（DCMF），a Frequent Semantic Subgraph Discovery（FSSD）process with minimum support as 1% results in 136 frequent patterns of herb communities, including the pattern ｛FGD-K，FGD-M，FGD-A，FGD-C｝that appears in 1474 evidences. This result supports that formula FGD is a frequently-used pattern in TCM. We integrate DCMF with the Database of Structured TCM Literature（50035 records in the experiment）and perform another FSSD process on the dataset with minimum support as 5%, with a constraint that the discovered patterns should include members of FPD. The result is a set of 147 patterns（Figure 5），which reveal that（1）the FPD is indeed frequently associated with concepts related to "nurture the *qi*"; and（2）the FPD is also frequently associated with concepts related to cardiovascular system diseases（CVD）. This evidence is coherent with TCM pharmaceutics theory, which claims that CVD is caused by the insufficiency of *qi*, and FPD's action is to nurture the *qi*, and therefore FPD is beneficial for CVD.

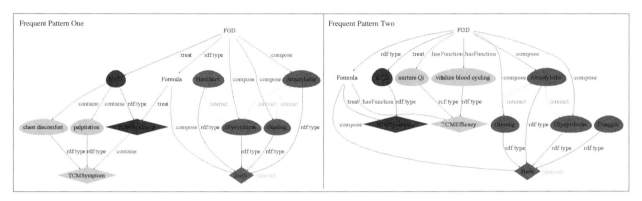

Figure 5　Discovered patterns can be annotated with domain knowledge based on semantic associations of concepts, and visualized as a semantically-enriched graph to facilitate human interpretation. The *Pattern One*, including four herbs and two symptoms, is interpreted by the fact that the formula *FGD* composed of these herbs frequently treats the syndrome *KYD* containing these symptoms. The *Pattern Two*, including four herbs and two drug efficacies, is interpreted by the fact that the formula *FGD* composed of these herbs has these two drug efficacies.

A global herb-drug interaction network can be mapped by inserting statements for all frequent herb-drug interactions into a semantic graph model. The nature and frequency of interactions involving these drugs are discovered through semantic association queries. The statement represents a pair of terms as subject and object, the type of interaction as predicate, and frequency as weight. In the clustering process, we first delete a certain number of centrality nodes, and then a certain number of centrality edges. We first delete nodes with closeness centrality exceeding a predefined threshold, because these nodes are seen as not exclusively belonging to any local community, and eliminating these nodes can help to reveal the local communities. We then delete the edge with the max betweenness centrality recursively until the population is separated, because these edges are seen as connecting local communities, and therefore eliminating these edges can also help to reveal the local communities. In the resulting network（Figure 6），most nodes（99.3%）participate in the largest connected components, and there is also a big drug community（pink colored on the left）that consists many biggest hubs in the network, including the four herbs in FGD, revealing that drug hubs tend to cluster together in TCM domain. The clustering results is evaluated by domain experts as correctly reflecting the TCM clinical practice.

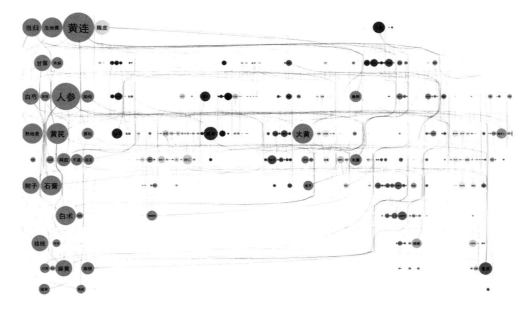

Figure 6 Global network of frequent herb-drug interactions, with drugs represented by nodes with size/font proportional to degree, interactions represented by edges, and drug communities represented by distinct colors.

4 User Evaluation

TCM domain experts accepted our Semantic Web solution with positive reactions. They are amazed by the Semantic Web's ability to address the semantic heterogeneity of databases, and praised the mapping tool for its simplicity and efficiency of database registration, which saved them considerable time as newly developed databases were frequently integrated into the data center. They found the semantic portal' functionalities very intuitive to use, in that it conforms to their cognitive style and thinking strategy. In semantic search, they tend to use the concept ranking functionality to refine their queries, when the resulting entries were overwhelmingly large. They found machine-learned patterns and rules interesting, especially when rendered as diagrams and semantically-enriched graphs. They realized that all herbs are connected through decentralized orchestration of formulae in their hands, and developed a series of discussions in interpreting frequent drug pairs and drug communities. They realize that machine learning methods essentially simulate their methodology of discovering novel formulae, with the difference that the past methodology is based on human observations and experiences, while the present methodology utilizes computational power to accelerate the process of discovery.

5 Conclusion

We presented an in-use Semantic Web platform supporting large-scale database integration, information retrieval, and knowledge discovery for Traditional Chinese Medicine domain. Underlying mechanisms, including semantic query and search, and semantic graph mining are described, and semantic-based tools are introduced. The project contributes to the preservation and modernization of TCM as intangible cultural heritage, and demonstrates the Semantic Web's ability to connect data from interrelated domains for interdisciplinary research.

Acknowledgements

This work is funded in part by China 973 subprograms No. 2003CB316906 and No. 2003CB317006; China NSF programs No. NSFC60503018, No. NSFC60525202, and No. NSFC60533040; and National Key Technology R&D Program No. 2006BAH02A01.

References

Brandes U. A faster algorithm for betweenness centrality. Journal of Mathematical Sociology, 25(2):163C177, 2001.
Chen, H. J. *et al*. 2006. From Legacy Relational Databases to the Semantic Web: an In-Use Application for Traditional Chinese Medicine. In 5th ISWC 06, Athens, GA, USA, November 5-9, LNCS 4273.

Feng Y. *et al*. 2006. Knowledge discovery in traditional Chinese medicine: State of the art and perspectives. Artificial Intelligence in Medicine, Volume 38, Issue 3, November 2006, Pages: 219-236.

Girvan M and Newman M. 2002. Community structure in social and biological networks. PNAS, 99:7821C7826, 2002.

Han J. *et al*. 2007. Frequent pattern mining: current status and future directions. Data Min. Knowl. Discov., 15(1): 55C86.

Cheung Kei-Hoi. *et al*. 2005. YeastHub: a semantic web use case for integrating data in the life sciences domain. Bioinformatics 21: i85-i96.

Neumann E K. *et al*. What the semantic web could do for the life sciences. Drug Discovery Today: BIOSILICO, 2(6): 228C236, 2004.

Prud'hommeaux E and Seaborne A. 2007. SPARQL Query Language for RDF-W3C Working Draft 26 March2007. http://www.w3.org/TR/rdf-sparql-query/.

Smith B. *et al*. 2007. The obo foundry: coordinated evolution of ontologies to support biomedical data integration. Nature Biotechnology, 25:1251C1255. Sougata Mukherjea. 2005. Information retrieval and knowledge discovery utilising a biomedical Semantic Web. Brief Bioinform 6: 252-262.

Stephens S. *et al*. Applying semantic web technologies to drug safety determination. IEEE Intelligent Systems, 21(1): 82C86, 2006.

WHO(World health organization), WHO traditional medicine strategy. http://www.who.int/medicines/publications/ traditionalpolicy/en/index.html, 2002.

2.2　学位论文摘要

　　本节摘录了中医药与语义网络知识图谱方向 2004—2019 年共 24 份学位论文资料信息(其中博士学位论文 6 份,硕士学位论文 18 份)。

2.2.1　Web 语义查询与推理研究

陈华钧(指导教师:吴朝晖、潘云鹤)
2004 年博士学位论文

　　随着信息资源共享的需求越来越迫切和互联网逐渐成为信息共享的支撑平台,以语义 Web 为代表的语义技术,以其严格的逻辑基础和标准化的技术路径,正逐渐成为未来 Web 信息系统的一项支撑技术。语义 Web 技术为 Web 信息系统提供了规范化的语义表达框架,以支持数据语义的明确表达。其目的一方面是要在尽可能的程度上实现数据的无缝集成、服务的动态组合和资源的自动发现;另一方面还缩小了人的认知域与计算机的处理域之间的距离,以实现用直观的语义对 Web 信息资源进行操作。

　　Web 语义查询与推理是语义 Web 需要实现的基本功能。本论文试图对这一问题进行系统性的研究。本论文的研究内容和主要贡献如下。

　　(1)基于视图的 Web 语义查询(answering queries using view in semantic web)。首先我们阐述了"视图"对实现分布式 Web 语义查询的重要性;然后结合 RDF 模型的特点,给出了 RDF 语义视图的形式化描述与定义;并系统地研究了在开放式世界假设下,基于语义视图的 Web 语义查询问答与语义查询重写;证明了基于视图的语义查询问答问题与 RDF 语义查询的包含推理问题之间的等价性;并给出了一个 RDF 语义查询包含算法和查询重写算法。

　　(2)上下文相关 Web 推理(Web Context and Contextual Reasoning)。首先我们阐述了上下文(context)对于 Web 语义建模的重要性;然后基于局部模型语义理论(Local Model Semantic)研究了上下文相关 Web 推理(Web Contextual Reasoning)的基本实现方法;并结合分布式描述逻辑的研究,设计了一个支持上下文相关 Web 推理的分布式 Tableaux 算法。更进一步,我们还基于类比相似的方法,研究了基于案例的推理在语义 Web 中的特点和实现方法,并提出和设计了基于 RDF 的 CaseML 案例表达语言。

　　(3)语义 Web 的网格体系架构及基于语义 Web 技术的数据库网格原型设计与实现。结合网格计算的思想,我们提出了一个面向语义 Web 的知识网格服务体系,以支持 Web 语义查询、语义映射和推理;基于该知识网格服务体系,我们实现了一个基于语义的数据库网格原型系统,称为 DartGrid,介绍了三种最基本的知识服务在数据库资源的模式集成和协同共享中所起的作用。DartGrid 基于语义 Web 若干技术标准,在网格平台 Globus 上开发。我们详细介绍了其核心组件的设计与实现,这包括语义浏览器、Q3 语义查询语言、本体服务、语义注册服务和语义查询服务。特别地,还介绍了关系模式向 RDF/OWL 模式的转化方法,以及 Q3 语义查询向 SQL 关系数据库查询的转化实现方法。

2.2.2　基于本体论的中医药一体化语言系统

方青(指导教师:吴朝晖)

2004 年硕士学位论文

传统中医药学历经数千年的发展,已经形成了完备的知识体系。但近年来随着信息化的深入,传统中医药学在发展过程中不够规范的弊端也逐渐突显出来,愈来愈多的应用开始受制于术语问题。目前的中医药数字资源缺乏知识层次的表达,也没有统一的术语定义标准,这给信息利用和共享造成了困难。

现有的医学术语系统缺乏知识的工程化,而本体论作为一种概念化的说明,采用框架系统对客观存在的概念和关系进行描述,能够表达复杂的概念关联关系,是一种有效的医学知识表达的手段。

本文针对医学术语系统面临的问题,提出了建立基于本体论的一体化语言系统的方案,目的是将现有的数字资源有效利用起来,以开放、简便的方式提供给用户使用。本文主要做了以下几个方面的工作。

(1)在本体论工程研究基础上,设计并开发了中医药本体论。针对中医药学领域知识建立概念集合和语义集合,定义本体的类以及层次结构,实现概念和语义的规范存储。

(2)在中医本体论的基础上提出中医药一体化语言系统原型,将本体知识库作为术语规范和通用编码模式的特性,设计基于本体查询的概念、语义服务,帮助用户获取综合性或特定性的中医药信息。

2.2.3　基于语义的中医药专家综合决策系统 DartSurvey

景鲲(指导教师:吴朝晖、陈华钧)

2006 年硕士学位论文

以急性传染病、中毒等为主的突发性公共卫生事件,对人们身体健康与国家正常政治经济秩序危害极大。为了解决这些问题,中医药领域专家必须要参与到问题处理、决策与规划活动中来。所以研究与建立快速、准确、科学、有效的公共卫生突发事件临床救治综合决策系统,是科学应对公共卫生突发事件,保障公众健康和国家利益的必然要求。

在本文中,我们设计和开发了针对中医药领域的综合决策系统 DartSurvey,用以协助领域专家进行决策,进而找到最优解决方案。在 DartSurvey 中,我们采用语义技术解决中医药领域知识分散、无统一标准的问题,并且对系统中的数据进行元信息描述,使得 DartSurvey 中所引用的基础数据、平台数据和讨论数据均有很好的重用性。同时 DartSurvey 中综合了 Brainstorming、Delphi Method、Analytic Hierarchy Process 等多种信息分析与决策的方法来辅助专家找到最优解决方案。

同时,本文还提出了一种新型语义 Web 浏览,替换了现在广泛流行的无意义的 HTML/XHTML 标记。语义 Web 浏览不仅给网页增加了语义信息,而且在浏览速度上也有很大的改进,也为语义 Web 的广泛发展提供了强有力的支持。本文将给出其核心设计与实现细节,同时还将介绍语义网站建设工具 DartFrontPage 的核心设计。

另外,本文还设计开发了一个面向复杂本体的浏览、查询与检索的工具 DartIE。它被用来辅助

DartSurvey 中的语义 Web 浏览。DartIE 的浏览模式非常丰富,可以动态并直观地把 DartSurvey 中的本体数据及其关系信息反馈给专家,同时它还允许专家对本体数据进行查询与检索。

最后,本文将介绍 DartSurvey 和 DartIE 的协同工作,同时会给出具体的案例来解释这一协作过程,然后还将介绍 DartSurvey 在中医药一体化语言系统中的应用。

2.2.4 中医药本体工程及相关应用

汤萌芽(指导教师:吴朝晖、陈华钧)

2007 年硕士学位论文

中医药作为中华文明的瑰宝,其知识体系的庞大和复杂也是众所周知的。因此规范中医药术语成了中医药学科研究和发展的重中之重。在利用这些规范化的数据指导自然语言知识处理工作的背景下,中医药一体化语言系统(Traditional Chinese Medicine Language System,TCMLS)应运而生。

本文首先介绍了支持基于本体开发的在线加工平台——语言系统,在该系统中,采用 Web 2.0 的相关技术,利用 Spring 的框架进行开发,目的是提供高质量的数据加工系统,同时提供一个具有良好用户体验的平台。目前,语言系统已经成为世界上最大的中医药本体,共采集 16 个一级类目,编录 12862 个类,收录词条数为 81811 个。

基于语言系统的外围工具也初现雏形。支持语言系统的 RDF 和 OWL 导出势在必行;同时支持语言系统的可配置的数据导出,旨在根据用户的偏好和实际需求,将数据扁平化,导出所需数据;另外,整合中医药领域的多个标准数据,提供一个可视化的查询和检索平台。

基于语言系统的应用一直是中医药领域发展的一个难题。经过长时间的探索,我们尝试了在不同方向对语言系统进行应用。在本文中将介绍语言系统在中医药共享和共建两大平台上的应用,同时介绍语言系统在中医药领域的中文分词中的贡献。这些应用是对中医药本体科学利用的大胆尝试,希望借此总结经验教训使得中医药本体有更光明的应用前景。

总的来说,本文阐述了中医药领域本体一体化语言系统从开发到应用的一个历程。

2.2.5 语义万维网的不确定知识表示与信任计算

郑骁庆(指导教师:吴朝晖)

2007 年博士学位论文

万维网(World Wide Web)的出现改变了人们的交流方式和商业模式,并逐渐成为人们通向知识经济和知识社会的核心支撑技术。语义万维网(Semantic Web)扩展了现有的万维网技术,通过制定相应的标准和规范,对网络资源以计算机更易处理的方式加以表示,并利用智能技术来发挥这种表示方法的潜在优势,实现诸如信息抽取、知识融合和基于知识搜索等高层功能与应用。

在语义万维网技术的层次结构中,目前较为成熟的部分(至底向上)有 XML(可扩展标记语言)、RDF/RDFS(资源描述框架及其模式)和 OWL(本体论语言),而在 OWL 之上的逻辑层和证明层(规则语言及其推理)相关标准的制定工作仍处于需求征询阶段,信任层则还处于研究阶段。

本文的研究是围绕语义万维网技术的逻辑层、证明层和信任层展开的,主要内容与贡献如下。

（1）针对单独采用描述逻辑（RDF/OWL 的逻辑学基础）或霍恩规则进行知识表示与推理的局限性，以及目前描述逻辑和霍恩规则结合推理算法并不同时具备可判定性和合理性的问题，利用"约束逻辑"的消解原理，提出了描述逻辑 ALCNR 和霍恩规则相结合的可判定推理算法，并且证明了约束消解算法的合理性和完备性。

（2）提出了适合于语义万维网的混合知识表示系统 ArtiGent，该系统由三个组成部分：描述逻辑 ALCNR、一组霍恩规则和事实集合。利用概率逻辑的思想，提出了在 ArtiGent 系统的霍恩规则和事实部分中引入概率不确定性的推理算法，并将这种不确定推理转化为求解相应的线性优化方程。

（3）针对语义万维网技术的信任层，提出了基于贝叶斯分析的"封闭"和"开放"信任计算模型。模型充分考虑了信任计算过程中涉及的五大关键因素——计算成本、机会成本、服务费用、咨询费用和效用，并且提出了平衡这些成本和得益的方法。模型具有坚实的数学理论依据和概率论上合理的解释，综合各种来源的信息能够为用户提供反映其偏好的一组个性化计算结果，从而辅助用户理性决策。

（4）ArtiGent 系统的描述逻辑断言和事实部分可以来源于关系数据库，并将语义数据库网格作为数据库集成和访问的基础平台。为了解决语义数据库网格系统查询效率较低的问题，以及数据库网格结点在设计、通信和执行方面的异质异构性与自治性对查询优化造成的困难，设计了适合于语义数据库网格的查询优化器，并且提出了相应的代价模型和查询优化算法 DG-QOA。该算法具有动态性、并行性和启发式的特点，启发式方法用于限制查询执行策略的搜索空间，并行性用来减少查询的响应时间，而动态性则能保证依据精确的统计和系统信息来确定后继的查询执行序列。

（5）对代表性的知识表示方法进行了综述与概括，指出了它们各自的特点和相互之间的关系，并讨论了知识表示的基本要求。以近期一些主要的研究工作和成果为依据，本文认为，面向网络、运用本体论和面向对象思想、具备可判定性，并且结合两种或两种以上知识表示方法的混合知识表示系统是目前和将来的研究重点。

2.2.6　基于图像语义和内容的半自动标注系统

丁艳春（指导教师：姜晓红）
2008 年硕士学位论文

十多年来，随着数字技术的迅速发展，每天都有来自军用与民用数以亿计的新的图片产生。为了有效地利用这些信息，我们就不得不找到一种可以有效浏览、搜索及索引这些图像的管理组织方式。一般的图像检索可以分为两类：一类是基于语义的，另一类是基于内容的。基于语义的图像检索，是指用户可以通过一些图像附加的诸如标题、关键字或者描述符的文本信息，利用文本匹配的方法得到想要的图像。例如用户输入关键字"房子"，系统返回所有标注"房子"的图像。然而由于传统的标注方法一般是人为对图像进行文字标注，其效率相当低。基于内容的图像检索，是指用户可以通过一些图像内在的特征信息，诸如颜色、纹理或者形状等，利用特征向量匹配的方法得到想要的图像。例如用户给予系统一座房子的轮廓图，系统返回所有与该图特征向量较为近似的图像。然而由于现有技术的局限，基于内容的搜索有时很难为用户找到真正想要的图像。

在本次的毕业论文中，我们将提出一种新的半自动图像标注框架。有这样的一个用户场景：用户输入关键字查询想要找的图像,系统根据基于语义的方式返回搜索结果。用户对当前显示的搜索结果根据自己的信息需求给出他们是否相关的判断,并反馈给系统。系统对反馈得到的图像做基于内容的搜索,并将结果图像与其对应的标注做相应的调整。这就是一个基于图像语义和内容的半自动标注系统的简要流程。通过这样的一个搜索-反馈的循环过程,数据库中图像标注的覆盖率和准确率都将会逐步地得到提高。这样的一个算法,与基于语义的搜索相比效率更高,与基于内容的搜索相比精度更高。此外,我们还将此算法应用到本次毕业设计的作品 Image Annotation 1.0 中,并得到一个较为满意的试验结果。

2.2.7　面向大规模本体重用的子本体模型研究

毛郁欣(指导教师:吴朝晖)
2008 年博士学位论文

本体作为语义 Web 的知识表示基础,在构建基于语义的系统或应用中发挥着至关重要的作用。随着本体规模的增长,系统处理和利用本体的效率会降低。对于大规模的领域本体,语义 Web 应用通常只需要利用其中的部分内容。从目前语义 Web 和本体的研究来看,还缺乏比较有效的模型与方法,来支持在语义 Web 应用中对大规模本体的重用。为了构建和推广面向语义 Web 的应用,有效地管理和利用已有的大规模本体已经成为一个十分现实和迫切的需求。

基于上述背景,本文着重探讨了面向大规模本体重用的子本体模型,主要研究内容和贡献包括以下几个方面。

(1)针对语义 Web 应用在利用本体时存在的局部性,提出了子本体的表示方法。将来自大规模本体的上下文相关的模块表示为子本体,给出了子本体的形式化表示,并定义了针对子本体的对象操作。语义 Web 应用能够根据需要动态地抽取子本体,创建特定的子本体知识库。将缓存机制与本体重用相结合,利用子本体缓存作为系统的局部知识库,支持对大规模本体的动态重用。

(2)对面向子本体的推理问题进行了研究。提出了子本体中的基本推理任务,通过特定的子本体推理算法,将本体的推理问题转化为子本体的推理问题,能从一定程度上降低推理的复杂性,提高推理的效率。给出了基于子本体表示的 Tableau 算法,支持模块化的本体推理。证明了面向子本体的 Tableau 算法相对源本体而言是半判定的,并给出了保持一致性的扩展推理算法。

(3)针对子本体知识库的优化问题,提出了基于遗传算法的优化方法。该方法对传统的遗传算法进行扩展,提出了基于语义的遗传算法 SemGA,使用基于三元组的非二进制编码方式将子本体表示为染色体,根据语义关系执行遗传算子。利用 SemGA 进行动态演化,从而达到优化知识库的语义结构的目的。与一般的缓存策略相比,基于演化的方法在效率上和性能上都有比较明显的优势。

(4)面向分布式的 Web 资源,提出了基于子本体的资源集成与管理方法。该方法利用本体语义对分布式的 Web 资源进行集成,通过在资源模式与本体之间建立语义映射,实现以子本体为单位的资源管理。将资源匹配过程转化为资源请求与子本体之间的概念匹配,利用遗传算法进行资源优化,满足动态变化的资源请求。模拟实验的结果表明,该算法能进一步提高资源匹配和重用的效率。

基于上述工作,同时还设计并实现了一个子本体原型系统 DartOnto,支持面向中医药领域的大规模本体重用。通过实例进一步说明了如何应用子本体模型创建中医药知识服务,解决大规模领域本体的重用问题。

2.2.8　面向中医药的分布式语义搜索系统

付志宏(指导教师:姜晓红、陈华钧)

2010 年硕士学位论文

随着 Internet 的快速发展以及信息技术在各个科学领域的普及,在同一科学领域的不同机构,数据的表现方式呈现出不同的特点,数据之间的共享以及集成成为对数据资源进行有效利用的难题。针对目前的这一难题,在实验室原有 DartSearchV3 的基础上,提出了新的分布式语义搜索系统的解决方案。本文主要介绍了该系统的具体设计以及详细实现过程。

首先,本文首先简要回顾了目前搜索引擎技术的发展现状以及面临的难题,并对实验室的原有相关工作 DartGrid 和 DartSearchV3 进行了简单介绍;随之介绍了在分布式语义搜索系统中将应用到的两个开源软件工具 Lucene 和 Hadoop;最后,通过分析中医药领域数据集成及搜索的新需求以及原 DartSearchV3 存在的缺陷,提出了分布式语义搜索系统的解决方案,并介绍了该系统的具体设计以及详细实现过程。

本文的核心内容在于对新的分布式语义搜索系统的总体设计,混合语义索引的构造算法,多个数据中心数据的语义集成技术,以及如何利用 Hadoop 进行分布式索引与搜索技术等进行详细分析与设计,并着重对混合语义索引的构建过程以及在 Hadoop 集群中分布式索引的管理与搜索任务的调度分发进行详细介绍。

最后,本文还简要分析了在未来的工作中,新的分布式语义搜索系统将要发展的几个方向。

2.2.9　中医药知识工程应用

宓金华(指导教师:姜晓红、陈华钧)

2010 年硕士学位论文

知识工程是人工智能的一种实现方法,为那些需要专家知识才能解决的应用难题提供求解的手段,它在中医学领域中的应用方兴未艾。本文介绍了浙江大学 CCNT 实验室与中国中医科学院在知识工程领域的合作项目——DartOnto 平台。DartOnto 平台围绕中医药知识工程的需求开发出:中医基础本体,通过重用和调整历史本体树并映射已有数据库创建,作为中医药知识来源为上层应用服务;五行本体模型,描述中医五行基础理论,并对其开发应用系统实现五行理论的展示和推理;温病本体模型,作为公共卫生领域本体,对疾病和治疗的本体表达进行深入探索,并对其开发应用系统以指导疫病的防治;OntoTool 工具,可视化地整合已有数据库和语义网络本体;DartWiki 语义维基,作为中医基础本体最主要的上层应用,提供中医药实例查询信息内容,为中医药领域知识共享提供服务。

2.2.10　面向中医药的多元语义搜索引擎

杨克特(指导教师:陈华钧、姜晓红)

2010 年硕士学位论文

随着万维网的迅速发展以及信息技术在各个科学领域的普及,数据的表现方式在同一科学领域的不同机构中已呈现出不同的特点,数据之间的共享以及集成成为对数据资源进行有效利用的难题。为了快速而准确地获取特定领域的科学数据,面向领域的搜索引擎应运而生。针对目前的这一需求,在实验室 DartSearch 与 DartQuery 的基础上,提出了新的面向中医药领域的多元语义搜索引擎系统。本文主要介绍该系统的设计与实现。

首先,本文简要回顾了目前搜索引擎技术的发展现状和面临的难题,并对实验室原有的相关工作 DartSearch 和 DartQuery 进行了简单介绍,对存在的问题进行了分析。随之介绍了与系统相关的全文检索技术、搜索结果排序机制以及开源搜索引擎的发展现状,并对系统中用到的两个开源工具 Lucene 和 Nutch 进行了简单介绍。

本文的重点主要体现在以下三个方面。首先,提出了搜索引擎系统的整体设计,对系统涉及的模块、架构以及所采取的技术进行了详细的介绍。其次,提出了多元语义数据索引方法,该方法能够集成中医药领域多种来源的异构异质数据,并且具有足够的灵活性来兼容以后新添加的数据类型。最后,提出了基于本体的搜索结果排序算法,该算法在考虑本体重要性的基础上,综合用户查询与结果的匹配度,对结果进行排序。此方法符合用户对搜索结果的预期,具有较好的实际效果。

论文最后还对搜索系统进行了展示,并扼要地分析了此系统将来可能面临的问题,提出了搜索系统的发展方向。

2.2.11 基于中医药本体的语义关系发现及验证方法

张小刚(指导教师:陈华钧、姜晓红)
2010 年硕士学位论文

中医药语言系统(Traditional Chinese Medical Language System,TCMLS)是世界上规模最大、数据最全的领域本体之一,在中医药科研和应用的多个领域发挥着重要的推动作用。但是,随着数据量不断扩大,TCMLS 的建设难度也在不断提高,其中存在的种种数据质量问题也制约着它的进一步发展和应用。更好地利用现有的领域知识,推动中医药本体建设的进一步完善和发展,对于 TCMLS 的建设乃至整个中医药信息化工作,都有着重要的意义。

在本文中,我们从中医药本体建设工作中面临的实际问题出发,通过分析中医药领域本体与领域文献数据特征,提出了一种基于中医药领域本体和领域文献的语义关系发现与验证方法。该方法在利用现有的领域本体的基础上,使用关联规则分析来提取中医药文献中隐含的语义关系,并可以对现有的语义关系进行验证。在此基础上,我们又引入了概率知识,提出一种基于概率的语义关系发现方法,这种方法可以利用挖掘过程中的概率信息来分析和优化结果,并使用基于概率的 RDF 来保存抽取过程中得到的概率数据,从而提高了结果的信息量和区分度。我们在实践中对这两种方法进行了检验,并取得了较为理想的应用效果。

2.2.12 基于 Linked Open Data 的语义关联发现及其应用

郑清照(指导教师:杨莹春、陈华钧)
2010 年硕士学位论文

语义网(Semantic Web)的目标是通过在网页内容上附加形式化的语义信息,让机器也能够理解网页的内容。随着语义网技术逐渐成熟,人们根据互联数据(Linked Data)的原则在语义网上发布、连接结构化数据,最终产生互联数据。开放互联数据社区的成立极大地促进了互联数据的发布。已经发布的互联数据集覆盖领域广泛,有地理信息、人口资料信息、在线社区、科学出版物、音乐等。互联数据为从分布式数据源中发现事物之间潜在的关系提供了巨大的可能。随着越来越多的互联数据的发布,如何在互联数据上进行语义关联发现成为研究的关键问题。

语义关联是语义数据模型中实体之间二维关系的知识表示形式。语义关联发现基于现有的语义关联,使用算法推导出更深层次的语义关系。然而现有的语义关联发现方法都是基于集中式的知识库的,这不符合互联数据的分布式特点,也使得现有的方法可扩展性较差。因此,研究设计一种符合互联数据分布式特点、可扩展性较好的语义关联发现方法是非常必要的。

针对上述问题,论文提出并设计实现了一个多代理协作的分布式语义关联发现框架。具体内容包括:①提出一种新的知识表示模型,介绍了假设、证据、证据图等知识元素的表示方法,该知识表示模型有助于多个代理之间进行知识交换;②提出了一种新的多代理协作式语义关联发现机制;③设计实现了两类代理,即目录代理和挖掘代理,并对代理提供的服务给出了详细的规范定义;④设计实现了语义关联发现的核心算法,并研究分析了算法可以采用的不同策略;⑤对该语义关联发现框架进行模拟实验,做性能分析,并将它应用于 DBLP 和 DBPedia 数据集,结果表明多代理之间协作进行语义关联发现是可行的。

2.2.13　基于 OWL 的中医理论语义模型及应用

梁欣颖(指导教师:陈华钧)
2012 年硕士学位论文

知识模型就是将知识进行形式化和结构化的抽象,是知识工程发展和应用的基石。它在中医学领域中的发展方兴未艾,而该领域的知识工程也在发展中。本文介绍了由中国中医科学院提供理论知识,浙江大学 CCNT 实验室提供科学方法的合作项目——温病知识模型、中医基础理论模型及其应用。其中,温病本体模型对疾病和治疗的本体表达进行了深入探索,并在该模型的基础上开发相应的应用系统用以指导温病的防治;个案加工平台则是对温病本体模型的一个实践方面的补充,为温病个案分析系统提供了数据来源;温病个案分析系统则是建立在个案加工平台和温病本体模型基础上的一个应用,探索了温病治疗体系的理论的继承和发展。中医基础理论针对阴阳学说和五行学说,描述了其基础理论,并对其开发应用系统实现中医领域内的文献检索、模型展示和养生指导。

2.2.14　基于语义的移动 Mashup 技术及应用

彭志鹏(指导教师:陈华钧)
2012 年硕士学位论文

近年来 Web 服务技术得到快速发展,它具有分布式、模块化、基于网络、自描述等特性,为互联网应用提供了统一的服务注册、发现、绑定和集成机制;而 Mashup 则主要是通过整合不同数据源的 Web 服务并结合 AJAX 的交互性等,为用户提供互联网应用。随着移动设备硬件性能的不断提升,移动互联网也在飞速发展,将移动设备上的用户数据信息如位置信息、通讯录等与互联网上的 Web

服务进行结合就可以生成许多新颖的以用户个人信息为中心的 Mashup 应用,这正是移动 Mashup 技术与应用的研究出发点。

本文提出基于语义的移动 Mashup 应用生成系统:MMAI(Mashup-based Mobile App Inventor)系统,该系统不仅使移动 Mashup 应用的开发不再局限于专业的编程人员,而且让不懂技术但富有想法的普通用户能够将自己的 Mashup 想法转化为一个可安装执行的移动 Mashup 应用程序。用户无须编写任何程序,只需要关注应用所需的功能,然后使用系统提供的交互界面选择功能对应的手机服务或者 Web 服务并进行简单的配置即可。MMAI 系统使用 OWL-S 服务资源描述框架对移动服务和 Web 服务进行统一描述,并使用语义推理器对服务进行语义匹配和服务推荐,同时建立 Mashup 工作流模型,使最终生成的移动 Mashup 应用在执行过程中能够得到更好的控制并能够与用户交互。

2.2.15　知识服务:语义 Web 在中医药领域的应用研究

于彤(指导教师:吴朝晖、陈华钧)

2012 年博士学位论文

语义 Web 是对当前 Web 架构的系统性重构和扩展,使 Web 支持结构性数据的发表、共享和关联,进一步提高 Web 的有序性、交互性和智能性。经过十余年的发展,语义 Web 的标准化建设取得了长足的发展。资源描述框架、Web 本体语言、SPARQL 查询语言、RIF 规则语言等基础性规范的制定使得语义 Web 从一个构想发展成为一套相对完整的技术体系。在可以预见的未来,语义 Web 将应用在生物医学、文化遗产、电子政务和社交网络等多个领域。语义 Web 是真正实用还是空中楼阁,将取决于这些应用的成败。因此,选择一个特定的领域进行语义 Web 的应用研究是合理而迫切的。

中医药是适合语义 Web 实施的领域。中医药的信息化过程中实现了全面的数据库群,也暴露了术语系统缺失、数据孤岛和缺乏深度利用等问题。为解决这些问题,该领域的专业人士基于语义 Web 技术,构建了中医药电子科学环境——TCM-SESE,其中包括中医药本体平台、中医药语义查询平台和中医药语义搜索平台等。TCM-SESE 取得了良好的示范性效果,但尚未充分发挥语义 Web 的全部潜能。

本文旨在引入国际最新的语义 Web 技术,对 TCM-SESE 进行进一步的改进和扩展,解决中医药信息化建设中面临的核心问题,促进中医药与现代科学之间的相互交叉、渗透、融合,为中医药信息学的发展做出贡献。本文的核心工作是中医药知识服务平台的构建。本文针对中医药信息化的核心问题,兼顾现代服务业的发展趋势,提出了"知识即服务"的理念,并在中医药领域具体实施。

本文首先针对中医核心思维模式进行了语义建模。笔者认为,"取象比类"是贯穿中医知识体系的思维模式,与中医其他的思想方法共同构成了中医"象思维"。本文追溯"象思维"的思想源流,并将其与认知语言学中的"隐喻"以及工程领域中的"设计模式"进行比较,在此基础上,提出一套与之相适应的建模方法,即语义模式。语义模式是面向语义 Web 的设计模式体系,其作用是指导领域知识的语义建模以及语义 Web 应用系统的开发。本文提出了语义模式的理论框架以及应用、归档、交流与传播的一系列方法,建立了语义模式名录,并从中医"象思维"建模等中医药领域问题出发,验证了这些语义模式的可行性和有效性,评估了它们的应用价值。

在中医药知识服务平台的具体实施中,重点解决了三个核心科学问题。

(1)中医药领域知识的本体建模。针对中医药领域知识的复杂性、模糊性和争议性,提供了基于本体技术的知识建模方法。通过构建中医药领域本体,对中医药理论知识进行辨认、梳理、澄清和永久保真处理。本体建模的对象包括阴阳、五行、脏腑、证候、草药、方剂等基本概念,以及五行学说、藏象学说、辨证论治和方剂配伍等理论学说。最终,将这些知识模型整合为一个包括多个模块的示范性本体。

(2)中医药领域知识的语义融合。针对中医药领域缺乏一体化的术语系统和知识模型的问题,构建基于本体的知识库,实现语义百科服务,支持中医药领域的术语资源和知识遗产的有序组织与有效管理。将中医药一体化语言系统和一系列国家、国际标准术语系统转化为语义 Web 本体,实现了中医药术语系统的语义融合。针对五行、温病、中药方剂和文献等核心领域开发了示范性知识库,并基于中医药术语系统实现了一系列示范性知识库的整合。

(3)面向结合医学的知识关联。针对中医药领域的知识孤岛现象,基于语义 Web 技术,提出一种面向关联数据的知识关联框架。设计了中医药知识与相关知识(如现代生物医学知识)进行关联的方案,使中医药知识接入全球互联的知识网络之中,在中西医结合医学中发挥更大的作用和影响力。

最后,综合论述了知识服务平台系统的总体架构、实施方案以及各个子系统的情况。在中医药知识服务平台的基础上,提供了一系列中医药智能应用的原型系统,演示知识展示、语义查询、语义搜索等功能。实现了五行模型演示、中医临床决策支持和中医方剂配伍规律发现等中医药领域的应用。这些智能应用能够改进中医药领域知识资源的利用效果,辅助中医药领域专家完成知识发现和决策支持等任务。

2.2.16　DartReasoner 面向海量数据的语义推理

郑耀文(指导教师:陈华钧)

2012 年硕士学位论文

近年来,语义网受到愈来愈多的关注,而语义推理一直都是语义网的核心问题,当前已经开发出了多个推理机,但其在查询推理性能上无法完全满足工业界应用。与语义查询相比较,关系型数据库发展至今相对比较成熟,工业界使用的数据也多存放在关系型数据库中,同时语义网研究中也有对语义数据资源与数据库数据资源的双射研究。通过结合元数据映射和关系型数据库的查询性能,对语义查询进行语义扩展并翻译成数据库查询,可以有效减小查询推理的规模。利用传统数据库查询技术可以提升关联查询性能,并使得现有的存储在数据库中的数据能够享受到语义查询的便利。

本文主要研究基于查询翻译的推理算法,设计并实现了基于该算法的推理引擎 DartReasoner,通过将元数据映射关系转换为语义映射图,并结合翻译算法将 SPARQL 查询转换为多个 SQL 查询,从而利用成熟的关系型数据库技术,在空间和时间开销中提升性能。

面对海量数据推理问题,本文尝试利用分布式推理算法解决具有多个前项式的 OWL2 属性链推理规则,设计并实现属性链的分布式推理算法。

2.2.17 语义图推理及中医药应用研究

顾珮嵚(指导教师:吴朝晖、陈华钧)

2013 年博士学位论文

自语义网的概念被提出以来,由 W3C 组织倡导和支持的语义网标准化建设已经取得了长足的发展,一系列包含资源描述框架 RDF、网络本体语言 OWL、SPARQL 查询语言、RIF 规则语言等的基础规范得以制定。在学术界的努力下,产生了一大批高质量的领域语义知识库,以及非结构化数据的语义标记、链接数据集和元数据描述等。由于语义数据的描述性和互联性,我们把这些领域的知识模型和语义描述的集合称为语义图(Semantic Graph)。语义图构成了领域知识的形式化表述,并被应用到生物医学、电子政务、社交网络和信息检索等多个领域,参与或主导知识表达、决策支持、人工智能等多种智能应用,并发挥着越来越重要的作用。语义图推理是用来保证语义图的质量,进行语义图的整合,以及进一步发展智能推理的重要处理手段之一。语义图推理除了可以检测语义图的一致性和完整性之外,还可以通过建模领域知识规则,应用推理技术完成领域知识推论,进而辅助自动化决策、知识挖掘和关联发现。

本文以语义图推理的三大实用性科学问题为研究内容。首先,表达能力有限的语义本体语言无法满足领域应用中的某些复杂因果关系建模,因此扩展语义因果表达能力对于领域知识建模和知识型应用非常有必要。再次,某些知识型领域,比如医学或者电子控制,常涉及多个因素对结果的影响以及模糊术语的大量使用,比如多、少、高、低等。当前的网络本体语言并不提供支持非精确描述以及推理的能力,这使得这些领域的知识建模和知识辅助应用进展缓慢。因此研究如何建立领域中的模糊描述建模和模糊推理是领域深度应用需要解决的核心问题。最后,带有领域知识的异域异构语义图之间的无缝信息整合,不仅需要通用一致的知识表达标准,而且需要对多个领域知识的交叉理解和大规模同步处理的能力,这是语义图的一大发展趋势和迫切需要解决的问题。本文重点解决三个核心科学问题。

(1)面向因果循环的因果语义图建模及推理。针对领域应用中的因果复杂关联性,提出了基于网络本体技术和因果语义规则的因果语义图建模方法,刻画领域知识中的概念、属性以及个体之间的因果关系。然后,提出了基于因果语义规则的语义推理方法,根据条件假设生成或者获取隐含的知识推理结果。在实际应用案例中,针对中医思维中的人与自然的相关关系和因果关系,对中医基础五行理论知识进行了辨认和梳理,创建了一个全面完整的中医五行语义图,采用因果语义推理引擎对中医五行诊疗进行推理,展示其内在的思维过程,或可用于诊疗建议。最后,基于 Web 开发技术研制了一个在线的中医五行知识展示系统。

(2)面向不精确主观描述的模糊语义图建模及推理。针对领域应用中的主观不精确描述,提出了扩展自模糊描述逻辑的模糊语义图建模方法,通过隶属函数来表述模糊术语的语义含义、模糊相关关系等。然后,提出了基于模糊描述逻辑的模糊语义图推理引擎,最终可以返回实例查询、包含性检测等的查询结果及其模糊度。在实际应用案例中,针对中医药诊疗案例中典型的自然语言术语表达和中医药诊疗结果中的不确定性,基于模糊语义图方法为现代中医病例术语定义了合理的不确定范围,针对症状、症候、疾病、中药提出了模糊表达方法,实现了中医药术语的形式化解释。同时,基于示范性中医诊疗模糊语义图的研究开发了两个在线中医自动诊疗演示系统,从本体主导和本体辅助的不同方向展示了模糊语义推理在决策支持中的作用。

(3)面向大规模语义图整合需求的弹性语义推理。针对大规模多语义图整合的数据量超载和跨语义图语义关联挖掘的实际问题,基于语义链接数据技术,提出了弹性推理的概念,即基于分布式计算的思想提供弹性扩展计算资源和存储资源的能力,通过分散迭代语义推理的任务,达到同步在多个计算节点上推理大规模语义图的目的。在实际应用案例中,为了挖掘中西医之间的已有研究成果的关联,收集各个领域的语义数据并进行标准化,在中西医领域专家的协助下制定关联传递规则,设计了中医药知识与相关现代生物医学知识进行关联的分布式语义推理算法。目的是使中医药知识接入全球互联的知识网络,使得中西医结合医学发挥更大的作用和影响力。最后,研制了一个基于开放共享原则的中西医关联搜索引擎,为全球用户提供快捷方便的资源关联、科普教育和科研交流的平台。

最后,综合论述了中医药开放语义平台的总体架构、实施方案以及各个子系统的情况。在中医药开放语义平台的基础上,实现了中医基础理论知识展示、中医临床决策支持和中西医关联发现等中医药领域应用案例。结论处总结了当前推理方法的不足之处,并展望了语义推理和中医药信息化的未来发展趋势。

2.2.18　面向大规模知识图谱的弹性推理研究方法研究及应用

陈曦(指导教师:陈华钧、吴朝晖)
2017 年博士学位论文

知识图谱可以被看作人类刻画和认知世界的一个载体,是人工智能的重要分支,它可以对现实世界的事物及其相互关系进行形式化描述,以刻画和揭示实体之间的语义关系,进而模仿人类的思维方式,进行逻辑推理。知识图谱的推理技术是知识图谱最核心的技术之一,是由一个或几个已知的判断推理出未知结论的过程。广义的推理包含语义查询和语义推理,本文所指的推理是广义范围的推理技术。近年来,随着知识抽取技术不断发展以及数据来源不断丰富,知识图谱的规模正在迅速增长,当前知识图谱默认已被用来代表各种海量知识图谱。伴随着知识图谱规模的增长,知识图谱呈现出结构复杂多样性、数据动态变化性以及查询实时响应性等多种特性,面对知识图谱所呈现的新特征和挑战,传统的语义推理方法和工具缺乏相应的对策,这极大地限制了知识图谱技术的进一步推广和发展。研究如何高效地在大规模知识图谱上实施弹性语义推理成为一个重要研究课题。

本文从大规模知识图谱语义推理所面临的挑战出发,研究了面向大规模知识图谱弹性语义推理的若干实用性科学问题,研究内容主要包括以下几个方面。

(1)针对大规模知识图谱复杂知识结构的挑战,研究基于 OWL 属性链的弹性语义关联推理方法。

(2)针对大规模知识图谱查询实时性的挑战,研究基于分布式内存的弹性语义查询推理方法。

(3)针对大规模知识图谱流式动态性的挑战,研究基于规则的弹性语义流推理方法。

(4)基于上述的方法和经验,设计实施了两个实用的面向大规模知识图谱弹性语义推理系统:基于 Spark 的大规模知识图谱规则推理系统和领域相关的大规模中西医知识图谱关联发现系统。

2.2.19　一种基于 Spark 的语义推理引擎实现及应用

黄崛（指导教师：陈华钧）

2017 年硕士学位论文

近些年在知识图谱蓬勃发展的大背景下，与之相关的语义 Web 的数据规模也呈现爆发态势。如何在大规模语义 Web 数据上有效地进行语义推理是研究者们面临的棘手问题。具体来说，在大规模语义 Web 数据上实施语义推理时，计算量巨大、消耗时间长都是突出的问题，特别是当应用复杂规则逻辑进行推理时，情况更是如此。传统单机环境下的语义推理引擎无法应对大规模知识图谱下的推理，缺乏可扩展性方面的考虑，难以满足在数据规模上日益增长的语义关联数据的推理需求。从分布式角度来看，已有的基于 Hadoop MapReduce 实现的语义推理框架由于欠缺推理算法相关的网络通信和磁盘 I/O 等的优化，推理效率依然较低。

本文针对上述问题，围绕分布式内存计算平台 Spark，研究以下几个方面的内容。首先，设计一个良好模块化且推理规则可配置的完整分布式推理引擎架构。接着，研究现有的单机和分布式语义推理算法，基于 Spark 框架对相关算法进行分布式的实现，并针对 Spark 的原理和特点做相应的优化。将基于 Spark 实现的推理引擎与现有的传统分布式推理引擎在推理效率上进行对比实验。实验结果表明，本文设计的基于 Spark 的语义推理引擎在推理效率上要远好于以 Hadoop MapReduce 为代表的推理实现，同时兼具了高可扩展性。最终将本系统应用到物联网领域，适应于实时和流式的语义数据流处理与推理场景。

2.2.20　中医药症状的中文分词与句子相似度研究

毛宇（指导教师：姜晓红）

2017 年硕士学位论文

中医药是中国传统医药，也是中华民族的文化瑰宝。随着医学技术的发展，中医药由于其整体性、动态性、辨证性等特征，越来越被人们重视。信息技术、人工智能的不断突破，也为中医药的发展提供了新思路。目前国家已将中医药信息化列在国家信息化发展战略纲要中。由于中医药信息化起步较晚、长期投入不足，中医药信息化的研究总体滞后。本文结合自然语言处理技术，对中医药信息化过程中的中医药症状，进行了深入的研究。本文重点研究了中医药症状分词和中医药症状句子相似度计算，具体贡献如下。

(1)研究了中医药症状的数据特征。在大量的观察实验和互联网搜索的基础上，将中医药症状总结成表达各异、理解不同、表述不清、单字成词、部分字词用法特殊、用字不规范、词典不完善这七大特征。

(2)研究了中文分词的主要算法、技术难点以及评价指标。分析了每种算法的优点和缺点。针对已有分词算法的不足和中医药症状数据的特征，设计了一种基于双向条件概率统计模型和相对位置的中医药症状分词算法。通过与互信息模型、二元文法模型、正向条件概率模型、双向条件概率模型比较，本文的方法在准确率和召回率上分别平均提高了 13.39% 和 17.88%。

(3)研究了汉语句子相似度计算的主要算法、技术难点以及评价指标。分析了每种算法在中医药环境下的优缺点。改进了已有的词语相似度计算方法。提出了中医药症状词语的分级概念,按照症状词语的重要性将其分为六个等级。综合词语相似度和词语重要性两个指标,改进了原来基于语义向量的句子相似度计算方法。新方法较传统方法在句子相似度打分的准确率上提高了 11%。

(4)为使中医药算法可以方便地被中医药领域的研究者使用,本文从中医药信息化角度出发,设计并实现了一个完整的、易用的、可扩展的中医药数据挖掘平台。该平台将所有算法看成一个算子,用户通过组合不同的算子来进行实验。

2.2.21　基于组合特征的网页主题块识别算法

张思(指导教师:姜晓红)

2017 年硕士学位论文

在当今的互联网时代,Web 是信息的重要来源,网页则是展示信息的重要媒介。网页传递着各种信息,但是其中有大量噪音信息严重影响了 Web 信息的自动化挖掘和采集。如何准确地识别出网页的主题信息成为计算机科学的研究热点。

本文对各种 Web 页面主题信息识别的技术进行了分析和总结,针对仅利用视觉特征或文本特征来识别 Web 页面主题信息算法的不足,提出了一种基于组合特征的主题块识别算法。实验证明,本算法有效地提高了网页主题信息识别的准确率和稳定性。本文的主要研究内容和贡献如下。

(1)实现并改进了 VIPS 算法。改进了网页分块规则,对网页块尺寸阈值采用动态调整的方式来调整分块粒度,使得分块后的网页块语义更加完整。

(2)借鉴 BM25 算法的思想,提出了计算网页块内容与主题相关性的算法模型 BBM25。BBM25 以网页块为基本单位,从关键词的权重、网页块中关键词的词频、网页块的文本内容长度等几个方面来考虑。

(3)提出了基于组合特征的主题块识别算法。对网页分块后,本文首先利用 SVM 根据网页块的视觉特征预测网页块是否为主题块,然后利用 BBM25 算法计算每个网页块内容与主题的相关性权重值,将权重值与寻找的最佳阈值进行比较,从而判断网页块是否为主题块,最后将这两种方式相结合,综合利用网页块的视觉特征和文本特征来判断其是否为主题块。通过实验,本文将基于组合特征的主题块识别算法和基于视觉特征、基于文本特征的主题块识别算法进行了对比,验证了本文提出的基于组合特征的主题块识别算法的准确性和稳定性。

2.2.22　一种基于表示学习的知识图谱融合算法与系统实现

罗丹(指导教师:陈华钧)

2018 年硕士学位论文

近年来,随着语义网的发展,越来越多的结构数据以知识图谱的形式公开发布,并广泛应用于信息检索、推荐系统、问答系统等领域。知识图谱作为语义数据的重要组成部分,通常包含大量相互重合的 RDF 三元组信息,然而只有少量实体之间存在等价链接。所以,如果要同时使用多个相互关联的知识图谱,就必须将实体进行对齐或者合并,其中的关键技术就是实体融合。由于不同知识图谱之间存在着数据的语义不均一性,实体和属性的表示有许多变种和歧义,这给实体融合技术带来了巨大的挑战。

实体融合算法主要基于语言学特征、层次结构、属性值域、辅助数据源、机器学习、知识表示学习等。一般地,基于语言学相似度的算法比较难于应用在大规模的数据集当中,机器学习相对灵活,但是依赖于训练数据和优化算法,知识表示学习能够脱离实体的文本信息,根据 RDF 三元组之间的结构特征对实体进行编码。传统的实体融合工具提供的匹配算法通常非常有限,不能满足用户的多样性需求,且缺少友好的用户界面,对于普通用户来说,使用门槛较高。

本文提出了一个基于知识表示学习的双向监督迭代融合算法,将实体和属性映射到了同一个低维的向量空间。与传统方法相比,该算法避免了对知识图谱的糅合操作,并实现了跨语言知识图谱实体融合。同时,还实现了一个基于 Web 的实体融合工具,提供了良好的交互界面以及详细的操作指南,实现了高效的在线融合计算与数据传输。该工具提供了多种融合算法,包括语言学距离度量、基于正样本的机器学习以及知识表示学习。

2.2.23　基于知识图谱的医疗问答系统

杨笑然(指导教师:李石坚)
2018 年硕士学位论文

随着互联网的发展,互联网医疗科普搜索需求急剧增加,但互联网上现有的医疗科普网站不仅导航过于专业,让普通用户无法快速找到所需的内容,而且缺乏针对性,无法根据用户的不同问题给出具有针对性的回答。为了缓解这一矛盾,基于知识图谱技术,本文设计并开发了一种基于知识图谱的医疗问答系统,通过运用自然语言处理相关技术,对医疗电子病历中的自有文本提取知识,构建知识图谱;在知识图谱的基础上,运用语义搜索和问答系统相关技术,提供医疗语义搜索和医疗智能问答服务。本系统可以直接理解用户的意图,用户不用在专业网站中寻找自己所需的信息;同时,本系统可以根据用户的不同输入做出具有针对性的回答。本文的贡献如下。

(1)设计并实现了针对非结构化数据的医疗知识图谱构建系统,从命名实体识别、关系抽取和知识融合三个方面进行了详述。

(2)设计并实现了基于知识图谱的医疗语义搜索模型,从搜索意图分类、实体相似度匹配两个方面进行了详述。

(3)设计并实现了基于知识图谱的医疗问答系统,提供医疗命名实体识别、医疗关系抽取、知识图谱可视化、医疗语义搜索和医疗智能问答服务。

2.2.24　基于关键语义信息的中医肾病病情文本分类问题研究

陈广(指导教师:姜晓红)
2019 年硕士学位论文

随着人工智能的快速发展以及国家政策对中医药的大力扶持,中医药信息化、智能化迎来了新的契机,也为改变目前中医药发展较慢这一困境创造了新机遇。本文以某中医院提供的中医病情文本数据为基础,对中医智能辨证问题开展了研究。针对中医病情文本特点,提出了基于关键词的中医病情文本关键语义信息提取方法,然后在深入了解中医辨证的基础上,将中医肾病辨证问题抽象成一个有监督的多分类问题,使用深度学习对中医肾病病情文本进行分类,最后构建了中医药智能服务平台。论文主要贡献如下。

(1)深入分析了中医病情文本的特点,使用文本 N-Gram 片段的信息熵等指标进行领域词识别,进一步提升了分词精度。

(2)基于中医病情文本特点,提出了一种基于病位的中医病情文本关键词提取算法(TF-IDF-DP),为获得病情文本关键语义信息打下了基础。

(3)在病情文本关键词的基础上,提出了一种基于关键词的中医病情文本关键语义信息提取方法(DKSIEK),完成症状词、病位词、症状严重程度词及症状有无关联等关键语义信息提取。实验结果表明,该方法不仅能够有效提取关键语义信息,还起到抑制噪音的作用。

(4)深入调研了深度学习文本分类方法,全面系统地将其应用到中医肾病病情文本分类中,并给出了 4 种深度学习分类模型。结合关键语义信息,提出了一种融合病情文本关键语义信息的分类方法,同时考虑到中医辨证的特点,进一步提出基于 two stage 的分类方法。实验结果表明,深度学习方法的分类 F1 值在 89% 左右,改进的两种方法分别能够有效提升分类 F1 值 2.6% 和 3.6%。

(5)深入调研分析了互联网已有的中医药服务平台,结合实验室在中医药方面的基础,设计并实现了以中医智能辨证为中心,知识搜索、图谱搜索和中医问答为辅助的中医药智能服务平台。

2.3 学术论文摘要

本节摘录了中医药与语义网络知识图谱方向 2003—2015 年共 23 篇主要学术论文(分别发表在 *IEEE Transactions Knowledge and Data Engineering*、*Briefings in Bioinformatics*、*Journal of Biomedical Informatics*、《中国数字医学》、《中国医学创新》、*ICTAI* 等国内外期刊和会议论文集上)。

2.3.1 On Case-Based Knowledge Sharing in Semantic Web

Huajun Chen, Zhaohui Wu
首发于 *ICTAI*,2003:200-207

Human experience is a special kind of knowledge, which captures previously experienced, similar problem situations (case) for human problem solving. This paper describes a case-based approach for knowledge sharing and management with regard to the semantic web settings. We define a RDF-based Case Markup Language (CaseML) for experience knowledge representation and develop a generic architecture for the case-based reasoning in the open, distributed environment with the emphasis on the integration of case knowledge with web ontologies. An application scenario from Traditional Chinese Medicine field is introduced to evaluate our methodology. With our application experience, we claim that, in contrast with logic-based knowledge representation formalisms, our case is more suitable for knowledge sharing in the semantic web, because case-based reasoning is similarity-based and there is weak demand on semantic consistent in such reasoning processes.

2.3.2 互联网 Ontology 语言和推理的比较和分析

高琦,陈华钧
首发于《计算机应用与软件》,2004,21(10):73-76

本文从描述逻辑和语义互联网两个角度,比较与分析几种 Web 本体描述语言(RDF/RDFS,

DAML＋OIL 和 OWL)的表达力和相关的推理,介绍它们的不同应用。然后总结出推理的分类,说明推理在本体建设、维护和应用中的作用。

2.3.3 Semantic Browser: An Intelligent Client for Dart-Grid

Yuxin Mao, Zhaohui Wu, Huajun Chen
首发于 *ICCS*,2004,*LNCS* 3036:470-473

In this paper, we propose a generic architecture of Semantic Browser for Dart-Grid, which is an intelligent Grid client and provides users with a series of Semantic functions. Extensible plug-in mechanism enables Semantic Browser to extend its functions dynamically. Semantic Browser converts various format of semantic information into uniform semantic graph with Semantic Graph Language (SGL). A semantic graph is composed of operational vectographic components. An application of Semantic Browser on Traditional Chinese Medicine (TCM) is also described.

2.3.4 A Computational Trust Model for Semantic Web Based on Bayesian Decision Theory

Xiaoqing Zheng, Huajun Chen, Zhaohui Wu, Yu Zhang
首发于 *APWeb*,2006,*LNCS* 3841:745-750

Enabling trust to ensure more effective and efficient agent interaction is at the heart of the Semantic Web vision. We propose a computational trust model based on Bayesian decision theory in this paper. Our trust model combines a variety of sources of information to assist users with correct decisions in choosing the appropriate providers according to their preferences expressed by prior information and utility function, and takes three types of costs (operational, opportunity and service charges) into account during trust evaluating. Our approach gives trust a strict probabilistic interpretation and lays solid foundation for trust evaluating on the Semantic Web.

2.3.5 Knowledge Fusion in Semantic Grid

Xiaoqing Zheng, Zhaohui Wu, Huajun Chen
首发于 *GCC*,2006:424-431

Just as the Web is shifting its focus from information and communication and emphasizes the need to the reuse of knowledge as a huge distributed knowledge base, the Semantic Grid in which information and services are given well-defined meaning extends the current Grid to enable software agents, users, and programs to work in cooperation. How to process the different sources of information, in particular, to combine a variety of sources of knowledge to assist users with effective reasoning or collaborative problem-solving, is one of the greatest barriers in realizing the above vision. Against this background, we propose a knowledge fusion and an integration approach based on statistical decision theory and Bayesian analysis for the Semantic Grid.

2.3.6 Dynamic Sub-Ontology Evolution for Traditional Chinese Medicine Web Ontology

Yuxin Mao, Zhaohui Wu, Wenya Tian, Xiaohong Jiang, William K. Cheung
首发于 *Journal of Biomedical Informatics*,2008,41(5):790-805

As a form of important domain knowledge, large-scale ontologies play a critical role in building a large variety of knowledge-based systems. To overcome the problem of semantic heterogeneity and encode domain knowledge in reusable format, a large-scale and well-defined ontology is also required in the traditional Chinese medicine discipline. We argue that to meet the on-demand and scalability requirement, ontology-based systems should go beyond the use of static ontology and be able to self-evolve and specialize for the domain knowledge they possess. In particular, we refer to the context-specific portions from large-scale ontologies like the traditional Chinese medicine ontology as *sub-ontologies*. Ontology-based systems are able to reuse sub-ontologies in local repository called ontology cache. In order to improve the overall performance of ontology cache, we propose to evolve sub-ontologies in ontology cache to optimize the knowledge structure of sub-ontologies. Moreover, we present the sub-ontology evolution approach based on a genetic algorithm for reusing large-scale ontologies. We evaluate the proposed evolution approach with the traditional Chinese medicine ontology and obtain promising results.

2.3.7　基于子本体的领域知识资源管理

毛郁欣,陈华钧,姜晓红

首发于《计算机集成制造系统》,2008,14(7):1434-1440

　　为实现按需动态的基于语义的知识资源管理,本文提出一种基于本体语义的动态演化方法。该方法改变了静态利用本体的方式,考虑资源重用的局部性,将来自大型本体的上下文相关的知识集合表示为子本体。通过建立语义映射,将知识资源的模式统一映射到子本体上,利用子本体的语义,将异质异构的知识资源集成到一个缓存中。同时,基于遗传算法,提出了一种子本体演化方法。针对子本体的语义结构和特征,在遗传算法中采用基于语义的参数编码和适应值评价,从而实现了动态、自适应的知识资源管理。此外,设计了相应的模拟实验,基于一个中医药本体,验证和评价了所提方法的有效性。

2.3.8　Intelligent Search on Integrated Knowledge Base of Traditional Chinese Medicine

Zhihong Fu, Huajun Chen, Tong Yu

首发于《东南大学学报(英文版)》,2009,25(4):460-463

　　To semantically integrate heterogeneous resources and provide a unified intelligent access interface, semantic web technology is exploited to publish and interlink machine-understandable resources so that intelligent search can be supported. TCMSearch, a deployed intelligent search engine for traditional Chinese medicine (TCM), is presented. The core of the system is an integrated knowledge base that uses a TCM domain ontology to represent the instances and relationships in TCM. Machine-learning techniques are used to generate semantic annotations for texts and semantic mappings for relational databases, and then a semantic index is constructed for these resources. The major benefit of representing the semantic index in RDF/OWL is to support some powerful reasoning functions, such as class hierarchies and relation inferences. By combining resource integration with reasoning, the knowledge base can support some intelligent search paradigms besides keyword search, such as correlated search, semantic graph navigation and concept recommendation.

2.3.9 Subontology-Based Resource Management for Web-Based e-Learning

Zhaohui Wu, Yuxin Mao, Huajun Chen

首发于 *IEEE Transactions Knowledge and Data Engineering*, 2009, 21(6):867-880

Recent advances in Web and information technologies have resulted in many e-learning resources. There is an emerging requirement to manage and reuse relevant resources together to achieve on-demand e-learning in the Web. Ontologies have become a key technology for enabling semantic-driven resource management. We argue that to meet the requirements of semantic-based resource management for Web-based e-learning, one should go beyond using domain ontologies statically. In this paper, we provide a semantic mapping mechanism to integrate e-learning databases by using ontology semantics. Heterogeneous e-learning databases can be integrated under a mediated ontology. Taking into account the locality of resource reuse, we propose to represent context-specific portions from the whole ontology as subontologies. We present a subontology-based approach for resource reuse by using an evolutionary algorithm. We also conduct simulation experiments to evaluate the approach with a traditional Chinese medicine e-learning scenario and obtain promising results.

2.3.10 Ontology Based Semantic Relation Verification for TCM Semantic Grid

Xiaogang Zhang, Huajun Chen, Jun Ma, Jinhuo Tao

首发于 *ChinaGrid*, 2009:185-191

Traditional Chinese Medicine (TCM) Semantic Grid is an application of Semantic Grid technique in TCM domain. It comprises TCM ontology and TCM Databases as data resources and Dart Search, Dart Query etc. as TCM applications. This paper reports an ontology engineering component of the TCM Semantic Grid. Although ontology engineering has gained significant progress, ontology construction still mainly depends on manual work and tends to be mistaken prone. In this paper, we introduce a semantic relation verification method based on both domain ontology and domain publications. A modified vector space model is used to extract semantic relations from domain publications, which is particularly useful when the semantic relation cannot be extracted directly. Association rule learning method is used to distinguish significant relations from trivial ones. Further verification method is used to give user recommendations of relation types. We use Traditional Chinese Medicine Language System, domain ontology for Traditional Chinese Medicine, and relevant publications to validate our approach. But our method is not limited to this field. In fact, any data source that can be extracted into relevant instance pairs is applicable.

2.3.11 A Semantic Bayesian Network for Web Mashup Network Construction

Chunying Zhou, Huajun Chen, Zhipeng Peng, Yuan Ni, Guotong Xie

首发于 *GreenCom&CPSCom*, 2010:645-652

With a mashup network in which a link indicates that two applications are mashupable, building a mashup can be simplified into network navigation. This paper presents an approach that constructs a Web mashup network by learning a semantic Bayesian network using a semi-supervised learning method. An RDF model is defined to describe attributes and activities of applications. To process all information sources on the

Semantic Web, a semantic Bayesian network (sBN) is proposed where a semantic subgraph template defined using a SPARQL query is used to describe the information about the graph structure. The sBN offers more powerful abilities to process the information sources on Semantic Web, especially the graph structure. To improve the learning performance, a semi-supervised learning method that makes use of both labeled and unlabeled data is proposed. We ran the approach on a data set containing 100 applications collected from the website Programmableweb. com and 3077 links checked manually. The results show that the approach outperforms the PRL and the rule-based methods, and the semi-supervised learning method achieved big improvements in recall and $F_{0.5}$, compared with the direct learning method.

2.3.12　GRAPH: A Domain Ontology-Driven Semantic Graph Auto Extraction System

Chunying Zhou, Huajun Chen, Jinhuo Tao
首发于 *Applied Mathematics & Information Sciences*,2011,5(2):9-16

This paper presents sGRAPH—a domain ontology-driven semantic graph auto extraction system used to discover knowledge from text publications in traditional Chinese medicine. The traditional Chinese medicine language system (TCMLs), composed of an ontology schema and a knowledge base containing 153692 words and 304114 relations, is used as the domain ontology. The sGRAPH comprises two components: a user interface that interacts with users and the domain ontology-based semantic graph extraction algorithm. This algorithm is divided into five steps: text processing, semantic graph extraction, graph identification, keyword-based semantic graph search and the selectable enrichment to the knowledge base. When the knowledge base of TCMLs is used, the domain-specific words are extracted from sentences more accurately; the hierarchical structure of the ontology can also be used to help identify the extracted graphs. The algorithm not only can extract relations between words that have already been annotated by relations in the knowledge base, but also can predict the relations between words that have never been annotated by relations. The sGRAPH was developed and evaluated by extracting semantic graphs from 2000 publications which predicted 6778 relations that have never been found.

2.3.13　Semantic Web Meets Integrative Biology: A Survey

Huajun Chen, Tong Yu, Jake Y. Chen
首发于 *Briefings in Bioinformatics*,2012,14(1):109-125

Integrative Biology (IB) uses experimental or computational quantitative technologies to characterize biological systems at the molecular, cellular, tissue and population levels. IB typically involves the integration of the data, knowledge and capabilities across disciplinary boundaries in order to solve complex problems. We identify a series of bioinformatics problems posed by interdisciplinary integration: (i) data integration that interconnects structured data across related biomedical domains; (ii) ontology integration that brings jargons, terminologies and taxonomies from various disciplines into a unified network of ontologies; (iii) knowledge integration that integrates disparate knowledge elements from multiple sources; (iv) service integration that build applications out of services provided by different vendors. We argue that IB can benefit significantly from the integration solutions enabled by Semantic Web (SW) technologies. The SW enables scientists to share content beyond the boundaries of applications and websites, resulting into a web of data that is meaningful and understandable to any computers. In this review, we provide insight into how SW technologies can be used to build open, standardized and interoperable solutions for interdisciplinary integration on a global basis. We present a rich set of case studies in system biology, integrative neuroscience, bio-pharmaceutics and translational medicine, to highlight the technical features and benefits of SW applications in IB.

2.3.14 OWL Reasoning over Big Biomedical Data

Xi Chen, Huajun Chen, Ningyu Zhang, Jiaoyan Chen, Zhaohui Wu
首发于 *ICBD*,2013:29-36

Recently, the emerging accumulation of biomedical data on the Web (e.g. vast amounts of protein sequences, genes, gene products, drugs, diseases and chemical compounds, etc.) has shaped a big network of isolated professional knowledge. Embedded with domain knowledge from different disciplines all regarding to human biological systems, the decentralized data repositories are implicitly connected by human expert knowledge. Lots of biomedical data sources are published separately in the form of semantic ontologies represented by Web Ontology Language (OWL) syntax, which is naturally based on linked graphs. When we are faced with such massive, disparate and interlinked data, biomedical data analysis becomes a challenge. In this paper, we present a general OWL reasoning framework for the analysis of big biomedical data and implement a MapReduce-based property chain reasoning prototype system. OWL reasoning method is ideally suitable for problems involving complex semantic associations because it is able to infer logical consequences based on a set of asserted rules or axioms. MapReduce framework is used to solve the problem of scalability. In our experiment, we focus on the discovery of associations between Traditional Chinese Medicine (TCM) and Western Medicine (WM). The results show that the system achieves high performance, accuracy and scalability.

2.3.15 Ontology-Oriented Diagnostic System for Traditional Chinese Medicine Based on Relation Refinement

Peiqin Gu, Huajun Chen, Tong Yu
首发于 *Computational and Mathematical Methods in Medicine*,2013:1-11

Although Chinese medicine treatments have become popular recently, the complicated Chinese medical knowledge has made it difficult to be applied in computer-aided diagnostics. The ability to model and use the knowledge becomes an important issue. In this paper, we define the diagnosis in Traditional Chinese Medicine (TCM) as discovering the fuzzy relations between symptoms and syndromes. An Ontology-oriented Diagnosis System (ODS) is created to address the knowledge-based diagnosis based on a well-defined ontology of syndromes. The ontology transforms the implicit relationships among syndromes into a machine-interpretable model. The clinical data used for feature selection is collected from a national TCM research institute in China, which serves as a training source for syndrome differentiation. The ODS analyzes the clinical cases to obtain a statistical mapping relation between each syndrome and associated symptom set, before rechecking the completeness of related symptoms via ontology refinement. Our diagnostic system provides an online web interface to interact with users, so that users can perform self-diagnosis. We tested 12 common clinical cases on the diagnosis system, and it turned out that, given the agree metric, the system achieved better diagnostic accuracy compared to nonontology method—92% of the results fit perfectly with the experts' expectations.

2.3.16　TCMSearch: An In-Use Semantic Web Infrastructure for Traditional Chinese Medicine

Tong Yu, Meng Cui, Haiyan Li, Shuo Yang, Jinghua Li, Huajun Chen, Peiqin Gu, Yu Zhang
首发于 *International Journal of Functional Informatics and Personalized Medicine*, 2013,4(2):103-125

In this paper, we present an information infrastructure named TCMSearch, which integrates a plurality of databases in traditional Chinese medicine (TCM) domain and provides a unified view of TCM knowledge assets through a web portal. TCMSearch was developed based on the Semantic Web, which refers to a bundle of technologies enabling a higher level of web intelligence, including resource description framework (RDF), expressive ontologies, web-accessible repositories, query and reasoning engines, and information extraction techniques. At the foundation of TCMSearch is the unified traditional Chinese medicine language system (UTCMLS), a large-scale TCM ontology that achieves a comprehensive coverage of the TCM domain. TCMSearch can serve TCM practitioners with knowledge assets covering a broad range of topics including basic theories, diagnostics, diseases, therapeutics, acupuncture and moxibustion, medicinal treatments and so on. It demonstrates the advantages of the Semantic Web in preserving cultural diversity and promoting cross-cultural and interdisciplinary dialogues.

2.3.17　基于语义 Web 的中医临床知识建模

于彤,崔蒙,吴朝晖,陈华钧,姜晓红,杨硕,张竹绿
首发于《中国数字医学》,2013,8(11):81-85

　　中医信息学界已开始关注语义 Web 技术,但对于如何使用该技术进行中医临床知识建模尚无定论。本文以"郁怒"的中医临床诊疗为例,分析中医辨证论治的思维过程,探讨基于语义 Web 技术对中医临床知识进行建模的方法,为致力于将中医药和语义 Web 结合起来进行研究的中医药信息学家提供参考。

2.3.18　面向中药新药研发的语义搜索系统

于彤,陈华钧,李敬华
首发于《中国医学创新》,2013,10(33):158-160

　　为解决中药新药研发中的信息集成和检索问题,设计并实现了语义搜索系统 TCM Search。为实现分布式、异构数据库的语义集成和一致性访问,提出语义视图,来定义关系型数据库与领域本体之间的模式映射。该系统根据关系型数据库的语义视图,将用户提出的语义查询重写为结构查询语言(SQL)查询,再分派给各个关系型数据库,最终将查询结果进行语义封装。它还基于本体构建文本内容的语义索引,从而实现了基于概念的内容检索。这些本体驱动的方法,使该系统与关键词搜索系统相比,具有更高的查准率与查全率。该系统已得到成功部署,它基于一个大型中药领域本体,

通过 Web 方式为中药领域专家提供智能搜索服务。

2.3.19　中医"象思维"的 OWL 语义建模

于彤,陈华钧,吴朝晖,顾珮崟,崔蒙,张竹绿

首发于《中国数字医学》,2013,8(4):29-33

　　"象思维"是中医的核心思维模式,在阴阳、五行、藏象等中医基础理论中贯穿始终。中医"象思维"的语义建模和计算模拟,对建设面向中医药领域的语义 Web 以及构建辅助中医临床实践的"智能体"起到了基础性作用。究其本质,中医"象思维"与认知语言学中的"隐喻"具有相似性,都可以抽象为概念网络中模式的涌现和匹配过程。本文基于语义 Web 技术对中医"象思维"进行语义建模,并结合阴阳理论加以阐释。

2.3.20　中医药语义维基系统研发

于彤,陈华钧,李敬华

首发于《中国医学创新》,2013,10(34):143-145

　　语义维基是语义 Web 技术与维基系统相结合的产物,它既保持了维基系统在社会化知识工程方面的优势,又强化了对结构性数据的支持。中医百科是通过语义维基技术构建的中医药知识共享网站,它基于中医药领域本体来整合中医药领域的知识与作品,向网络用户提供百科全书式的知识服务。本文对语义维基技术进行了简要介绍,并阐述了中医百科的后台技术和交互方式,以期为中医药信息化领域的研究和开发人员提供参考。

2.3.21　BioTCM-SE: A Semantic Search Engine for the Information Retrieval of Modern Biology and Traditional Chinese Medicine

Xi Chen, Huajun Chen, Xuan Bi, Peiqin Gu, Jiaoyan Chen, Zhaohui Wu

首发于 *Computational and Mathematical Methods in Medicine*, 2014:1-13

Understanding the functional mechanisms of the complex biological system as a whole is drawing more and more attention in global health care management. Traditional Chinese Medicine (TCM), essentially different from Western Medicine (WM), is gaining increasing attention due to its emphasis on individual wellness and natural herbal medicine, which satisfies the goal of integrative medicine. However, with the explosive growth of biomedical data on the Web, biomedical researchers are now confronted with the problem of large-scale data analysis and data query. Besides that, biomedical data also has a wide coverage which usually comes from multiple heterogeneous data sources and has different taxonomies, making it hard to integrate and query the big biomedical data. Embedded with domain knowledge from different disciplines all regarding human biological systems, the heterogeneous data repositories are implicitly connected by human expert knowledge. Traditional search engines cannot provide accurate and comprehensive search results for the semantically associated knowledge since they only support keywords-based searches. In this paper, we present BioTCM-SE, a semantic search engine for the information retrieval of modern biology and TCM, which provides biologists with a comprehensive and accurate associated knowledge query platform to greatly facilitate the implicit knowledge discovery between WM and TCM.

2.3.22　基于 Open Linked Data 的中西医关联发现云平台

顾珮嵚,吴朝晖,陈华钧,陈曦
首发于《中国数字医学》,2014,9(5):88-92

　　本文提出了一个用于中西医关联发现的云平台——BioTCM Cloud。该平台构建在大量的开放链接数据(Linked Data)的基础上,旨在满足跨领域知识整合的需要。面对海量的链接数据,本文提出了基于 MapReduce 框架的分布式语义推理框架,用于解决基于领域规则的知识推理问题。以中医草药为案例,分布式语义推理可以建立中医药和西医之间的关联,以促进中西医之间的沟通和数据共享。

2.3.23　大型中医药知识图谱构建研究

于彤,刘静,贾李蓉,张竹绿,杨硕,刘丽红,李敬华,于琦
首发于《中国数字医学》,2015,10(3):80-82

　　知识图谱(Knowledge Graph)是以"语义网络"为骨架构建起来的巨型、网络化的知识系统,能捕捉并呈现领域概念之间的语义关系,使各种信息系统中琐碎、零散的知识相互连接,支持综合性知识检索以及问答、决策支持等智能应用。本文将探索如何构建面向中医药领域的知识图谱,实现中医药知识资源的有效整合,给中医药工作者和百姓提供全面、及时、可靠的知识服务。

2.4　学术著作

　　本节主要介绍了中医药与语义网络知识图谱方向于 2017 年由科学出版社出版的"中医药信息学丛书"中的一部《中医药知识工程》,摘录了该著作前言和一级目录信息。

2.4.1　中医药知识工程

于彤,陈华钧,姜晓红
首发于科学出版社,2017

前言

　　中医药根植于中华文化,源于中国传统哲学,是中华民族非常宝贵的知识遗产。近年来,中医药知识工程成为中医药知识遗产保护和知识创造的一种新模式。中医药工作者开始建立各种面向中医药领域的知识工程平台,支持跨学科、跨组织、跨地域的协作式知识加工,建成了一系列的领域本体、知识库及智能系统,推动群体性的知识创新活动,加速知识转化过程,促进知识的传播。

　　在中医药领域中实施知识工程项目是颇具挑战性的任务。中医药领域的知识相当复杂,对知识工程有独特的需求。传统中医实践者分布于世界各地,为知识的协同加工和共享制造了障碍。中医药知识工程领域还有尚未解决的技术难题。因此,有必要对中医药知识工程的原则、最佳实践方法和核心技术进行系统的总结。《中医药知识工程》对近年来在知识工程领域中所积累的实践经验进行了总结,介绍了中医药知识工程的原理和基本内容,阐述了中医药知识建模、知识融合、知识发现

与知识服务的核心方法和关键技术,并结合实际应用案例介绍了知识工程的实施过程。全书共分为 8 章。

第 1 章为绪论。本章介绍中医药领域背景和中医药信息化建设的历程,讨论中医药信息学的内涵和外延,阐述中医药知识管理的过程与方法,具体阐述了中医药知识工程的概念、意义、价值、发展历程、研究范畴和发展前景。

第 2 章为知识工程技术。知识工程已经成为知识管理中不可或缺的关键技术,也是当前计算机科学领域的一个研究热点。本章介绍知识工程的基本概念、基本方法、发展历史、研究重点和应用领域,论述知识表示与推理、知识获取、知识运用、知识发现和语义网等方面的背景知识与研究情况。

第 3 章为中医药知识分析与建模。"取象比类"是贯穿中医知识体系的思维模式,与中医其他的思想方法共同构成了中医"象思维"。本章追溯"象思理"的思想源流,并将其与认知语言学中的"隐喻"进行比较分析,进而对中医"象思雄"进行语义建模。在此基础上,讨论阴阳、五行、证候,临床等方面知识的建模方法。

第 4 章为中医药知识获取。知识获取是任何知识管理和知识工程的基础性工作。在中医药领域中,知识获取是一项复杂的工作,被公认为知识处理过程中的一个"瓶颈"问题。本章介绍通过大量专家虚拟协作和文本挖掘这两种主要的知识获取方法,来突破中医药领域的知识获取瓶颈。

第 5 章为中医药知识组织与存储。近年来,随着知识创新步伐的加快和中医药信息化工作的推进,在中医药领域中积累了数字化文献、多媒体档案、数据库、知识库等多种形式的知识资源。如何采用信息技术对海量的中医药知识资源进行合理组织和有效存储,以利于知识的检索与应用,成为一个重要的问题。本章首先介绍中医药知识库的总体情况,包括构建方法和应用范围等,再分别介绍文献库、数据库、知识组织系统、本体、知识图谱这 5 种广义的知识库,阐述它们的特点、功能和中医药应用。

第 6 章为中医药知识发现。中医团体开展了将各种知识发现方法(如频繁模式发现、关联规则发现、聚类分析、复杂网络分析等)引入中医药领域的若干探索,用于研究方剂配伍规律,辅助中医开具中药处方,解释中医证候的本质,以及辅助基于中医药的新药研发。本章讨论知识发现方法在中医药领域的各种应用,介绍知识发现在其中发挥的作用和应用的效果。

第 7 章为中医药语义网的构建与应用。针对中医药领域的知识孤岛现象,基于语义网技术,提出一种面向关联数据的知识关联框架。它基于本体实现中医药知识资源的融合,实现语义搜索、语义维基、决策支持和知识发现等应用,使中医药知识接入全球互联的知识网络之中,在中医药研究和医疗保健中发挥更大的作用和影响力。

第 8 章为中医药知识服务。中医药是知识驱动型领域,如何促进中医药知识资源的深度共享与广泛传播,使全球中医、学者都能充分利用这座知识宝库,是非常重要的问题。该领域急需新颖的知识服务模式,使蕴含于数据库中的知识存量得到有效利用。在分析中医药领域特点和需求的基础上,提出知识服务的概念和性质,阐述中医药知识服务平台的技术特点、体系结构、服务模式,讨论发展中医药知识服务的价值和意义。

本书对中医药知识工程的实施有指导作用,可作为中医药信息学、人工智能、知识工程等领域的科技工作者及研究人员的参考书。中医药知识工程的项目实施人员,以及有志从事中医药学与计算机技术交叉研究的科研工作者,都可以从本书中得到启发。

本书出版过程中得到了"国家人口与健康科学数据共享平台——中医药学科学数据中心"项目资助,特此表示感谢。

目录

2.5　发明专利

本节摘录了中医药与语义网络知识图谱方向 4 项相关发明专利(其中 2 项于 2013 年得到授权,另 2 项于 2019 年得到授权)。

2.5.1　基于浏览器的本体 3D 可视化和编辑的系统及方法

陈华钧,王超,顾珮嵚,吴朝晖

专利号:ZL201110048281.4;授权公告号:CN102110166B;授权公告日:2013-07-31

本发明公开了一种基于浏览器的本体 3D 可视化和在线编辑系统及方法。它基于 3D 树形展示和 B/S 架构的思想,通过用户在前台上传本体文件,由后端应用本体数据平台对本体文件进行分析处理,在前台采用 Silverlight 技术在浏览器中将本体文件的结构以 3D 树形式展示,并在浏览器中提供相应的对本体文件进行删除、加工、更新等动态 3D 操作的在线工具,极大地方便了用户对本体的结构可视化及可视化编辑。本发明能支持多用户通过浏览器随时随地进行 OWL、RDF 本体文件的结构可视化、可视化结果保存和通过可视化操作对本体文件进行再加工。

2.5.2　一种基于 3D 技术的中医五行模型在线展示的实现方法

陈华钧,吴朝晖,王超,顾珮嵚

专利号:ZL201110053929.7;授权公告号:CN102129514B;授权公告日:2013-07-31

本发明公开了一种基于 3D 技术的中医五行理论在线展示的实现方法。它基于中医五行理论和 B/S 架构的思想,使用户通过浏览访问,获取对中医五行理论更为形象直观的认识,通过对五行理论中相关知识的数据化,将所得结果以 3D 立体空间模型的形式展示出来(包括五行生克模式与中土模式的相互转换、五行元素与五脏间的变换、脏器生理活动、脏器阴阳失衡病理的展示及变化)。本发明首次实现了五行理论中平面五行生克模式与中土模式在三维空间中的结合,将二者合为同一个空间体系。

2.5.3 一种基于 Deepdive 的领域文本知识抽取方法

陈华钧,陈曦,张宁豫,吴朝晖

专利号:ZL201710326192.9;授权公告号:CN107169079B;授权公告日:2019-09-20

本发明公开了一种基于 Deepdive 的领域文本知识抽取方法,包括:①获取知识库构建系统所需的原始文本,并且对其进行预处理;②对预处理后的文本进行实体连接,找到与预设特定关系对应的目标实体,并生成满足实体-关系-实体的三元组,组成候选关系实体对集;③采用弱监督的方法,对多个候选关系实体对进行学习和标注,生成 Deepdive 工具的训练样本;④将训练样本输入至 Deepdive 工具中,对 Deepdive 进行训练,并输出概率值大于阈值的候选关系实体对,组成提取的知识库。本发明能够用于完成领域知识库的构建工作,具有很强的扩展性,对非结构化数据的利用和提取工作具有很高的实用价值。

2.5.4 一种基于 Spark 的大规模知识图谱语义查询方法

陈华钧,陈曦,张宁豫,吴朝晖

专利号:ZL201710326554.4;授权公告号:CN107247738B;授权公告日:2019-09-06

本发明公开了一种基于 Spark 大规模知识图谱语义查询方法,包括:①将每一个三元组中的实体、关系分别替换成为相应的 ID;②基于类别与关系构建分层的子图索引,并将其存储于 HDFS 文件中;③将 SPARQL 查询所涉的操作通过 Spark 操作元语进行翻译;④根据每个三元组模式的特征分配不同的得分函数,确定 SPARQL 查询中每个三元组模式的执行顺序;⑤根据三元组模式的执行顺序,Spark 操作元语执行查询与链接,并将其链接结果通过映射表进行解析后返回。本发明支持海量语义数据的高效查询,具有很强的扩展性,对基于大规模语义数据的查询应用具有很高的实用价值。

第3章　中医药数据挖掘与知识发现

知识发现是人工智能与数据库、统计学、机器学习等技术的交叉技术,能从海量数据中获取有效、新颖、有潜在应用价值的知识。而自20世纪80年代开始,中医药工作者采用数据库技术对中医药知识进行了梳理和采集,建设了大量中医药科学数据资源,实现了大量中医药知识遗产的数字化。

在中国千年文化发展史中,中医药形成了大量"主客融合的体验"及"包含本质的现象"等经验知识,同时中文古籍描述的单字多义、异字同义问题,导致了辨证论治、中药性味归经和方剂功效的不确定性与模糊性的特点。中医还强调人、自然、社会综合的信息系统性和整体性,重视系统内各因素间的相关性。

中医药智能计算研究团队基于大数据的数据挖掘和知识发现技术,为在知识密集型的中医药大数据中挖掘和发现潜在的中医药隐性知识提供了有力的工具,为中西医结合研究、跨领域的中医药新药发现、中医辨证诊疗提供了理论分析和研究支持。

在中医药数据挖掘与知识发现研究中,我们着重从以下几个方面进行了研究。

(1)数据挖掘与知识发现技术与理论研究

主要目的是为在中医药领域开展相关的知识挖掘研究做好相关数据挖掘和知识发现技术的基础理论和技术研究。我们早在2000年就起步研究知识发现技术,对20世纪90年代知识发现方法进行分类,从九个维度上进行优缺点分析比较,见文献[1];探讨了粗集理论在数据挖掘方向的应用、具体实现并开发了原型系统,见文献[2];研究了文本挖掘相关的挖掘算法,包括文本分类、基于最大频繁模式的挖掘以及基于相关性的模式挖掘,见文献[3-10];研究了知识发现解空间的压缩方法,以及知识发现的可靠性问题,见文献[11-12];在2006年就综述了基于数据库的知识发现技术在中医药领域的应用情况,见文献[13];基于语义网格的模型、方法与应用总结在两本专著中,见文献[14-15]。

[1]陆伟,吴朝晖.知识发现方法的比较研究[J].计算机科学,2000,27(3):80-84,89.

主要调研分析了20世纪90年代以来的KDD方法,按方法不同分为五类,并从描述能力、伸缩性、精确性、鲁棒性、抗噪性等九个维度比较评价了五类方法的优缺点和不同的适用领域。

[2]陆伟.基于粗集理论的数据挖掘方法的研究[D].杭州:浙江大学,2000.

主要研究了粗集理论在KDD中的具体应用,探讨了具体的实现方法,并且结合其他KDD方法构建了一个完整的KDD系统原型——RoughMiner。实现了粗集理论的基本概念和方法,提供了包括数据准备、数据挖掘、知识检验和评估、结果表现等步骤在内的完整的KDD处理流程。

[3]周雪忠,吴朝晖.文本知识发现:基于信息抽取的文本挖掘[J].计算机科学,2003,30(9):63-66.

主要综述了文本挖掘技术,归纳了文本挖掘在信息抽取方面的应用以及面向特定子语义领域的实践和应用。介绍了文本挖掘的概念和过程,分析了关键技术及其应用和趋势,总结了中文文本挖掘的技术特点。

[4] Zhou X,Wu Z. Distributional character clustering for Chinese text categorization[C]// Eighth Pacific Rim International Conference on Artificial Intelligence(PRICAI'2004),LNAI 3157,2004:575-584.

主要提出了一种新的分布字聚类的特征提取方法,并将其用于中文文本分类,避免了分词操作。通过混合聚类评价函数和平分聚类算法改进字聚类质量。实验结果表明分布字聚类方法是一种有效的降维聚类方法,有效降低了特征空间维度,保证了聚类高性能。

[5] Feng Y,Wu Z,Zhou Z. Multi-label text categorization using k-nearest neighbor approach with M-similarity[C]// 12th International Conference of String Processing and Information Retrieval (SPIRE'2005),LNCS 3772:155-160.

主要研究了多标签文本分类问题。论文将文本视为符号序列,在传统的 k-最近邻方法(kNN)基础上,提出了一种多标签懒惰学习方法 kNN-M。灵活的顺序半敏感测度 M-相似性能够利用文本中的序列信息,并在 kNN-M 中用该方法来评估文本在寻找近邻时的贴近度,此外还能解决传统的文本表示方法的词序信息丢失问题。

[6] Zhou Z,Wu Z. Mining frequent maximum patterns with constraint[J]. Journal of Fudan University(Natural Science),2004,43(5):746-749.

主要研究了基于约束的最大频繁模式的挖掘技术,给出了基于约束的频繁最大模式的定义和基于约束的频繁最大模式挖掘算法,解决了频繁模式挖掘的效率问题。

[7] Zhou Z,Wu Z,Wang C, et al. Efficiently mining maximal frequent mutually associated patterns[C]// Second International Conference on Advanced Data Mining and Applications (ADMA'2006),LNAI 4093:110-117.

主要提出了一种新的最大频繁互关联模式挖掘的新方法。该方法利用关联测度的向下封闭性,在不丢失信息的情况下,显著减少了模式的生成数量,同时提高了挖掘效率。

[8] Zhou Z,Wu Z,Wang C, et al. Efficiently mining mutually and positively correlated patterns[C] // Second International Conference on Advanced Data Mining and Applications (ADMA'2006),LNAI 4093:118-125.

主要研究了相互关联且正相关的模式发现,提出了一种新的相关性兴趣度测度。为了提高挖掘效率,将关联与正相关结合起来,在挖掘过程中不仅使用关联度量,而且还使用了正相关度量。结果表明,互为正相关模式挖掘是一种既能反映项目间关联关系又能反映项目间正相关关系的模式挖掘方法。

[9] Zhou Z,Wu Z,Wang C, et al. Efficiently mining both association and correlation rules [C]// Third International Conference on Fuzzy Systems and Knowledge Discovery (FSKD' 2006),LNAI 4223:369-372.

主要研究了在挖掘过程中将关联与相关结合起来,以发现关联规则和相关规则。提出了一种既有关联又相关的新概念,并给出了一种发现所有关联且相关频繁模式挖掘算法。

[10] Zhou Z,Wu Z,Wang C,*et al*. Mining both associated and correlated patterns[C]// 6th International Conference on Computational Science(ICCS'2006),LNCS 3994:468-475.

主要研究了在关联且相关关系挖掘中的相关关系评价方法。提出了一种新的兴趣度度量——相关自信度(corr-confidence)。这个度量不仅有合适的上下界用于估计模式的相关程度,而且适用于长模式的挖掘。

[11] 吴朝晖,张宇,陈华钧.一种基于复杂网络的压缩空间高效搜索方法:200810121364.X[P]. 2010-11-10.

主要提出了一种基于启发信息的压缩空间搜索算法。该方法将一个巨大、松散、带有极大冗余信息的原解空间,压缩成一个计算机可处理的、集中的、带有高启发信息的另一个解空间,从而保证最大可能地找出一组较优解。

[12]封毅.中医药知识发现可靠性研究[D].杭州:浙江大学,2008.

主要研究了中医药知识发现可靠性问题。基于知识发现整个生命周期的各个阶段的可靠性因素分析,提出了知识发现可靠性框架 PBRF-KD,研究了结构相关的可靠性因素的优化方法,以及表达相关的可靠性因素的优化方法。

[13] Feng Y,Wu Z,Zhou X,*et al*. Knowledge discovery in traditional Chinese medicine: state of the art and perspectives[J]. Artificial Intelligence Medicine,2006,38(3):219-236.

主要综述了 2006 年前基于数据库的知识发现技术(KDD)在中医药领域的研究状况。主要从四个方面总结了研究成果:中药配方的知识发现、中医症候的知识发现、中药材的知识发现以及中医辨证诊断的知识发现。分析了现有研究中存在的问题,指明了未来研究方向。

[14] Wu Z,Chen H,Semantic Grid:Model,Methodology,and Applications[M]. Springer, 2008.(英文版)

[15] 吴朝晖、陈华钧.语义网格:模型、方法与应用[M].浙江大学出版社,2008.(中文版)

主要研究了语义网格的关键技术,对语义网格中的语义表达和知识表示方法、数据集成和管理、基于语义的流程组合与服务拼接、信任管理和问题求解以及基于语义网格的数据挖掘和知识发现展开了深入分析和研究,最后综合理论探索和应用研究,探讨了语义网格中的各种技术如何被实际应用到医学信息化领域。

(2)基于中医药文献的数据挖掘

主要目的是利用数据挖掘和知识发现技术在中医药领域进行潜在中医药知识的发现,包括中药复方配伍规律发现、方剂药物组配规律发现、中药成分分析、功能基因组学分析以及中医智能辨证。早期的数据挖掘技术包括了中医药文献的主题自动标引,如文献[16]。然后采用模式挖掘、相关性挖掘技术对中药方剂进行了配伍规律、药物组配、中药功效、成分分析等研究,如文献[17-26]。为提高知识发现的速度性能,研究了并行知识发现算法,见文献[27-29]。后期则研究基于主题模型的中医药隐含知识的发现和智能诊断,如文献[30-33]。

[16] 周雪忠,崔蒙,吴朝晖.基于文本挖掘的中医学文献主题自动标引[J].中国中医药信息杂志,2003,10(1):72-74.

主要研究了利用计算机技术实现中医文献的自动或半自动标引技术。面向文献的题名和文摘,采用基于机器学习的信息抽取和文本分类等文本挖掘方法,研究中医文献主题的自动标引,介绍了实现中医文献主题自动标引的系统框架、功能分析,还介绍了模糊词识别和概念语义组配算法。

[17] 周雪忠. 文本挖掘在中医药中的若干应用研究[D]. 杭州:浙江大学,2004.

主要利用文本挖掘技术对基于文献的中医药信息进行了知识挖掘研究,研究了基于字特征的中文文本分类方法,以及中医药文献信息抽取方法。提出了文献临床复方药物组成和科属配伍知识发现,研究了中医术语与关系抽取以及中医证候和基因相关关系的知识发现。

[18] 陆伟,王雁峰,吴朝晖. 中药复方组成规律的关联规则发现系统[J]. 浙江大学学报(工学版),2001,35(4):370-373,407.

主要提出了基于数据立方体的关联规则发现方法,在2500条中药复方信息的数据库上,根据用户的设定,用提出的方法发现治疗某一特定疾病的所有复方中不同单方之间的关联规则。

[19] 蔡越君. 数据挖掘技术及其在中药配伍系统中的应用研究[D]. 杭州:浙江大学,2003.

主要研究了数据挖掘技术在中药配伍系统中的应用。提出了利用高频集发现算法,发现常用的单味药合用模式;利用贝叶斯训练器和分类器,实现中医症候的初步诊断;开发了一个计算机系统Formula,集成了中药药对发现算法、中医症候诊断以及计算机辅助的组方。

[20] 周忠眉,林宝德,肖青. 古代方剂与新药方剂高频药组配情况分析[J]. 漳州师范学院学报(自然科学版),2004,17(1):19-21.

利用高频集方法,挖掘古代方剂与新药方剂的高频药对,探讨古代方剂与新药方剂高频药组配异同情况。

[21] 周忠眉. 数据挖掘在方剂配伍规律研究应用的探讨[J]. 漳州师范学院学报(自然科学版),2003,16(4):31-35.

主要探讨了数据挖掘技术在中药方剂配伍规律研究方面的应用。给出了一个应用案例:用频繁模式挖掘研究中医处方中症状与药物的联系。指出了频繁药集的一些研究思路。

[22] 何前锋,崔蒙,吴朝晖,等. 方剂中配伍知识的发现[J]. 中国中医药信息杂志,2004,11(7):655-656.

利用高频集挖掘的方法,对中国方剂数据库、中药新药品种数据库、中药成方制剂标准数据库中各方剂药物组成数据进行了分析,并使用中国中药药对数据库中的药对组成与从各方剂数据库中所得到的高频用药组合之间的数据进行了比较分析。

[23] 何前锋,周雪忠,周忠眉,等. 基于中药功效的聚类分析[J]. 中国中医药信息杂志,2004,11(6):561-562.

用数理统计和数据挖掘技术,对中药库中的大量数据进行分析,研究组成方剂的单味药,从对单味药按照功效进行分类入手,逐步由简到繁探索方剂的配伍规律。

[24] 周忠眉. 中医方剂数据挖掘模式和算法研究[D]. 杭州:浙江大学,2006.

主要研究了中医方剂的数据挖掘模式和算法。提出了最大频繁关联挖掘模式和挖掘算法、关联且相关频繁模式挖掘和挖掘算法、互为正相关频繁模式挖掘和挖掘算法以及关联且相关的规则挖掘算法,提出了新的兴趣度度量相关自信度,解决了挖掘长模式的度量问题。集成所有方剂挖掘模式和算法,研发了方剂药物组配模式分析和方剂功效分析系统。

[25] 吴朝晖,于彤,封毅,等. 用于分析中医方剂药物组配规律的泛化关联规则挖掘方法 200710156365.3[P]. 2012-06-06.

主要提出了一种结合关联规则挖掘和领域知识表示的泛化关联规则挖掘方法。利用领域知识库所提供的术语系统和领域规则完成数据挖掘过程,将挖掘结果以提案形式提交领域知识库,由领域专家验证评价。该方法可在发现新的中医方剂与药物中发挥作用。

[26] 刘明魁. 几种机器学习算法的改进及其在中药成分分析中的应用[D]. 杭州:浙江大学,2012.

主要研究了几种机器学习算法在中药成分分析、成分与证候的关系分析上的应用。提出了根据疾病历史抽取疾病集合和频次以及 TF-IDF 权重计算方法,设计了中药成分之间的相似度计算方法,用改进的 K-medoids 方法对中药成分进行聚类分析。提出了基于中药成分 IDF 值的黑名单算法,提高了黑名单的自动化和可解释性。

[27] Liu Y, Jiang X, Chen H, *et al*. MapReduce-based pattern finding algorithm applied in motif detection for prescription compatibility network[C]// 8th International Conference on Advanced Parallel Processing Technologie(APPT'2009),LNCS,2009:341-355.

为解决复杂网络模体发现过程中模式发现的高计算代价问题,设计实现了一种基于 MapReduce 的并行模式发现算法。实验表明,算法在大规模网络中发现较大模式的有效性和高可扩展性。将该方法应用于方剂网络用于发现常用的方剂配伍模式,可为方剂配伍规律发现提供可能性。

[28] 秘中凯,姜晓红,雷蕾. 一种稳定的并行分布式频繁集挖掘算法及其应用[J]. 计算机应用与软件,2011,28(3):83-85,124.

主要提出了一种 P-FIM 并行分布式频繁集挖掘算法,利用 Map/Reduce 框架和集群环境提高算法鲁棒性和负载均衡能力。实验表明,算法具有良好的稳定性和可扩展性。应用此算法,可实现 512 万条中医药方剂数据记录上的中医药数据相关性分析。

[29] 刘洋. 基于 MapReduce 的中医药并行数据挖掘服务[D].杭州:浙江大学,2010.

主要研究了海量数据挖掘技术问题。针对单机系统的计算能力限制问题,研究了基于 MapReduce 的中医药并行数据挖掘服务框架,实现了可视化交互平台和可编程的 Web Service 服务。开发了针对单图的频繁模式并行发现算法和简化点式互信息算法,并应用于中医方剂配伍研究和临床数据研究。

[30] 姜晓红,严海明,商任翔,等. 基于 LDA 主题模型的中医药数据挖掘方法:201310276021.1 [P].2017-03-29.

主要提出了一种基于 LDA 主题模型的中医药数据挖掘方法。确定处方-主题和主题-药剂两组先验后,确定 LDA 模型中的主题数目,用 Gibbs 采样方法对 LDA 模型求解,将求解结果映射到四元组,即可建立处方-主题-药物的可视化结构网络,从而发现中医药处方和药物之间的隐含关系。

[31] 商任翔. 基于主题模型的中医药隐含语义信息挖掘[D]. 杭州:浙江大学,2013.

主要研究了利用 LDA 主题模型对大量中医处方的数据挖掘技术,提出了 Gibbs-LDA 算法,用

中医药智能计算

以分析中医药处方数据,并将主题模型训练出来的知识用 RDF 进行描述,融合到中医药语义知识网格中,并通过语义网格图可视化算法形象展示中医药作用机理。

[32] 付钊. 基于文本语义分块的中医病情分类问题研究[D]. 杭州:浙江大学,2018.

主要研究了中医病情文本分类问题,提出了基于分块向量的病情文本相似性计算方法,根据描述的病位划分文本块、病位权重区分主次症状,提出了一种融合病情非文本特征的多维度中医病情分类方法,以实现中医的智能辨证。

[33] 姜晓红,付钊,陈广,等. 一种中医病情文本相似度的计算方法:201810359667.9[P]. 2020-07-07.

主要提出了一种中医病情文本相似度的计算方法。以文本语义分块为最小粒度,表示病情文本特征,按照所描述的病位划分为文本语义分块,并对不同分块设置不同的权重以区分主次症状,加权得到两段病情文本的相似度。克服了传统文本相似度计算方法或丢失语义信息,或不能突出主次病医的缺点。

(3)基于互联网链接数据的集成数据挖掘

主要目的是利用中医药文献数据库的数据,同时充分利用互联网上大量的链接数据进行中医药与现代生物医学基因组学之间的跨学科知识发现研究。包括构建基于中医症状的基因网络,从全新的视角分析中医症状与基因功能之间的关系;用综合图挖掘技术和本体推理技术进行跨领域的网络数据分析,应用于疾病-致病基因分析、基因-蛋白质相互作用分析、药物有效性分析以及中药材和中药互作用分析。研究了面向链接数据、超数据的集成挖掘方法。

[34] 周雪忠,吴朝晖,刘保延. 生物医学文献知识发现研究探讨及展望[J]. 复杂系统与复杂性科学,2004,1(3):45-55.

对生物医学文献知识发现的研究内容、研究成果以及基于文本挖掘的关键技术进行了系统的分析和阐述。分析中医药学数据的特点,提出了基于文本挖掘的中医证候分子生物学知识发现研究。该方法的特点是综合利用中医药学文献和 MEDLINE,能够获得创新的证候与基因相关知识。

[35] Wu Z, Zhou X, Liu B, et al. Text mining for finding functional community of related genes using TCM knowledge[C]// 8th European Conference Principles and Practice of Knowledge Discovery in Database (PKDD'2004),LNAI 3202,2004:459-470.

主要提出了一种面向 MEDLINE 新的文本挖掘方法,用来发现功能基因组,即时间和空间上的分子交互作用网络。利用中医症候群以及 50000 个中医文献书目记录自动聚集相关基因。基于与相同的症候群相关的基因会有种间关系的假设,用有效的自举法在中医药文献中抽取疾病名称,通过术语共现从 MEDLINE 的摘要和题目中发现疾病-基因关系。研究结果表明,从症候群角度研究功能基因组学是一种自上而下的新研究思路。

[36] Zhou X, Liu B, Wu Z, et al. Integrative mining of traditional Chinese medicine literature and MEDLINE for functional gene networks[J]. Artificial Intelligence Medicine,2007,41(2):87-104.

主要研究了在中医药文献和在线检索系统 MEDLINE 上的功能基因网络集成挖掘技术。介绍了以 50000 条 TCM 文献记录为知识资源构建的基于文献的基因网络。通过从 TCM 文献中抽取的

138

症状-疾病关系以及从 MEDLINE 上抽取的疾病-基因关系,发现症状-基因关系。基于气泡自举、关系权重计算,实现了一个原型系统 MeDisco/3S,其具有命名实体和关系抽取、在线分析处理、集成挖掘功能。通过原型系统发现了 200000 对症状-基因关系。

[37] Chen H,Ding L,Wu Z,et al. Semantic web for integrated network analysis in biomedicine[J]. Briefings in Bioinformatics,2009,10(2):177-192.

综述了利用语义网技术来表示、集成和分析不同生物医学网络中的知识的研究现状。介绍了一种新的概念框架结构——语义图挖掘技术,综合利用图挖掘技术和本体推理技术来实现网络数据分析。用四个案例(疾病-致病基因分析、基因-蛋白质相互作用分析、药物有效性分析、草药-药物相互作用分析)验证了语义图挖掘技术在知识挖掘上的有效性。

[38] Zheng Q,Chen H,Yu T,et al. Collaborative semantic association discovery from linked data[C]// 10th IEEE Informational Conference on Information Reuse & Integration(IRI'2009),IEEE,2009:394-399.

主要提出了一种在语义网上针对链接数据的多代理语义关联挖掘框架。多个代理通过发布互依赖假设和证据,提升证据网络中的链接和不同知识元素来发现潜在的关联关系。通过模拟实验,验证了我们的多代理协同挖掘框架很适合于跨领域的关系挖掘任务。

[39] 周春英. 超数据集成挖掘方法与技术研究[D]. 杭州:浙江大学,2012.

主要研究了超数据集成挖掘的三个关键技术:超数据准备、超数据集成挖掘以及基于云计算框架的超数据集成挖掘原型系统。解决了超数据的高关联性、分布性和海量性给超数据集成挖掘带来的问题。

(4)基于中药生产过程大数据的知识发现

主要目的是利用知识发现技术研究中药自动化生产过程中产生的大量实时工艺控制数据、质量控制数据,发现影响药品质量的关键工艺参数,进而实现工艺质量指标的预测、参数调优和在线反馈,提升中药产品的稳定性和一致性。

[40] 李金昌. 中药生产工艺的智能优化研究[D]. 杭州:浙江大学,2018.

主要研究了中药生产过程中的关键工艺参数筛选算法、工艺质量指标预测算法、工艺参数优选方法以及工艺在线反馈等重要生产过程控制技术,利用统计分析、数据挖掘方法,实现中药生产过程的实时监控和工艺智能优化,以提升中药生产的可靠性和产品稳定性。

[41] 吴朝晖,包友军,姜晓红,等. 一种获取多维数据稳定性的方法和系统:201510100623.0[P]. 2018-04-17.

主要提出了一种获取多维数据稳定性的方法和系统,具体包括多维数据的降维、均值分析、距离向量计算和显著性分析,计算超半径 $r1$ 和 $r2$。通过预设统计值判定稳定性。通过预设统计值判断稳定性,解决了工业生产领域中产品数据稳定性评估问题,确保产品质量均一性。

(5)数据挖掘系统和平台

主要目的是研究适用于 TCM 领域的数据挖掘系统和平台,助力中医药研究人员在中医药文献、网上资源等获取潜在的中医药知识。具体工具包括:自动文本分类系统 Bow_TCM、文本挖掘系统 MeDisco/3T、中医临床数据库、中医药数据查询和搜索平台、DartSpora 数据挖掘平台等。

［42］Chen J，Zhou X，Wu Z. A multi-label Chinese text categorization system based on boosting algorithm［C］// 7th International Conference on Information Technology（CIT'2004），2004:1153-1158.

主要提出了一种基于中文字特征和 Boosting 算法的多标签的中文文本分类系统。系统在 TCM-MED 数据集上通过了 Reuters-21578 基准测试程序的检验和专家验收。实验结果表明，基于多标签中文文本分类的 boosting 算法性能比基于其他分类方法的算法性能更高。

［43］陈君利. 文本分类技术及其在中药文献中的应用［D］. 杭州:浙江大学,2005.

基于 CMU 的 Bow 系统,开发了多标签中文文本自动分类系统 Bow_TCM;应用多标签中文文本自动分类方法进行中医药文献自动标引;开发了中医证候分子生物学在线挖掘原型系统,通过 MEDLINE 和中医学证候群找出中医证候与基因蛋白质可能的关联。

［44］Zhou X，Liu B，Wu Z. Text mining for clinical Chinese herbal medical knowledge discovery［C］// Discovery Science（DS'2005），LNAI 3735,2005:396-398.

主要研究开发了一个基于中医药文献数据的文本挖掘系统 MeDisco/3T,从文献中抽取临床中医药配方数据,通过频繁项分析发现中草药的相关规律知识。用此系统获取了 18000 例中医临床配方,并发现了其中的频繁中草药药对以及中草药配伍规则。

［45］何前锋. 中医方剂数据挖掘平台研发［D］. 杭州:浙江大学,2005.

主要设计开发了中医药方剂挖掘平台,具体介绍了平台的整体框架和主体功能、数据预处理方案、方剂挖掘分析模块的原型开发,以及方剂挖掘平台应用于数据管理、关联规则分析、单味药与功效聚类分析。

［46］于彤. 中医临床数据仓库的设计与构建［D］. 杭州:浙江大学,2006.

主要设计实现了一个面向中医临床研究的示范性数据仓库系统。首先根据中医临床数据特点进行数据模型设计,开发了一套面向中医临床领域信息的 ETL 工具,实现数据模式转换和一致性规则。开发了基于 Web 的 OLAP 平台,实现报表生成和多维分析。

［47］Ma J，Chen H. Complex network analysis on TCMLS sub-ontologies［C］// 3rd International Conference on Semantics，Knowledge and Grid(SKG'2007),IEEE,2007:551-553.

TCMLS 是全球最大的中医药本体。论文用复杂网络方法研究了 TCMLS 子本体。结果表明,由概念和实例构成的网络具有小世界的模式和无尺度特征,而且少数概念驱动了大量的实例,可推论本体网络结构与类的分层结构类似。

［48］Wu Z，Yu T，Chen H，et al. Information retrieval and knowledge discovery on the semantic web of traditional Chinese medicine［C］// 17th International Conference on World Wide Web（WWW'2008),IEEE,2008:1085-1086.

首次将语义网技术用于中医药信息和知识资源的集成管理和利用。构建了最大的中医药语义本体,并将其作为统一的知识表达方法;开发部署了基于本体的查询和搜索引擎,将大量异构的关系数据库映射到语义网,实现了跨数据库的语义查询和搜索。通过语义集成,建立了中草药和药物相互作用网络,通过语义图挖掘方法实现了该网络上有趣的模式发现和解释。在与 TCM 相关的药物利用、发现和安全性分析上的实践证明,平台和相关底层技术是有效的。

［49］吴毅挺. DartSpora 数据挖掘平台的构建及其在中医方剂领域的应用［D］. 杭州：浙江大学,2008.

主要设计实现了面向中医药领域的数据挖掘平台 DartSpora。采用 AJAX 技术,基于 GWT-Ext 开源框架和 Rapid Miner 软件原型,设计实现了实验管理模块、DartGrid 模块、数据库连接管理模块、用户管理模块等。整合了 DartSpora 与 DartGrid,提供基于语义集成的分布式数据库访问;同时提供了中医方剂领域的数据挖掘实验案例。

［50］吴朝晖,吴毅挺,秘中凯,等. 基于操作流的异步交互式数据挖掘系统及方法：200810060418.6［P］. 2012-12-05.

主要提出了一种基于操作流的异步交互式数据挖掘系统。该系统由基于语义集成的分布式数据库模块、操作符参数模块、用户管理模块、Rapid Miner 内核模块、Web Service 模块组成,提供了一套在 Web 环境下利用现有分布式数据库快速开发和实施数据挖掘系统的解决方案。

［51］秘中凯. 中医药数据挖掘平台与服务［D］. 杭州：浙江大学,2010.

主要研究了面向领域的数据挖掘服务平台的设计实现技术。用 SOA 和 Web 2.0 技术基于 Rapid Miner 实现 DartSpora 2.0 平台的系统框架,支持挖掘方案的定制服务,提供针对第三方平台的挖掘方案 API;将给予 MapReduce 框架的并行数据挖掘算法集成到平台中,支持并行数据挖掘。

［52］Bao Y,Jiang X. An intelligent medicine recommender system framework［C］// 11th IEEE Conference on Industrial Electronics and Applications（ICIEA'2016）,IEEE,2016：1383-1388.

基于数据挖掘技术设计实现了一种药物推荐系统框架。基于诊疗数据集,实验测试评估了多个推荐算法的准确性、模型效率和模型可扩展性。还提出了一种错误检测机制,以保证推荐结果的准确性和服务质量。

3.1　代表性学术论文全文

本节选取了中医药数据挖掘与知识发现方向的 2 篇代表性学术论文《知识发现方法的比较研究》和"Knowledge Discovery in Traditional Chinese Medicine State of the Art and Perspectives"全文（分别于 2000 年和 2006 年发表于期刊《计算机科学》及 *Artificial Intelligence in Medicine*）。

知识发现方法的比较研究

陆伟,吴朝晖

首发于《计算机科学》,2000,27(3):80-84,89

Abstract

Knowledge Discovery in Database(KDD)is a rapid emerging research field. This paper gives an analysis and comparison for methods used in Knowledge Discovery in Database. Our aim is to discuss how to utilize those methods properly in order to construct an efficient KDD system.

Keywords

KDD; model recognition; machine learning; rough set

1 引　言

从已有信息中发现模式或规律是信息处理技术的本质所在。长期以来,为了实现这个目标人们从不同领域、不同角度提出各种方法。典型的如:从数学角度提出的数理统计方法、从模拟生物神经结构角度提出的神经网络技术、从知识角度提出的机器学习方法等。与上述方法不同的是,KDD 并不是研究某种具体的方法,而是根据用户的需要和领域的特点,利用已有的技术形成一个完整的系统,在有限的计算资源下从大型数据库中自动地发现知识。因此我们认为,KDD 着重于系统的实用性,其主要目的是使上述方法适用于大型数据库以及根据领域特性适当地利用它们。

本文主要从方法论的角度对 KDD 作一个初步的介绍。通过对 KDD 中各常用方法的介绍和比较,来讨论当前 KDD 各方法在不同应用背景下的优缺点。

2 KDD 概述及比较研究框架

KDD 在不同应用领域有多种不同的定义,目前,比较为大家所接受的定义是由 Fayyad 等[1]给出的定义:

KDD 是从目标数据集合中识别出有效的、新颖的、潜在有用的,以及最终可理解的模式的非平凡过程。

整个 KDD 的过程可大致分为:数据准备、数据挖掘、知识评估和表现。数据准备阶段主要包括数据选择、数据清理和数据预处理。本质上,数据准备阶段也是一种粗粒度的模式发现过程(如预测空数据、概念层次变化和维数简约等),因此我们将要讨论的各种方法也适用于该阶段。数据挖掘阶段是整个 KDD 过程的核心,首先要确定需要从数据中发现什么类型的知识,数据挖掘任务可以是总结描述、分类、聚类、关联规则发现或序列模式发现等。确定了开采任务后,就要决定使用什么样的开采方法。由于领域对挖掘任务的约束条件千差万别,同时作为挖掘算法一部分的目标数据和领域知识本身存在着多种异质的表达方式,因此需要根据实际的挖掘任务和领域特点,来选择合适的挖掘算法。目前流行的 KDD 方法来源于多个领域,典型的如数理统计、机器学习、模式识别、神经网络、数据库技术等。数据挖掘往往可以发现相当数量的模式,因此一个完整的 KDD 系统应该能对发现的模式进行评估,挑选出其中能够成为知识的模式。本文对 KDD 各方法的比较研究框架基于以下九个标准：

- 描述模型的能力：该方法是否能够从数据中挖掘出复杂的模型；
- 可伸缩性：该方法对目标数据集合的大小的敏感度，即是否适合于大型数据库；
- 精确性：该方法挖掘出的模型是否精确；
- 鲁棒性：该方法对非法输入、错误数据以及环境因素的适应能力；
- 抗噪音能力：当目标数据中存在数据丢失、失真等情况时，该方法是否能够自动恢复正确的值或仅仅将噪音过滤；
- 知识的可理解性：该方法发现的知识是否能够为人所理解，是否能够作为先验知识被再利用；
- 是否需要主观知识：该方法在挖掘过程中，是否依赖于外部专家的主观知识；
- 开放性：该方法是否能够结合领域知识来高效发现知识；
- 适用的数据类型：该方法是否只适用于数值类型的数据或符号类型的数据或者皆可。

下面，将在该框架下对各类方法作简单的介绍。

3　统计模式识别方法

统计模式识别方法指运用数理统计的方法，在样本空间中抽取出模式。模式可以是对样本的分类、聚类、回归估计和分布密度估计。下面介绍统计模式识别中的几种方法：

1）几何分类

利用样本在样本空间的几何分布状况，找到类与类之间的分割由面，在此基础上进行分类或聚类。典型的算法如：距离分类法、感知器、LMSE 梯度法和势函数法。该类方法的关键在于：在搜索空间中找到分割曲面，同时保证曲面与类之间的距离足够大，避免出现过分偶合（over-fit）。

几何分类器的优点在于不依赖条件概率分布密度知识，但它所能处理的只是确定可分的模式，当样本集聚的空间发生重叠现象时，寻找分类曲面的迭代过程将加长或产生振荡。

2）概率分类法

其基本思想是利用贝叶斯法则从样本数据中获得各个模式的后验概率，从后验概率出发，运用风险函数，求出具有最小风险的贝叶斯模式分类器，所谓风险函数是指将属于 y_i 类的样本 X 决策为 y 类（记为 a_j）风险，记为 $\lambda(a_j \mid y_i)$。因此将样本 X 决策为 y_1 类的总风险为：

$$R(a_j \mid X) = \sum_{y_i}\lambda(a_j \mid y_i)P(y_i \mid X)$$

分类器选择决策风险 $R(a_1 \mid X)$ 为最小的类，作为样本 X 的分类。每个类的先验概率 $P(y_i)$ 代表系统对任务的先验知识；条件概率 $P(X \mid y_i)$ 的分布形式可以根据先验知识来估计，而函数的参数向量可以从训练数据中估计出（估计的方法可以是最大似然估计、贝叶斯估计等方法）。

概率分类器的优点是训练样本不必几何可分，对噪音和畸变不敏感等；但它需要用户提供先验概率和条件概率分布形式，即使采用密度函数的参数估计，也仍然较粗糙，因此分类器的性能受主观知识的影响较大[2]。

3）动态聚类分析

聚类分析是在训练集中无导师信号情况下根据样本数据自身的分布特点来进行分类。动态聚类是聚类分析中常用的方法之一。其基本过程是：

- 随机选择若干样本为聚类中心;
- 按某种聚类准则,如最小距离准则,使其余样品向各中心聚集,得到一种聚类模式;
- 评价该聚类的优劣,若满意则结束算法,否则按照一定的策略重新选择样本作为聚类中心,重复上述步骤。其中选择聚类中心的策略可以是选择已有聚类的几何中心或选择离中心最远的边界点。

比较著名的动态聚类算法有 K 均值算法和 ISODATA 算法。

4)贝叶斯网

贝叶斯网是一种用于描述对象之间的概率关系的有向非循环图模型,在数据挖掘领域中,主要用于发现对象间的因果关系[3]。贝叶斯网中的每个结点表示变量或状态,两点之间的有向弧表示结点之间的依赖关系。网络的结构实际上描述了变量之间的条件独立性(两点之间若不存在弧,表明两个变量条件独立),而每个变量都有相应的局部概率分布。以此为基础,可以计算出整个变量集合或变量子集的联合分布密度,一个典型的贝叶斯网如图 1 所示。

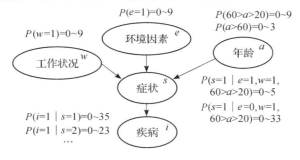

图 1 用于描述疾病原因的贝叶斯网

在知识挖掘中应用贝叶斯网方法主要是根据样本数据来修正网络的结构和局部条件概率分布。这可以分为两种情况:(1)当网络结构已知时,分析的目的是根据数据集合计算出每个弧所对应的后验条件概率分布。(2)当网络结构不确定时,分析的目的是能够根据数据集合从候选的网络结构中选择最合适的结构。无论是第一种情况还是第二种情况,都需在模型空间中搜索最优。其中的评价函数可以是:最大后验概率(MAP)、贝叶斯信息标准(BIC)、贝叶斯因子(BF)等。

贝叶斯网络应用于知识挖掘领域的优点是:抗噪音能力强,能够处理不完全的数据;可以发现隐藏在数据中的因果模型;可以很容易地结合领域知识,比如用概率来表达因果关系的强弱,先验的因果知识以候选贝叶斯网的形式出现。但其缺点在于:模型的复杂度随网络中节点的增加而呈指数级增长;通常只能找到较优解并且取决于所用的领域知识和启发性规则。

总之,统计模式识别方法具有良好的理论基础,描述模型的能力较强,可伸缩性、精确性、鲁棒性、抗噪音能力和开放性都较好,比较适合于数值信息。但大部分方法需要对概率分布作主观假设,因此需要主观知识支持;并且发现的结果多为数学公式,不易理解。

4 面向符号的机器学习方法

机器学习方法是采用人工智能技术来实现机器从客观世界中学习的能力。归纳学习是机器学习中最核心、最成熟的分枝,旨在从大量的经验数据中归纳抽取一般的判定规则和模式。归纳学习可以发现分类、聚类、归纳描述等模式。归纳学习又可以根据有无导师信号分为有导师学习和无导师学习。

1）有导师学习

有导师学习是事先由外部导师将训练例子分类，然后对这些带有导师信号的训练例子进行学习。有导师的学习也可以根据其学习策略分为以 AQ 系列为代表的覆盖算法和以 ID3 为代表的分治算法。

覆盖算法的基本思想是：对于给定的正例集和反例集，在由属性构成的概念空间中，找到一个能够覆盖所有正例和排斥所有反例的最佳概念描述。所谓最佳即在概念的充分完备性和概念的简明性上取得一致。最早的覆盖算法是 Michalski 的 AQ11 算法，其采用了自下而上的归纳方法，即在归纳过程中正例用于制导系统生成较概括的假设，反例用来减削不合适的假设。AQ11 算法的特点在于采用约束星和 LEF 评价函数来约束对概念空间的搜索[4]。覆盖算法除了上述的自下而上的策略之外，还有自上而下和双向策略。

AQ11 的后继算法在不同方面对算法作了改进，如 AQ15 增加了构造性学习、渐进学习和近似推理的功能，而 AE 系列引进了扩张矩阵技术，对降低算法的逻辑复杂度作了很大的改进[5]。覆盖方法是模拟人类的学习过程，因此所得出的知识较易为人理解，并且适合于符号数据，但因为需要对训练集作多遍扫描，大多数算法都是面向小训练集的。

分治方法的基本思想是用属性值对例子集合逐级划分形成树状结构，直到一个节点仅含有同一类的例子为止。分治算法的结果往往是一棵决策树。Quinlan 的 ID3 算法是分治方法中的典型代表。在 ID3 中使用了基于信息理论的启发式方法来选择属性，即根据每个属性的信息增益来衡量它对减少系统的不确定性的贡献[6]，以此来产生决策树。这样属性选择策略使得在剖分后的子树中对对象分类所要获得的信息最少。

在 ID3 之后出现了许多改进算法，它们主要从处理离散和连续量、处理大量数据、处理数据属性之间的关联关系使系统可利用非平行于轴的剖分面、处理非静态的训练集等方面进行了改进。如 ID4 是一种递增式方法，通过不断获得的新信息更新决策树，适用于动态的训练集；C4.5 可以同时处理具有离散和连续取值的属性，并且使用信息增益比来选择属性使系统能够在分支数目和一次剖分后的分类准确度上进行权衡；CART-LC 和 OC1 可以生成有斜剖分平面的决策树分类系统；SLIQ 则使用了一个特定的数据结构和 Gini 为分裂标准，使算法更加适合于大型的训练集。

决策树方法的优点是适合于符号数据、知识易理解、算法精确并且鲁棒性强。缺点是对连续量数据分类能力较弱，而且可能由于噪音的存在使得决策树过大。

2）无导师学习

此方法事先不知道训练例子的分类，算法通过学习能够对它们进行聚类。Michalski 等人的 CLUSTER/2 的基本思想与前述的动态聚类类似，但两者在实现上有三点不同[4]：

- 对于距离的定义：在 CLUSTER/2 中定义了对象之间的句法距离，用于衡量名词性实体之间的相似性。

- 对于搜索空间的约束：在 CLUSTER/2 中采用了约束星和 LEF 评价函数来实现对搜索空间的约束。

- 在 CLUSTER/2 中,对所得到的聚类评价准则为聚类和事件之间的适合度、聚类描述的简洁性、聚类之间的差异性和区分度等。

比较统计方法而言,概念聚类产生的结果比较容易理解,适合于名词性数据,但不适合于数值属性。同样概念聚类也需要对目标数据集进行多次扫描,因此不适合大训练集。

总之,面向机器学习的方法描述模型的能力较强,结果的可理解性、开放性较好,处理符号信息能力强。但它的精确性、鲁棒性和抗噪音能力一般,需要以算法的复杂度为代价,并且往往是面向经过整理过的小训练集,因此可伸缩性差。

5 神经网络方法

人工神经网络是一种典型的面向连接的学习技术。常用的人工神经网络有多种模型,每个模型有不同的倾向,如快速训练、快速联想和求最优解。就 KDD 而言,BP 网和 Kohonen 网应用最为广泛。

BP 网是由 Rumelhart 等人在 1985 年提出的,系统地解决了多层神经网络中隐层单元连接权的学习问题,并在数学上给出了完整的推导。BP 网采用多层前向的拓扑形状,由输入层、中间层和输出层组成。BP 网的学习策略为有导师学习,其学习过程由训练数据的正向传播和误差信号的反向传播两部分组成,并且这种过程不断迭代,最后使得信号误差达到允许的范围之内。

BP 网能在最小均方差的意义下实现对样本输入输出对的逼近,它的学习能力强。与传统的统计分析相比,BP 网可以同时逼近多个输出,可以满足多输入参数所造成的复杂情况并且实现简单。BP 网可以被用于分类、回归和时间序列预测等 KDD 任务中。

Kohonen 网络是一个由全互连的神经网阵列形成的无导师自组织和自学习网络。它采用前向拓扑结构,其结构为两层神经单元,分别为输入层和竞争输出层,并且两层之间全互连。Kohonen 网的基本思想是通过调整从输入结点到竞争层上结点的连接权值,建立向量量化器。当训练开始时,连续取值且未指定预期输出的输入向量依次加载到网络上,竞争输出层的单元互相竞争,竞争胜利的单元表示与输入模式相对接近,于是该单元以及临近其他点的权值也被修正,使得这部分区域对相应输入敏感。随着训练的继续,该区域的半径越来越小,拥有最大权值的区域就对应着向量空间的聚类中心,此中心的点密度函数大致就是输入向量的概率密度函数。网络中的权值将被组织得使拓扑上接近的结点对物理上的相似输入敏感。因此 Kohonen 网是一种逐步形成特征映射的算法。

与其他聚类方法相比,Kohonen 网的优点在于:可以实现实时学习,网络具有自稳定性,无须外界给出评价函数,能够主动识别向量空间中最有意义的特征,抗噪音能力强等。

此外可用于 KDD 领域中的人工神经网络模型还可以有:ART 网、循环 BP(Recurrent Back Propagation)网、RBF (Radial Basis Function)网络和 PNN(Probabilistic Neural Networks)网等。应能根据任务的特点来选择适当的网络模型,比如:发现的内容类别(如需要对时间序列预测时,用循环 BP 网要比普通的 BP 网好)、训练数据的类型、训练数据量以及对训练速度的要求(如当需要在线学习时,ART 和 RBF 的训练数据相对而言要更快)。

从 KDD 的角度来看,神经网络的模型描述能力强,精确性、鲁棒性和抗噪音能力都较好,一般不需要主观知识的支持。但它需要对数据做多遍扫描,训练时间较长,可伸缩性差;由于知识是以网络结构和连接权值的形式来表达的,因此结果的可理解性和开放性都很差;对于知识的可理解性,虽然可以通过观察输入和输出来分析网络内部的知识或者通过网络剪枝来简化网络的结构从而提取规则,但效果都不理想。

6　粗集理论和方法

粗集方法是近年来提出的用于对不完整数据进行分析、学习的方法。该方法与传统的统计分析和模糊集理论不同的是:后者需要依赖先验知识来定量描述不确定性,如统计分析中的先验概率、模糊集理论中的模糊度等;而前者只依赖数据内部的知识,用数据之间的近似来表示知识的不确定性。下面先简单介绍粗集理论中的一些基本概念[7]:

定义决策系统 $DS=(U,C,D)$,其中 U 是实体集合,C 是条件属性集合,D 是决策属性集合。C 的任意一个子集 B 在 U 上定义了一个等价关系:

$$IND(B)=\{(x,y)|a(x)=a(y),\forall a\in B\}$$

该关系也称为由 B 定义的不可分辨关系。对于 $x\in U$,它的 B 等价类定义为:

$$[x]B=\{y|(x,y)\in IND(B)\}$$

对任意几何 X,R 是 U 的一个不可分辨关系,X 的 R 下近似和上近似分别定义为:

$$\underline{R}X=\{x|x\in U:[x]_R\subseteq X\};$$

$$\overline{R}X=\{x|x\in U:[x]_R\bigcap X\neq\varnothing\}$$

$\underline{R}X$ 表示根据关系 R 能够确定地被分入 X 的元素的集合,$\overline{R}X$ 表示根据关系 R 有可能被分入 X 的 U 的元素的集合。对于 $B\subset C$,定义 B 相对于 D 的正域:

$$POSB(D)=U\{\underline{B}X|X\in U|IND(D)\}$$

其中 $U|IND(D)$ 为 D 对 U 划分所得到的等价类集合。$POSB(D)$ 实际上是那些可以根据属性集合 B 准确地被分入由属性 D 所确定的分类的元素的集合。设 $a\in C$,若有 $POS_C(D)=POS_{C-|a|}(D)$,则称 a 为 C 中 D 可省略。当 C 中每个元素都不为 C 中 D 可省略的话,称 C 为 D 独立。当 $C'=C-C''$ 为 D 独立,且 C'' 中的所有元素都是 D 可省略时,则称 C' 为 C 的 D 相对简约。从分类的角度来看,相对简约就是用一种分类来表达另一种分类必不可少的属性集合。

D 和 C 之间的依赖程度可以由关系间的分类近似质量来度量:$r=|POS_C(D)|/|U|$。$r=1$ 表示全可导,$r<1$ 表示粗可导。属性 a 对于由决策属性 D 导致的分类的重要性就等于从 C 中删除 a 后 C 对 D 的依赖程度的变化值。

粗集方法在 KDD 中的应用可以是:

● 知识简约:简约和相对简约在粗集中是非常重要的概念,它反应了一个决策系统的本质。通过对条件属性集合的简约,可以保证简化后的决策系统具有与原先系统一样的分类能力。从数据预处理的角度看,属性简约能去掉多余属性,从而提高系统的效率。

● 属性相关分析:粗集方法中的属性重要程度可以用来衡量该属性对分类的影响程度,它与 ID3 中的信息增益类似,可以证明两者在一定条件下是等价的[8]。

● 规则学习和决策表推导:在保证简化后的决策系统具有与原先系统一样的分类能力的前提条件下,通过使用知识简约和范畴简约,将决策系统简化并且找到最小(最短)决策规则集合,以达到最大限度泛化的目的。

总之,从 KDD 的角度来看,由于粗集方法中的决策表可以被视为关系型数据库中的关系表,因此粗集方法的伸缩性较强,鲁棒性和抗噪音能力都较强,知识的可理解性和开放性较好,比较适用于符号信息。此外,粗集方法可以对数据进行预处理,去掉多余属性,可提高发现效率,降低错误率。但是粗集方法的模型描述能力一般。

7 数据库技术

数据库技术是近年来发展得较为成熟的领域,如何利用已经相当成熟的数据库或数据仓库技术来为 KDD 服务是当前 KDD 研究领域中的一个热点。

1) OLAP 和数据仓库

数据仓库是一种为了实现决策支持的数据模型、存储决策所需信息的语义一致的数据存储机制。数据仓库中的数据是经过清洗、整理过的数据,它能够向用户提供一致的、完整的数据集合。因此数据仓库为 KDD 的算法提供了一个很好的数据平台,

数据仓库的主要功能是提供联机分析过程(OLAP)[9]。OLAP 提供的服务主要包括切片和切块、概念上升、概念下钻、旋转等。OLAP 是一种由用户驱动的、自上而下不断深入的分析工具。它有助于简化数据分析过程并且能够发现描述性的规则。但与 KDD 相比,OLAP 更多地依赖于用户提出问题和指导,并且它往往只用于对数据的总结描述。因此数据挖掘应用的广度和深度要大于 OLAP。但数据仓库为数据挖掘提供了经过整理的数据,同时 OLAP 的多角度、多层次的数据汇总能力为数据挖掘提供了良好的基础。

2) 面向属性的归纳(Attribute-Oriented Induction)

AOI 技术由 Han 提出[10]。该方法采用概念树爬升的技术来实现从关系表中归纳出高层次的总结性规则。AOI 的基本思路是:首先得到与任务相关的以关系表形式出现的数据集合,然后通过对每个属性采用爬升概念树的方法对该属性进行泛化直到该属性中的不同值的个数小于一定的泛化阈值为止,最后合并数据集合中一致的元组。泛化后的关系中的每个泛化元组可以被视为一条对原关系的总结性特征描述规则。如果有另一个关系作为对照的话,对两个关系利用相同的办法,可以得到关系之间的区别描述规则。

AOI 的优点在于过程简单,容易实现,并且在大型数据库上实现的效率较高,发现的知识易于理解,可以在多层次上发现知识,同时领域知识通过概念树的形式可以被容易结合进来。但它需要领域知识来构造每个属性对应的概念树并且定义泛化阈值,而且只能发现描述性知识。

总之,面向数据库的 KDD 方法的普遍优点在于:适合于在大型数据上的知识挖掘,伸缩性强;精确性、抗噪音和鲁棒性较好;对数值和符号数据都适合;知识的开放性和可理解性都较强。它的缺点在于:依赖数据模型,只能发现比较简单的描述性知识,用它来发现复杂模型较难。

综上所述,KDD 的各个方法的比较结果如表 1 所示。从表 1 可以看出,各个方法都有其优缺点和不同的适用领域,一个完整的知识发现系统应该能够根据实际需要充分地利用各方法的特点以达到扬长避短的目的。对不同方法的利用更多体现在知识发现过程的不同阶段,比如:

- 在数据选择阶段,粗集方法和统计方法都可以实现对属性的选择;

- 在数据清理阶段,回归方法或神经网络方法可以用于对缺值的预测,统计方法或利用元规则的约束推理可以用于清除噪音和数据修正;
- 在数据预处理阶段,统计聚类或神经网络聚类方法都可以用于对连续数值的离散化,OLAP或 AOI 方法可以改变原始数据的抽象层次;
- 在数据挖掘阶段,可以根据输入数据源的特点和任务的要求来选择合适的方法。

表 1　知识发现各方法特点比较

方法	描述模型的能力	伸缩性	精确性	鲁棒性	抗噪音能力	知识可理解性	是否需要主观知识	开放性	适合的数据类型
统计模式识别方法	强	强	强	强	强	较差	需要	较差	数值
面向符号的机器学习方法	强	较差	一般	一般	一般	强	不需要	强	符号
神经网络方法	强	较差	强	强	强	较差	不需要	较差	皆可
粗集方法	一般	强	一般	强	强	强	不需要	强	符号
面向数据库的方法	较差	强	强	强	强	强	不需要	强	皆可

参考文献

[1]Fayyad U M, *et al*. From Data Mining to Knowledge Discovery:An Overview. Advances in Knowledge Discovery and Data Mining. AAAI/MIT Press, 1996.

[2]沈清,汤霖.模式识别导论.国防科技大学出版社,1991.

[3]Heckerman D. Bayesian Networks for Data Mining-Data Mining and Knowledge Discovery, 1997(1):79-119.

[4]Michalski R. Machine Learning:An Artificial Intelligence Approach, volume 1. Morgan Kaufmann, Sam Mateo, California, 1984.

[5]洪家荣.归纳学习——算法 理论 应用.科学出版社,1997.

[6]Quinlan J R. Induction of Decision Trees. Machine Learning, 1986.

[7]Pawlak Z. Rough Sets Theoretical Aspects of Reasoning about Data. Kluwer Academic Publishers, 1991.

[8]曾黄麟.粗集理论及应用.重庆大学出版社,1998.

[9]Chaudhri S, Dayal U. An Overview of Data Warehousing and OLAP Technology. SIGMOD Record, 1997, 26:65-74.

[10]Han J, *et al*. Knowledge Discovery in Databases:An Attribute-Oriented Approach. In:Proc, of the 18th VLDB Conference. 1992:335-350.

Knowledge Discovery in Traditional Chinese Medicine: State of the Art and Perspectives

Yi Feng, Zhaohui Wu, Xuezhong Zhou, Zhongmei Zhou, Weiyu Fan

首发于 *Artificial Intelligence in Medicine*, 2006, 38(3): 219-236

Summary

Objective: As a complementary medical system to Western medicine, traditional Chinese medicine (TCM) provides a unique theoretical and practical approach to the treatment of diseases over thousands of years. Confronted with the increasing popularity of TCM and the huge volume of TCM data, historically accumulated and recently obtained, there is an urgent need to explore these resources effectively by the techniques of knowledge discovery in database (KDD). This paper aims at providing an overview of recent KDD studies in TCM field.

Methods: A literature search was conducted in both English and Chinese publications, and major studies of knowledge discovery in TCM (KDTCM) reported in these materials were identified. Based on an introduction to the state of the art of TCM data resources, a review of four subfields of KDTCM research was presented, including KDD for the research of Chinese medical formula, KDD for the research of Chinese herbal medicine, KDD for TCM syndrome research, and KDD for TCM clinical diagnosis. Furthermore, the current state and main problems in each subfield were summarized based on a discussion of existing studies, and future directions for each subfield were also proposed accordingly.

Results: A series of KDD methods are used in existing KDTCM researches, ranging from conventional frequent itemset mining to state of the art latent structure model. Considerable interesting discoveries are obtained by these methods, such as novel TCM paired drugs discovered by frequent itemset analysis, functional community of related genes discovered under syndrome perspective by text mining, the high proportion of toxic plants in the botanical family *Ranunculaceae* disclosed by statistical analysis, the association between M-cholinoceptor blocking drug and *Solanaceae* revealed by association rule mining, etc. It is particularly inspiring to see some studies connecting TCM with biomedicine, which provide a novel top-down view for functional genomics research. However, further developments of KDD methods are still expected to better adapt to the features of TCM.

Conclusions: Existing studies demonstrate that KDTCM is effective in obtaining medical discoveries. However, much more work needs to be done in order to discover real diamonds from TCM domain. The usage and development of KDTCM in the future will substantially contribute to the TCM community, as well as modern life science.

Keywords

traditional Chinese medicine; knowledge discovery; data mining

1 Introduction

As a complete medical knowledge system other than orthodox medicine, traditional Chinese medicine (TCM) plays an indispensable role in the health care for Chinese people for several thousand years. The holistic and systematic ideas of TCM are essentially different from the thinking modes based on Reductionism in Western medicine. With the development of modern science, people come to realize the limitations of Reductionism, and begin to lay more emphasis on the systematic thinking patterns, such as Systems Biology[1]. Based on the methodology of holism, TCM plays a unique role in advancing the development of life science and medicine. Meanwhile, with the dramatic increase in the prevalence of chronic conditions, the chemical medicines cannot totally satisfy the needs of health maintenance, disease prevention, and treatment. Human health demands the large-scale development and application of natural medicines, to which TCM experiences and knowledge can contribute a lot. The ever-increasing use of Chinese herbal medicine and acupuncture worldwide is a good indication of the public interest in TCM [2-6].

Countless TCM practices and theoretical researches in thousands of years accumulated a great deal of knowledge in the form of ancient books and literatures. In China, the domestic collection of the ancient books about TCM published before Xinhai Revolution (1911) reaches 130,000 volumes. Besides, thousands of studies on TCM treatments are published yearly in journals all around the world. There were more than 600,000 journal articles during the period of 1984—2005. With such a vast volume of TCM data, there is an urgent need to use these precious resources effectively and sufficiently. Besides, the last decade has been marked by unprecedented growth in both the production of biomedical data and the amount of published literature discussing it. Thus, it is an opportunity, but also a pressing need to connect TCM with modern life science.

Knowledge discovery in databases (KDD) is one proper methodology to analyze and understand such huge amounts of data. As an interdisciplinary area between artificial intelligence, database, statistics, and machine learning, the idea of KDD came into being in the late 1980s. The most prominent definition of KDD was proposed by Fayyad et al. [7] in 1996. In that paper, KDD was defined as "the nontrivial process of identifying valid, novel, potentially useful, and ultimately understandable patterns in data." This definition may also be applied to "data mining" (DM). Indeed, in the recent literature of DM and KDD, the terms are often used interchangeably or without distinction. However, according to classical KDD methodologies [7], data mining is the knowledge extraction step in KDD process, which also involves the selection and preprocessing of appropriate data from various sources, and proper interpretation of the mining results. Typical data mining methods include concept description, association rule mining, classification and prediction, clustering analysis, time-series analysis, text mining, etc. [8]. During the last two decades, the field of KDD has attracted considerable interest in numerous disciplines, ranging from telecommunications, banking and marketing to scientific analysis. It is also the case within medical environments. The discipline of medicine deals with complex organisms, processes and relations, and KDD methodology is particularly suitable to handle such complexity [9]. Besides, the advent of computer-based patient records (CPRs) and data warehouses contribute greatly to the availability of medical data and offer voluminous data resources for KDD. Also, the need to increase medical knowledge of human beings pushes researchers to carry out knowledge discovery, not only in CPRs and clinical warehouses, but also in biomedical literature databases. The creation of new medical knowledge with DM techniques is listed as one of the 10 grand challenges to medicine by Altman [10]. As Roddick et al. [11] indicates, the application of KDD to medical datasets is a rewarding and highly challenging area. Due to the ever-increasing accumulation of biomedicine data and the pressing demand to explore these resources, the methods of knowledge discovery are widely applied to analyze medical information during the decades. Reviews of KDD in the medical area from different perspectives can be found in refs. [9, 11-16]. However, the topic of knowledge discovery in TCM (KDTCM) is not covered in these reviews.

Considering the fast-growing number of researches carried out on KDTCM, it is also necessary and helpful to provide an overview of recent KDTCM researches. As a complementary medical system, TCM is quite different from Western medicine, both in practice and in theory. In view of the high domain specificity of KDD technology, it is more necessary to gain an insight into KDTCM. Motivated by these needs, this review paper focuses on the introduction and summarization of existing work about KDTCM. Because a great amount of KDTCM work is reported only in Chinese literature, the literature search is conducted in both English and Chinese publications, and the major KDTCM studies published in these materials are covered in this review. For each work, the KDD methods used in the study are introduced, as well as corresponding results. Particularly, some studies with interesting results are highlighted, such as novel TCM paired drugs discovered by frequent itemset analysis, the laboratory-confirmed relationship between CRF gene and *kidney YangXu* syndrome discovered by text mining, the high proportion of toxic plants in the botanical family *Ranunculaceae* discovered by statistical analysis, the association between M-cholinoceptor blocking drug and *Solanaceae* discovered by association rule mining, etc. The existing work in KDTCM demonstrates that the usage of KDD in TCM is both feasible and promising. Meanwhile, it should be noticed that the TCM field is still nearly a piece of virgin soil with copious amounts of hidden gold as far as KDD methodology is concerned. To ease gold mining in this field, the future directions of KDTCM research are also provided in this article based on a discussion of existing work.

The rest of this paper is arranged as follows. The prerequisite of applying KDD is the digitalization of the vast amount of data. Thus, an overview of currently available TCM data resources is firstly presented in Section 2. Subsequently, the review of KDTCM work is presented in four research subfields in Section 3, including KDD for the research of Chinese medical formula (CMF), KDD for the research of Chinese herbal medicine (CHM), KDD for TCM syndrome research, and KDD for TCM clinical diagnosis. Based on a discussion of these KDTCM studies, the current state and main problems of KDTCM work in each subfield are summarized in Section 4, and the future directions for each subfield are also presented. Finally, we conclude in Section 5.

2 State of the art of TCM data resources

Data availability is the first consideration before any knowledge discovery task could be undertaken. In this section, we introduce the current state of TCM data resources, especially those data resources focusing on TCM particularly.

As a significant part of complementary and alternative medicines (CAM), literature reporting TCM issues can be found in main CAM databases, such as CAM on PubMed (Complementary and Alternative Medicine subset of PubMed), AMED (Allied and Complementary Medicine Database), CISCOM (Centralised Information Service for Complementary Medicine), CAMPAIN (Complementary and Alternative Medicine and Pain Database), etc. A more comprehensive list of TCM databases can be found in ref.[17]. Currently, the primary data resources specific to TCM includes China TCM Patent Database

(CTCMPD) [18], TradiMed Database [19], TCM chemical database [20], and TCM-Online Database System [21]. CTCMPD has been established by Patent Data Research & Development Center, a subsidiary to the Intellectual Property Publishing House of State Intellectual Property Office (SIPO) of China. More than 19,000 patent records and over 40,000 TCM formulas published from 1985 to present are contained in CTCMPD [18]. TradiMed Database was built by the Natural Product Research Institute at Seoul National University, Korea. Based on various Chinese and Korean medical classics, TradiMed represents a combination of traditional medicine knowledge and modern medicine. So far, TradiMed contains information of 3199 herbs, 11,810 formulae, 20,012 chemical compositions of herbs, and 4080 diseases [19]. TCM chemical database was developed by National Key Laboratory of Bio-chemical Engineering at The Institute of Process Engineering, Chinese Academy of Sciences. This database contains detailed information of 9000 chemicals isolated from nearly 4000 natural sources used in TCM and provides in-depth bioactivity data for many of the compounds [20].

In this section, we place our emphasis on the TCM-Online Database System. To the best of our knowledge, currently TCM-Online Database System is the largest TCM data collections in the world. The prototype of TCM-Online was firstly built in the later 1990s. In 1998, the AdvanCed Computing aNd sysTem (CCNT) Lab in the College of Computer Science in Zhejiang University and China Academy of Traditional Chinese Medicine (CATCM) began to collaborate in building the scientific databases for TCM, and established a unified web accessible multi-database query system TCMMDB [22] that integrates 17 branches in the whole country. Through the input from nearly 300 scientists from more than 30 colleges, universities and academies of TCM, this system has already integrated more than 50 databases, including Traditional Chinese Medical Literature Analysis and Retrieval System, Traditional Chinese Drug Database, Database of Chinese Medical Formula, etc. TCMMDB was replaced by the grid-based system TCM-Grid [23] in 2002, which provides more powerful functions, such as dynamic registration, binding, associated navigation, etc. The TCM-Grid system was further extended to a semantic-based database grid named DartGrid in 2002. In present, these databases are available as TCM-Online Database System via website [21] and CD-ROM versions. Besides, a large-scale ontology-based Unified TCM Language System (UTCMLS) [24] has been developed to support concept-based information retrieval and information integration since 2001. All these efforts help to realize the organization, storage, and sharing of TCM data, which provides a feasible environment for the effective implementation of KDD technology.

Today, the TCM-Online Database System integrates more than 50 TCM-related databases. The main databases are listed as below.

2.1　Traditional Chinese medical literature analysis and retrieval system (TCMLARS) (Chinese/English)

The bibliographic system TCMLARS [25] has two versions. So far, the Chinese version has contained over 600,000 TCM periodical articles, while the corresponding number reaches 92,000 in English version of TCMLARS. The source material for the database is drawn from about 900 biomedical journals published in China since 1984. The main fields included in TCMLARS are similar with MEDLINE, such as title, author, journal title, publication year, abstract, etc. Besides, some fields specifically existing in TCM are also included, such as pharmacology of Chinese herbs, ingredients and dosage of formula, drug compatibility, acupuncture and Tuina points, etc. TCMLARS is considered as an important new asset in literature review and meta-analysis of Chinese herbal medicine by McCulloch *et al*. [26]. It also serves as a significant data resource for KDTCM, especially for the methods based on text mining.

2.2 Traditional Chinese Drug Database (TCDBASE) (Chinese/English)

This database also has Chinese and English versions. The Chinese version contains over 11,000 records, while the English version contains 545 records. Each record represents a single herb, or mineral drug, or other natural medicines, and provides the cited information. The data is derived from *Chinese Materia Medica Dictionary*, *Thesaurus of Chinese Herbs*, *Chinese Medicinal Materials*, *Manual of Composition and Pharmacology of Common Traditional Chinese Medicine*, etc. Main contents of TCDBASE include drug name, original source of medical materials, collection and storage of medical materials, parts of the plant/animal for medicinal use, chemical composition, physical/chemical properties, processing methods, dosage form, pharmaceutical techniques, pharmacokinetics, toxicology, compatibility of medicines, efficacy, adverse reactions and their treatment, etc. Such contents of TCDBASE make it an important collection for CHM research, as well as the KDTCM research related to CHM.

2.3 Database of Chinese Medical Formula (DCMF) (Chinese)

This database contains more than 85,000 formulae. Each record represents a single prescription and provides the cited information. Data is derived from modern publications such as *Pharmacopoeia of the People's Republic of China*, *Chinese Medical Formula Dictionary*, etc. The main contents of DCMF include formal name, efficacy, indication, usage, precaution, adverse reactions and its treatment, ingredients, modification of the prescription, dosage form and specifications, preparation, storage, compatibility of medicines, chemical composition, toxicology, etc. DCMF collects a comprehensive clinical cases using combinatorial medicines in thousands of years, and thus is particularly worth in-depth analysis by KDD technology, especially the approaches based on frequent itemset analysis and association rule mining.

2.4 Database of Chemical Composition from Chinese Herbal Medicine (DCCCHM) (Chinese)

This database contains over 4500 records. Each record represents a single chemical composition and provides the cited information. Data is derived from *Active Compositions of Chinese Herbal Medicine*, *Pharmacology of Traditional Chinese Medicine*, *Chinese Herbal Medicine*, etc. Main contents include formal name, chemical name, physical/chemical properties, molecular formula, chemical formula, origin, pharmacological action, efficacy, toxicity, adverse reactions, chemical category, functional category, etc. Although the information of 3D chemical structure is not included in this database, DCCCHM could still be used as an important data resource for CHM research and drug discovery from CHM.

2.5 Clinical Medicine Database (CLINMED) (Chinese)

This database contains information on more than 3500 diseases. The source material for the database was drawn from authoritative reference books and teaching materials of Chinese and Western medicine. The main contents of CLINMED include name of diseases, disease classification code by Western medicine/TCM, disease name definition by Western medicine/TCM, Western medicine/TCM etiology, pathology, pathological physiopathology, pathogenesis, diagnosis, Western medicine therapy, treatment of TCM, Chinese herbal medicine therapy, acupuncture and moxibustion, massage, integrated therapy of Western medicine and TCM, etc. CLINMED reflects the understanding and experience of treating diseases in today's China, involving both western medicine treatment and TCM therapy. As an effective avenue to combine Western medicine and TCM, multilevel knowledge discovery could be carried out based on the integration of data in both fields, and CLINMED could contribute in this trend.

2.6 TCM Electronic Medical Record Database (TCM-EMRD) (Chinese)

TCM Electronic Medical Record (EMR) contains the data of TCM clinical practice on inpatient and out-patient. Clinical daily practice takes a vital role for TCM research and theory refinement, because unlike modern medicine, almost no bench-side studies are performed in TCM. China Government has initiated several important programs since 2002 to collect the clinical TCM EMR data and the clinical data warehouse TCM-EMRD is built for potential decision support applications and TCM knowledge discovery. Currently, TCM-EMRD contains more than 3500 EMRs of inpatients. The main contents of TCM-EMRD include TCM Diagnosis, Chinese Medical Formula, the conceptual description of symptoms, etc. TCM-EMRD is especially ideal for clinical KDTCM studies because KDD is considered as the major purpose when establishing this database. Thus, special considerations are given to issues related to knowledge discovery, such as the quality of data, the standardization of terms, etc.

Other data resources within TCM-Online Database System include Database of Tibetan Medicines, Medical News Database, OTC Database, Database of State Essential Druggery of China, Database of Medical Research Awards in China, Database of Medical Product in China, TCM Pharmaceutical Industry Database, China Hospitals Database, Database of Paired Drugs (DPD), etc. The TCM-Online Database System, as well as other digitized TCM data resources, serves as the available data sources in various KDTCM researches, which can be seen in the following review section.

3　Review of KDTCM researches

3.1　Knowledge discovery for CMF research

One distinguishing feature of TCM lies in its emphasis on the usage of combinatorial medicines, in the form of CMF. A CMF is composed of selected drugs and suitable doses based on syndrome differentiation for etiology and the composition of therapies in accordance with the principle of formulating a TCM prescription. Except for very few single drugs of all the prescriptions used clinically, the great majority of them are compound drugs consisting of two or more drugs. The reasons are that the potency of a single drug is usually limited, and some of them may produce certain side effects or even toxicity. But when several drugs are applied together, ensuring a full play of their advantages and inhibiting the disadvantages, they will display their superiority over a single drug in the treatment of diseases. In this way, TCM uses processed multi-component natural products in various combinations and formulations. Due to the great diversity of candidate drugs to form a compound prescription, hundreds of thousands of Chinese medical formulae have been accumulated over thousands of years.

To use combinatorial medicines properly, one key issue is to realize the combination rules of multiple drugs. Compared with Western biomedicine, countless TCM practices in thousands of years accumulate numerous cases of combinatorial medicines as the form of formulae. These TCM formulae are valuable resources for research of drug compatibility. Besides, due to the tradition of usage of combinatorial medicines, the analysis of combination rules of multiple drugs exhibits much more significance in TCM than Western medicine. Therefore, the CMF research attracts more data miners than other subjects.

A breakthrough of herbal combination rule research lies in the analysis of paired drugs, which usually means a relatively fixed combination of two CHMs. In generalized definition of paired drugs, the number of medicines in paired drugs can be extended to three, four, etc. According to TCM theory, such combinations can increase their medical effectiveness, or reduce the toxicity and side effects of some drugs. A number of paired drugs have already been induced from practice and included in the Database of Paired Drugs as a part of TCM-Online Database System recently. However, such kind of valuable combinations could be revealed more and deeper. When two drugs are frequently used in combination with each other in practice, they are more likely to be paired drugs. Therefore, frequent item set analysis and association rule mining could be used to discover paired drugs [27-31]. As the most classical example of data mining, association rule mining aims at searching for interesting relationships among items in a given data set. It can serve as one proper KDD method to analyze combination patterns of multiple drugs in TCM. The first step in association rule mining, also the core issue in association rule mining, is to find frequent item sets, which means each of these item-sets will occur at least as frequently as a predetermined percentage in whole dataset. This method can be used to find frequent herb co-occurrences. In 2002, the classical association rule method was used by Yao *et al*. [27] to study 106 formulae for treating diabetes. The results indicate that different experts have similar ideas and principles for treating this disease, which helps to reveal the scientific rule in the composition of the TCM formulae for diabetes. This work also demonstrates that KDD is a powerful tool for acquiring knowledge and expressing TCM knowledge in an understandable way. In 2003, Jiang *et al*. [28] used basic frequent itemset analysis and association rule mining to analyze 1355 formulae for the treatment of spleen-stomach diseases from *the section of Prescriptions*, *Dictionary of Traditional Chinese Medicine*. The results of KDTCM in ref. [28] are found to correspond basically with the rules and characteristics of the compatibility of spleen-stomach formulae in TCM. Another association mining on spleen-stomach formulae was carried out by Li *et al*. [29] using an effective algorithm based on a novel data structure named indexed frequent pattern tree. However, the number of formulae used in experiment was not reported in that literature. To provide a powerful assist for TCM experts and KDTCM participants, Li *et al*. [30] developed a CMF data mining system named TCMiner in 2004. Several efficient algorithms were implemented for frequent itemset/ association rule mining in TCMiner.

The largest frequent itemset analysis in TCM field was carried out by He *et al*. [31] in 2004. In this study, the DCMF database in TCM-Online Database System, which contains 85,989 formulae collected in thousands of years, was used as the data source to discover potential paired drugs. To improve performance, FP-growth algorithm was applied to find frequent herb co-occurrences in DCMF without candidate generation. Besides, an important preprocessing step was carried out, that is, to remove *Radix Glycyrrhizae* from each formula. This is because *Radix Glycyrrhizae* is frequently used in all kinds of formulae (it can decrease or moderate medicinal side-effects or toxicity and regulate actions of all other herbs in one formula).

This research is also noteworthy in that all of the generated paired drugs are compared with DPD. The results of discovered top-15 herb co-occurrences with highest frequency are presented in Table 1. The frequency and content of these herb co-occurrences are listed in leftmost and rightmost columns, respectively. The middle column indicates whether these discovered herb co-occurrences exist in DPD. Those records with the field "Yes" substantiate the existing paired drugs statistically. More significantly, as is shown in Table 1, many frequent herb co-occurrences that do not exist in DPD could also be revealed, such as *Radix Angelicae Sinensis* and *Rhizoma Atractylodis Macrocephalae*. Such combinations are highly likely to be paired drugs, which are worthy of further analysis and verification by TCM experts. Actually, the above process of knowledge discovery essentially simulates what TCM researchers did to generalize novel paired drugs in the past. The only distinction is that past discovery is based on human observations and experiences, while KDTCM participants utilize powerful computers and efficient algorithms instead to accomplish this task, which greatly quickens the disclosure of new paired drugs and promotes the development of compatibility rule research.

Table 1　Top-15 discovered herb co-occurrences with highest frequency

Frequency of herb co-occurrences	Exist in DPD	Discovered frequent herb co-occurrences
5127	Yes	*Radix Ginseng, Rhizoma Atractylodis Macrocephalae*
4428	Yes	*Radix Angelicae Sinensis, Radix Ginseng*
4062	Yes	*Radix Angelicae Sinensis, Rhizoma Chuanxiong*
3523	No	*Radix Angelicae Sinensis, Rhizoma Atractylodis Macrocephalae*
3049	Yes	*Radix Ginseng, Radix Astragali*
2853	No	*Radix Ginseng, Poria*
2760	No	*Radix Angelicae Sinensis, Radix Sapshnikoviae*
2688	Yes	*Rhizoma Atractylodis Macrocephalae, Poria*
2678	Yes	*Radix Sapshnikoviae, Rhizoma Notopterygii*
2596	Yes	*Radix Angelicae Sinensis, Radix Astragali*
2522	No	*Radix Ginseng, White Poria*
2321	Yes	*Rhizoma Atractylodis Macrocephalae, Pericarpium Citri Reticulatae*
2210	Yes	*Radix Angelicae Sinensis, Radix Paooniae Alba*
2142	No	*Radix Ginseng, Radix Sapshnikoviae*
2127	No	*Radix Sapshnikoviae, Rhizoma Chuanxiong*

With the deeper understanding of frequent itemsets and association rules in TCM background, researchers realize that it is not enough to discover patterns using conventional methods. Although itemsets with very high frequency always indicate significant discoveries in many disciplines, this is not the case in TCM formulae, just as the condition of *Radix Glycyrrhizae* mentioned above. To overcome this limitation, Zeng *et al*. [32] introduced a new support (maximum support) into association mining. Based on this new bi-support, as well as a bitmap matrix technique to improve efficiency, a new association mining algorithm named BM_DB_Apriori was proposed in ref. [32]. The experimental results on 1060 formulae show that BM_DB_Apriori is much faster and more accurate than the baseline algorithm Apriori.

Another improvement is the consideration of correlated patterns in TCM. In the basic approaches of frequent itemset/association mining, we aim to find itemset/rule with minimum support and confidence. However, for TCM formulae, the interesting itemsets/rules always have low support but high confidence. Besides, considering a paired drug A and B, if A and B frequently coexist in formulae, but the existence of A cannot increase the likelihood of the existence of B, it shows that B is very likely a general drug used to moderate side-effects or regulate actions of all other herbs in many kinds of formulae (e.g., *Radix Glycyrrhizae*). As far as drug compatibility research is concerned, this is not what we are interested. To remedy this situation, Zeng *et al*. [33] proposed a new method to discover bidirectional TCM association rules in 2005. Similar idea was presented and formalized by Zhou *et al*. [34] in 2006, and the concept of both associated and correlated pattern was presented in that paper. A new interesting measure corr-confidence was proposed for rationally evaluating the correlation relationships. This measure not only has proper bounds for effectively evaluating the correlation degree of patterns, but also is suitable for mining long patterns. The experimental results on 4643 TCM formulae data demonstrate that the mining considering both association and correlation is a valid approach to discovering both associated and correlated patterns in TCM formulae.

One interesting extension of frequent itemset mining in CMFs appeared in 2005 [35]. Considering that most CHMs are natural products, the knowledge of botanical taxonomy could be introduced to analyze CMFs. Based on frequent itemset mining of paired drugs, as well as the mapping relation between CHM and botanical family, Zhou *et al*. [35] performed experiments to discover family combination rules of CHM in formulae. Over 18,000 CMFs from TCMLARS were collected and five subtypes of these CMFs were chosen according to the efficacy such as promoting blood circulation for removing blood stasis, invigorating spleen and replenishing *qi*, etc. The discovery process was carried out for each subtype, and many family combination rules got revealed. For example, *Radix Astragali-Radix Angelicae Sinensis* is a typical CHM pair with the efficacy of invigorating spleen and replenishing *qi*, and *Umbelliferae-Legaminosae* builds the core of CMFs with this efficacy, because the support of *Umbelliferae-Legaminosae* combination in CMFs with this efficacy is as high as 180%. Compared to CHM combination rules, family combination rules give a higher level of knowledge about the drug combinations, which would be of help to clinical CMF prescription practice and new drug development.

Both frequent itemset and association rule mentioned above can be classified as linear rule model. To explore and present the pattern of combinatorial medicines in different perspectives, researchers began to introduce other models. Considering that undirected graphical models is suitable for discovering causal relationships and associations between variables, Deng *et al*. [36] proposed a structural learning algorithm named Information-Based Local Optimization (IBLO) to analyze CHMs in 554 formulae for apoplexy patients. These formulae were collected from books about historic prescriptions of Chinese medicine. A graph including 40 most important herbs in these formulae was obtained by IBLO algorithm, from which we can see which CHMs are frequently used together. This method is noteworthy for TCM in that it extends the pattern of combinatorial medicines research from linear rule model to graph model.

The studies mentioned above share a common feature, i.e., they generally analyze CMFs without the consideration of herb dosage. The reason behind it might be that in TCM literature, especially in historical literature, the dosage information of each herb in one formula is quite fuzzy. In some cases, the dosage is a range value (e.g., 20-30 g). In many other cases, the dosage information is even missing. New knowledge discovery approaches are needed to analyze formulae with such fuzzy dosage information in historical literature.

One way of formula research with dosage is to study the dispensing ratio of different CHMs within one formula. Suppose a combination pattern of multiple CHMs is found to have therapeutic effects for a certain condition, the next issue is to determine optimal dispensing ratio of these CHMs. This task can be performed with the help of knowledge discovery techniques. In 2003, Xiang [37] proposed a three-stage voting algorithm for mining optimal herb dispensing ratio in formulae. This method was applied to obtain optimal *Radix Salviae Miltiorrhizae-Radix Notoginseng* dispensing ratio in the formulae to treat cardiopathy based on an animal model (dogs). Ten test groups including seven ratio groups (10/6, 10/3, 10/1, 1/1, 10/0, 0/10, and 1/10) and three comparison groups (groups of Western medicine, model of compound, and pseudo-surgery) were used in the experiments. The latter was designed to test the cardio-index of all samples. After extracting features about the therapeutic effects from time series samples, the three-stage voting algorithm works as follows: the preliminary vote generates the features of each test group and cardio-index by each sample; the metaphase vote obtains the value of the therapeutic effect by each feature of the given group and index; the final vote mines the optimal dispensing ratio. An optimal dispensing ratio 10/6 was finally obtained in the experiment, showing the effectiveness of this method.

Confronted with the voluminous amount of TCM literature, historically accumulated and recently published, text mining is another group of knowledge discovery methods which can be used in KDTCM. Text mining is defined as the discovery of novel, previously unknown information, by automatically extracting information from different textual resources. For research of CMF, this technique was applied by KDTCM participants [35, 38, 39] to extract knowledge of herbs and formulae from TCM literature. Cao *et al*. [38] developed an ontology-based system for extracting knowledge of CHMs and CMFs from semi-structured text. In this work, ontologies of CHMs and CMFs were developed, consisting of a set of classes and their relations. In addition to offering a terminology for describing classes and their instances, the attributes of a class also play the role of knowledge place-holders for the class and its instances, and they are to be filled in during the knowledge extraction process. To perform knowledge acquisition, an executable knowledge extraction language (EKEL) was proposed to specify knowledge-extracting agents based on the guidelines of the frame-oriented ontologies, and a support machine was implemented to execute EKEL programs. The authors reported that the system successfully extracted knowledge of more than 2710 CHMs and 5900 CMFs. A limitation of this work lies in the requirement of semi-structured text as input. A more general method of text mining, based on the idea of bootstrapping, was utilized by Zhou and co-workers [39] in 2004. Given a small set of seed words and a large set of unlabeled data, this approach can automatically iterate to extract the objective patterns and new seeds from free texts. Based on this bootstrapping method, as well as other components (e.g., TCM literature DB, data mining module), the authors developed a text mining system called MeDisco/3T (Medical Discover for Traditional Treatment in Telligence) [35]. In practice, MeDisco/3T was used in the family combination rule experiment [35] mentioned above, and the boot-strapping method was used as an significant step to extract CMF names, CHM components and efficacy descriptions from TCMLARS with high precision.

3.2 Knowledge discovery for CHM research

Apart from CMF research, knowledge discovery techniques could also be used in CHM research. Existing work in this aspect can be further divided into two subfields: KDD for the research of CHM characteristics and KDD for the research of CHM chemical compositions.

1) KDD for the research of CHM characteristics

As one of the core contents in TCM knowledge system, the completeness of theory of CHM characteristics largely determines the accuracy and scientificity of forming a CMF, and also the effectiveness and safety of this therapy. The therapeutic effects and side-effect/toxicity of drugs are often two sides of the same coin. The toxicity of drugs must be thoroughly understood in order to ensure safety, not only for orthodox medicine, but also for complementary and alternative medicine. Chen and Giu [40] applied computer-based statistical analysis to study the relevant factors of toxicity for 3906 kinds of common used CHM. Besides toxicity, seven other aspects of CHM data were collected, including nature and flavor, meridian tropism, processing method, botanical family, chemical compositions, medicinal part, and pharmacological effects. The relations between these factors and CHM toxicity were analyzed by statistical analysis, yielding some meaningful results. Among 1119 CHMs with toxicity information recorded in literature, only 3.3% is found to have high toxicity, providing an evidence for the safety of most CHMs. However, 59.7% of the CHMs with hot nature exhibit toxicity in varying degrees, showing that CHM toxicity is somehow related to the hot nature. It is also found that the botanical family of CHM is closely related to its toxicity. Among 108 kinds of CHMs belonging to *Ranunculaceae*, the proportion of CHMs with toxicity in varying degrees reaches as high as 42.6%. Moreover, 29.7% of *Ranunculaceae* CHMs exhibits high toxicity. Other families of CHMs with relatively large proportions of toxic ones include *Araceae* (14.2%) and *Euphorbiaceae* (11.3%). As for the factor of chemical compositions, alkaloid is noteworthy in that 71.8% of CHMs with alkaloid ingredients exhibit toxicity. This number is by far largest compared with other groups of chemical compositions in CHMs.

Another statistical analysis about CHM characteristics was performed by Yang [41] in 2005. In the study, 417 CHMs were collected from *Chinese Pharmacopeia*, from which 101 blood pressure-reducing CHMs were further selected. A comparison was made between these two groups of CHMs (101 group and 417 group) in aspects of four natures, five flavors and meridian tropism. The results show that most blood pressure-reducing CHMs are characterized by pungent nature and bitter flavor, mainly acting on liver and gallbladder meridians. Such knowledge is beneficial to the discovery of effective phytochemical components and the research of pharmacological properties.

The relation between CHM efficacy and other characteristics is a hot topic in CHM research. The usage of knowledge discovery approaches can partly help this research. Yao *et al*. [42] applied artificial neural network (ANN) and decision tree to classify 54 deficiency-nourishing CHMs into four groups (four subtypes of deficiency-nourishing efficacy) in 2004. Two quantification methods of CHM characteristics were used in the experiments, including two-valued quantification and multi-valued quantification. The classification results of KDD methods were compared with the records in TCM teaching materials as the evaluation. It is found that the classification accuracies of ANN equals decision tree (98. 11%) for multi-valued quantification, but ANN (96. 13%) outperforms decision tree (87. 10%) for two-valued quantification. The results show that different quantification methods of CHM characteristics have certain influence on the prediction of efficacy, and ANN outperforms decision tree in this task. However, the sample size in this experiment seems too small.

Besides statistical analysis and classification, clustering is another type of KDD approaches used in researches of CHM characteristics. Based on characteristics features, Zhou *et al*. [43] applied clustering to group 28 CHMs for relieving exterior syndrome in 2004. By this clustering method, the authors obtained quite a few identical results to the CHM theory. Although the sample size was also small (28 CHMs), the methodology is still worth recognition. Another larger scale of clustering was carried out by He *et al*. [44] in 2004. In this KDTCM study, TCDBASE in the TCM-Online Database System was used the data source, which contains information of more than 11, 000 CHMs. Different from the former experiment, this was an efficacy-based clustering, and the similarity of values in attribute *efficacy* was used to evaluate the closeness between CHMs. The clustering algorithm applied in the experiment was agglomerative approach, also known as the bottom-up approach. As a hierarchical clustering method, this algorithm starts with each object forming a separate group. It successively merges the objects or groups close to one another into larger and larger clusters, until certain termination conditions. By this clustering, the large number of CHMs in TCDBASE was clustered into different groups based on efficacy. Such kind of categorization is highly important for the research of CHM characteristics and the analysis of effective chemical components in CHM, because similar efficacies of different CHMs often indicate high closeness of characteristics, as well as the chemical ingredients contained. Furthermore, these clustering results can serve as valuable references for selection of substitute drug in formula-forming and design of novel CMFs.

2) KDD for the research of CHM chemical compositions

The substances that exhibit therapeutic effects are the chemical compositions of CHM. However, because the medicinal powers of CHM come from the cooperative effects of multiple active ingredients, the conventional research methodology that targets at only single ingredient is not enough. One probing method for this problem is to analyze CHM by knowledge discovery techniques at the level of chemical element. In 1998, Qi *et al*. [45] applied factor analysis and clustering to study the relationships between CHM characteristics and the contents of trace elements in CHM. 42 kinds of trace elements in 105 CHMs were determined and factor analysis was carried out. The results indicate that a 10-factor model can interpret the correlation of these trace elements. Besides, the information of trace elements was used in a hierarchy clustering to classify 105 CHMs into different nature groups. Compared with traditional knowledge of CHM nature, the trace-element-based clustering achieved the accuracy of 78. 1% , showing that trace elements are related to the nature of CHMs to a certain degree. A following study of trace elements was conducted by Qi *et al*. [46] in 2003. This time the information of trace elements was also used in a hierarchy clustering, but aiming at classifying 10 CHMs for treating exterior syndromes into different efficacy groups. The accuracy of classification in the experiment is 90% , partly revealing the correlation between efficacy and the amount of trace elements in CHMs.

The modern technique of fingerprint enables us to takes thousands of chemical compositions into account simultaneously, thus providing huge data resources for knowledge discovery. Due to its specificity, integrity, stability and quantifiability, the fingerprint method has been successfully used in identification and quality evaluation of traditional Chinese medicinal materials. This is an application where knowledge discovery approaches can contribute a lot. Typical data mining methods used in this field include primary component analysis (PCA), ANN, fuzzy clustering, etc. [47]. The main drawback of these methods is that extracted features are needed from original information to form the feature space. For fingerprint data, the dimensions of the feature space are up to 1000 after discretization, and the sample set is usually small. ANN is easy to suffer from overfitting on such small train set, while PCA method is more dependent on the statistical information after discretization. To solve this problem, a novel method based on nearest neighbor (NN) and genetic algorithm was presented by Zhang *et al*. [48] in 2004. A new measure, named corresponding-peak distance, was proposed to calculate the distance between samples directly for NN classifier, and genetic algorithm was used to optimize the parameters of NN classifier. Experiments on HPLC data of *Radix Ginseng* indicate that this hybrid method can effectively identify the medicine material of different harvest time or habitats.

Another KDTCM study with regard to CHM chemical compositions was conducted by Lu *et al*. [49] in 2005. TCM chemical database [20] was used as the data source in this study, and association rule mining was carried out to analyze the relations between CHM efficacy, botanical family, bioactivity of chemical compositions, and pharmacology of CHM extracts. Some meaningful rules were obtained in the experiments. For example, a bidirectional association rule was found between M-cholinoceptor blocking drug and *Solanaceae*. This rule indicates a large proportion of plants in *Solanaceae* (21.37%) contain ingredients with M-cholinoceptor blocking activity, and meanwhile, a large proportion of M-cholinoceptor blocking drugs (15.69%) can be found from plants in *Solanaceae*. Another interesting rule was found between *Ranunculaceae* and anti-hypertension drug. Such kind of rules found by knowledge discovery techniques is valuable for drug discovery process.

3.3 Knowledge discovery for research of TCM syndrome

Syndrome (*zheng*) is one of the core issues in TCM; it is a holistic clinical disease concept reflecting the dynamic, functional, temporal and spatial morbid status of human body. Considering the systematic knowledge accumulated from thousands of years' TCM clinical practice, which is valuable hypothesis for modern biomedicine research, it is of great importance to deepen the study of TCM syndrome. One idea of syndrome research in this post-genomic era is to study syndrome at molecular level. As an effective avenue to combine Western medicine and TCM, knowledge discovery could be undertaken based on the integration of literature and clinical data in both fields.

In a probing research connecting TCM with modern biomedicine, Wu *et al*. [39] proposed a text mining approach to identifying the gene functional relationships from MEDLINE based on TCM knowledge stored in TCM literature. The TCM literature used in this study comes from TCMLARS, which contains more than 600,000 articles from 900 biomedical journals published in China since 1984. There materials were treated by a simple but efficient bootstrapping method to extract syndrome-disease relationships. Besides, the term co-occurrence was used to identify the relationships between disease and gene from MEDLINE. Then the authors got the syndrome-gene relationships by one-step inference, i. e. , to compute the genes and syndromes with the same relevant disease. The underlying hypothesis behind this research was that the relevant genes of the same syndrome would have some biological interactions.

The relationship of *kidney YangXu* syndrome and related genes was taken as an example by the authors because *kidney YangXu* syndrome is an important syndrome involving caducity, neural disease and immunity etc. Moreover, through an experimental study of *kidney YangXu* syndrome at molecular level, Shen [50] found that *kidney YangXu* syndrome was associated with the expression of CRF (C1q-related factor). This laboratory-confirmed relationship, as well as other novel syndrome-gene relationships, was found revealable by the text mining method in ref. [39].

The authors compiled about 2. 5 million disease relevant PubMed citations and 1,479,630 human gene relevant PubMed citations in local database drawn from online MEDLINE. Meanwhile, about 1100 syndrome-disease relationships were obtained from TCM literatures published in 2002. Considering the bi-lingual issues, before searching MEDLINE, Chinese disease names were translated partially automatically to formal English disease names according to the TCM headings database, and manual check by TCM terminological expert was conducted when no TCM headings of disease existed. Filtering by total co-occurrence is above 10 or the number of relevant diseases is above 2, 72 genes related to *kidney YangXu* syndrome were discovered, in which CRH (corticotropin releasing hormone) was included. By querying gene databases, it was found that CRF was an alias name of CRH. Thus, it means the relation ship between *kidney YangXu* syndrome and CRF had already been discovered by the method. Furthermore, suppose the alias relation between CRF and CRH was not known, the authors showed that it was also capable to confirm the relationship between CRF and *kidney YangXu* syndrome by the next several steps. First, some important genes in *kidney YangXu* syndrome were selected, including CRP (C-reactive protein, pentraxin-related), CRH, IL10 (interleukin 10), ACE (angiotensin I converting enzyme), PTH (parathyroid hormone), and MPO (myeloperoxidase). Second, the PubGene [51] was searched for subset network using each of the above genes, and the corresponding subset networks were shown as Figure 1. The third step was analyzing the extracted knowledge. Now suppose that we do not know CRF is a relevant gene of *kidney YangXu* syndrome. By analyzing the six subset networks in the left part and the CRF subset network of Figure 1, we may conclude that CRF is somewhat relevant to *kidney YangXu* syndrome, because the subset networks, which reassembled with the gene nodes such as IL10, CRAT, CRF/CRH/ACE/MPO/PTH, etc. , constitute possible functional gene communities that contribute to *kidney YangXu* syndrome. No existing literature reporting the relationship between CRF and *kidney YangXu* syndrome was used to generate the novel knowledge. It is exciting that this simple demonstration has shown the primary text mining results will largely decrease the labor in molecular level syndrome research.

This work proposes a tool for the TCM researchers to rapidly narrow their search for new and interesting genes of a specific syndrome. Meanwhile, the work gives specific functional information to the literature networks and divides large literature networks to functional communities (e. g. , the community containing IL10, CRAT, CRH/CRF, etc. , genes for *kidney YangXu* syndrome), which cannot be identified in the current PubGene. Moreover, through syndrome perspective, the study gives an approach to having a subset selection or explanation of giant literature based gene network. The results demonstrate that syndrome can give a novel top-down view of functional genomics research, and it could be a promising research field while connecting TCM with modern life science using text mining and other knowledge discovery methods.

3.4 Knowledge discovery for TCM clinical diagnosis

Diagnosis is of crucial importance in any medical or healing system that works on the body. Unlike Western medicine, diagnostic methods in traditional Chinese medicine include four basic methods (called *si zhen* in Chinese): inspection, listening and smelling, inquiry, and palpation. The case history, symptoms, and signs gained through those four diagnostic methods are analyzed and generalized to find the causes, nature, and interrelations of the disease, and to provide evidence for further differentiation of syndromes. Although used in clinical practice for thousands of years, these diagnostic methods seem subjective and unreliable at present time. Thus, researchers begin to apply modern techniques to improve the objectivity of these methods. Knowledge discovery is one of the techniques that could contribute greatly in this process.

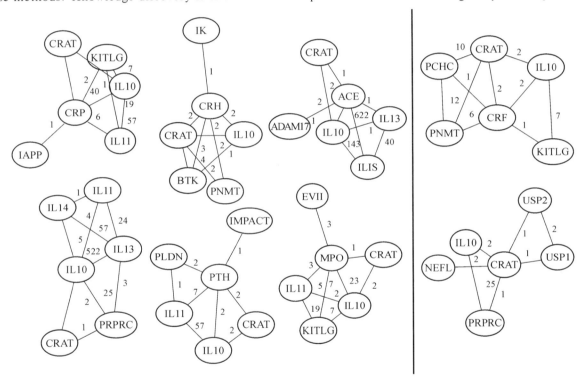

Figure 1   The six subset networks of each selected genes (left part of the vertical line). Gene CRAT, which in all of the six subset networks, may be a novel relevant gene of *kidney YangXu* syndrome. The right part gives the subset network of the already known relevant gene CRF, and the subset network of CRAT.

Among the diagnostic methods mentioned above, the examination of tongue is one of the most important approaches for getting significant evidences in diagnosing the patient's health conditions. However, the clinical competence of tongue diagnosis was largely determined by the experience and knowledge of the physicians adopting the tongue diagnosis, and was easily influenced by environmental factors. Therefore, it is necessary to build an objective diagnostic standard for tongue diagnosis. In the last decades, researchers have been developing various methods and computer-based systems to solve this problem. A recent review of studies in pattern recognition of tongue image was undertaken by Yue and Liu [52] in 2004. By analyzing these researches, we can find many cases where image-based knowledge discovery methods got used. A typical study involving knowledge discovery approaches was conducted by Pang *et al*. [53] in 2004. In this work, two kinds of quantitative features, chromatic and textural measures, were extracted from tongue images by digital image processing techniques, and Bayesian networks were employed subsequently to model the relationship between these quantitative features and diseases. Experiments on a group of 455 in-patients affected by 13 common diseases, as well as other 70 healthy volunteers, show that the diagnosis accuracy based on the previously trained Bayesian networks is up to 75.8%. In another study in 2005, Ying *et al*. [54] proposed eight characteristic quantity variables of tongue manifestations, including color, shape, wetness-dryness, etc. These features were treated by k-means clustering and ANN to predict the diagnostic result. An experiment was performed on 49 patients with cerebrovascular diseases and 39 health people, and the classification accuracies for k-means clustering and ANN based on the newly presented eight characteristics reach 87.5% and 92%, respectively.

Besides the diagnostic information obtained through tongue diagnosis, other measures, including all kinds of symptoms and signs, are also considered as potential important features in TCM diagnosis. Unlike Western medicine in which intervenes are performed only after crisis arises, TCM is characterized by diagnosing diseases at earlier stages and subsequently preventing greater problems from occurring by adjusting the imbalance in the body in time. Therefore, symptoms that are not characteristic features for certain diseases in biomedicine background are also used in TCM diagnosis in many cases. The rationality of this diagnostic idea is partly supported by a recent study conducted by Lu et al. [55] in 2005. In this work, correlation between CD4, CD8 cell infiltration in gastric mucosa, *Helicobacter pylori* infection and symptoms in 62 patients with chronic gastritis, were analyzed by logistic regression analysis and k-means clustering. The results indicate that an assemblage of eight non-digestive related symptoms (such as heavy feeling in head or body, thirst, cool limbs with aversion to cold, etc.) could increase the predicted percentage of CD4 and CD8 cell infiltration in gastric mucosa, including lower CD4 infiltration by 12.5%, higher CD8 infiltration by 33.3%, and also *non-H. pylori* infection by 23.6%. This study also demonstrates that the subjective symptoms could play an important role in the diagnosis and treatment of diseases.

Apart from the studies of subjective symptoms in TCM diagnosis, some novel objective parameters for syndrome differentiation were also proposed by researches, and usually these new parameters were further treated by knowledge discovery methods to establish the diagnoses. In a study conducted by Deng *et al*. [56] in 1996, the contents of 14 trace elements in hair of 163 cases of rheumatoid arthritis were used as the objective parameters in syndrome differentiation. Dynamic clustering was carried out based on these indexes, and the diagnostic results were compared with clinical diagnoses. Great consistency in this comparison was observed in the experiment, and the accuracy of clustering-based method reached as high as 95.70%.

The studies above show the power of subjective symptoms and objective parameters in TCM diagnosis. However, this does not mean that all subjective symptoms and objective parameters should always be taken into account simultaneously. A recent study undertaken by Li *et al*. [57] in 2005 showed that the selection of symptoms can influence the accuracy of diagnosis in 209 patients with *H. pylori* infection. 35 clinical presentations were observed in the experiment, including digestive symptoms (such as appetite, stomachache, nausea, etc.), general status (such as complexion, stool, etc.), spirit and psychological status (such as sleep, emotion, etc.), and pathogenic factors (such as smoking, alcohol, etc.). These parameters were analyzed by statistical methods and k-means clustering. In the experiment, the diagnostic accuracy based on 35 clinical presentations was 65.7%. It could be improved by 5.7% when only the assemblage of digestive symptoms was engaged, or by 8.6% when the pathogenic factors, general status and tongue observation were combined. The diagnostic accuracy could be decreased when only the general symptoms were engaged, or when the pathogenic factors were accompanied with some common digestive symptoms. We can conclude from this study that it should be cautious on the selection of symptoms in diagnosis.

Researches in the last decades showed that knowledge discovery methods combined with clinical experiments could greatly help to determine this selection. Existing KDD methods used in this task include factor analysis [58], clustering [58], rough set [59], Bayesian networks [60], latent class analysis [61], etc. In an original research conducted by Zhang *et al*. [58] in 2005, the methods of factor analysis and clustering were combined in the diagnosis of TCM syndromes in 310 patients with posthepatitic cirrhosis. The information of conventional four diagnoses was collected by the method of clinical epidemiological research, and these features were reduced and grouped by factor analysis. Based on these obtained common factors, clustering was carried out subsequently to form different groups of syndromes. The results indicate that the TCM syndromes in 287 of the 310 patients (92.58%) could be classified, and the 287 cases could be divided into seven categories of syndromes, showing the effectiveness of combing factor analysis and clustering. Rough set is another effective knowledge discovery method for attribute reduction, thus suitable for the selection of symptoms in TCM diagnosis. In 2001, Qin *et al*. [59] applied rough set in the diagnosis of rheumatoid arthritis. The results show that the diagnostic accuracy of rough set for rheumatoid arthritis is greatly higher than that of fuzzy set. Because of its powerful capacity of handling uncertainty, Bayesian network has become an attractive tool able to model the dependence and independence relationships among the variables in the domain with network. In a self-learning expert system constructed for TCM diagnosis in 2004, a novel hybrid learning algorithm GBPS* based on Bayesian networks was proposed by Wang *et al*. [60]. This efficient algorithm was applied to discover the dependence and independence relationships among symptoms and essential symptoms (named *key-elements*), and the results were represented by directed acyclic graphs. This explicit representation of Bayesian networks helps to gain an insight into TCM knowledge and explain the diagnosis and treatment of TCM experts. Besides Bayesian networks, this expert system also included other modules to extract knowledge from clinical data automatically, such as the module for mining frequent sets of key-elements. This data-driven nature made this system distinguishing from the rule-based expert systems developed previously.

Another interesting knowledge discovery study in TCM diagnosis was conducted by Zhang and Yuan [61] in 2006. Unlike other researches which focused on the selection of distinguishing symptoms, Zhang aimed at discovering the latent variables hidden in the TCM diagnosis. Considering that latent variable detection might lead to scientific discovery [62], Zhang proposed hierarchical latent class (HLC) models [63] to discover latent structures, and applied HLC models to discover the latent variables in TCM diagnosis of kidney deficiency syndromes [61]. In this study, 2600 cases of the elderly older than 60 years were investigated to collect 67 symptoms related to kidney deficiency syndromes. The HLC model was subsequently learned by a search-based algorithm proposed in ref. [64]. The resultant model was found to match the relevant TCM theories well, and diagnosis based on the model produced conclusions consistent with those by a group of experts. This indicates that latent structure models can help greatly in building an objective statistical foundation for TCM diagnosis.

4　Discussion and future directions

The previous sections aim at presenting a whole picture of state of the art of KDTCM researches. In this picture, a number of future research directions in KDTCM need to be highlighted. In this section, a discussion of these previous KDTCM studies is given, as well as a summary of the future directions in KDTCM.

Due to the preference and more understanding of combinatorial medicines, TCM community provides a large number of real-world cases using multiple drugs as the form of CMF over thousands of years. With the digitalization of these data and the development of computer science, it is very natural for the researches to introduce knowledge discovery techniques, especially the methods based on frequent itemset analysis and association rule mining, to discover compatibility rules of medicines in CMF data. These KDTCM researches are inspiring, with plenty of room for improvement. The extension from conventional methods to correlated pattern mining and graph model learning adapts to the features of CMF analysis better, however, most of these studies still stay at the level of analyzing formulae without the consideration of CHM dosage. The researches of optimal dispensing ratio for CHMs are noteworthy, but new knowledge discovery approaches are still needed to analyze formulae with the fuzzy dosage information in historical literature. Moreover, through experiments combined with knowledge discovery methods, the action target of different drugs in a formula could also be analyzed by observing how the dosage change of some drug could influence the curability of related syndrome and symptoms.

Besides dosage, current KDTCM researches in CMF also suffer from the exclusion of some other important attributes of CMF, such as efficacy and indication. As a complex drug system, a CMF involves a large number of effective ingredients, which cooperate with each other and contribute to the final holistic therapeutic effects. Meanwhile, there are complicated relations among ingredients, efficacy, indication, and other elements within this system. A variety of important relationships between these attributes in CMF, such as the correlation between ingredients and indication, between efficacy and indication, and between ingredients and adverse reactions, are still waiting to be disclosed with the aid of knowledge discovery methods.

As for the research of CHM characteristics, the relations between medicinal effects and toxicity, as well as the connections among four natures, five flavors, meridian tropism, botanical family and other elements, are of vast importance to TCM community. Existing KDTCM studies demonstrate that it is very helpful to apply knowledge discovery approaches in this subfield. For example, the strong connections between some botanical families and their toxicities (e. g., *Ranunculaceae*) discovered by knowledge discovery methods [40] are highly beneficial to toxicological research. Processing is the preparation of crude medicinal materials according to TCM theory, which mainly serves as the functions of reducing side effect/toxicity, and promoting therapeutic effects. Currently, there are few KDTCM researches conducted with regard to

167

processing methods. We believe that the future KDTCM studies in processing methods could help us to gain an insight into the traditional wisdom of TCM in treatment of herb toxicity.

Compared with other subfields, KDTCM studies in chemical compositions of CHM is a bit preliminary. The analysis of trace elements by knowledge discovery methods seems interesting, but is by far not enough. Due to its specificity, integrity, stability and quantifiability, the fingerprint technique has been successfully used in identification and quality evaluation of traditional Chinese medicinal materials, in which various knowledge discovery approaches are used to construct the classifies. However, it is worth noting that fingerprint technique also lays the foundation for data mining of spectra-effect relationship. Through analyzing the relativity of the variables generated by fingerprint and the ones related to CHM characteristics and effects, it is promising to aid the discovery of active ingredients in CHM with known and unknown pharmacological actions. To derive new chemical drugs from CHM, the main approach is to extract potential effective ingredients from Chinese herbs as lead compounds, and then design new chemical drugs by structural modification on the basis of these lead compounds. However, during the discovery of lead compounds from natural products, the conventional random screening method suffers from low efficiency. For CHM, the ingredients with similar efficacy always have resemblance in active group. Thus, by QSAR analysis and related methods, knowledge discovery techniques could be utilized to seek promising active groups with regard to some therapeutic effect, which are beneficial to directional screening. However, there are few KDTCM researches currently in this aspect. With the increasing availability of high quality 3D chemical structure data-bases and the development of KDTCM techniques, we believe that knowledge discovery will contribute greatly to the drug discovery in CHM.

Although the number of KDTCM studies in syndrome research is relatively small, it is very encouraging to see some studies connecting TCM with modern biomedicine in this subfield. In spite of the differences on methodology and technology, modern biomedicine and TCM share the same research subject, i. e., the diseases phenomena of human body. Thus, there are a lot of connections between biomedicine and TCM. For instance, on the one hand, the syndrome research could be carried out at molecular level. On the other hand, the syndrome could give a novel top-down view of functional genomics research, which is particularly required in this post-genomic era. It is proved that text mining could contribute greatly in this multidisciplinary research. Based on the integration of literature in both Western medicine and TCM, the syndrome-gene relationships, including some laboratory-confirmed relationships (e. g., CRF—*kidney YangXu* syndrome), are found discoverable by text mining. Moreover, through syndrome perspective, current KDTCM study gives an approach to having a subset selection or explanation of giant literature based gene network. As protein-protein interactions are central to most biological processes, the systematic identification of all protein interactions is considered as a key strategy for uncovering the inner workings of a cell. Thus, one aspect of future KDTCM work could focus on studying the protein-protein interactions using the knowledge of TCM syndrome.

In spite of the interesting KDTCM work above in functional genomics research, it should also be noticed that for TCM itself, currently the standard of classification hierarchy for specific syndromes and even the definitions for some syndromes have not reached consensus yet. Thus, the standardization and in-depth study of specific syndrome has become an urgent demand for development and research of TCM. This problem can also be partly solved by knowledge discovery approaches. For instance, information extraction could be carried out on the vast amount of TCM literature, which helps to discover the most frequently used terms to describe syndromes in practice. All variety of classification and clustering methods could be applied on syndrome data, which could provide useful guidance on how to form a classification hierarchy for syndrome. More KDTCM researches in the study of syndrome standardization can be expected in the future.

Apart from the above KDTCM directions mainly with regard to basic medical research, knowledge discovery techniques could also contribute to clinical TCM research. In practice, various kinds of data mining methods have already been used in TCM clinical diagnosis, including factor analysis, clustering, ANN, rough set, Bayesian networks, latent class analysis, etc. Among these methods, Bayesian networks have several advantages. The main reasons are as follows. First, a Bayesian network can be used to learn causal relationships, and hence can be used to gain understanding about a problem domain and to predict the consequences of intervention, which is particularly suitable for analyzing the complicated features obtained by TCM diagnostic methods. Second, prior knowledge in TCM can be easily represented in Bayesian networks. Third, it is found [65] that diagnostic performance with Bayesian networks is often surprisingly insensitive to imprecision in the numerical probabilities. As an extension of conventional Bayesian networks, HLC model can serve as a better tool to discover latent structures behind diagnostic observations in TCM. As is reported in ref. [61], currently the problem of HLC model lies in the performance, which is only capable to deal with 35 variables in 67 candidates. In the future, this bottleneck can be expected to be removed with the development of related algorithms.

Another aspect of clinical research in TCM is the clinical evaluation. So far there are hardly any knowledge discovery studies undertaken in this subfield. The reason probably lies in the unavailability of high-quality TCM clinical data sources in the past. However, the situation has been improving in recent years. The establishments of related real-world clinical databases, such as the TCM-EMRD mentioned in section 2, will be of great help to promote the usage of knowledge discovery in TCM clinical evaluation in the future.

5 Conclusion

With a history that spans thousands of years, TCM provides Chinese people with effective health undertakings. As a medical system based on holistic idea, which is totally different from orthodox medicine, TCM is a field worthy of in-depth analysis and research. What KDD is good at is searching the huge volume of data for meaningful patterns and knowledge, which is otherwise an almost impossible task to accomplish manually. Thus, KDD is a necessary technology to be applied in analyzing the great amounts of data in TCM. Based on an introduction to the current state of TCM data resources, this paper provides an overview of knowledge discovery research in TCM in recent years. Major studies in four subfields of KDTCM are reviewed, including KDD for CMF research, KDD for CHM research, KDD for TCM syndrome research, and KDD for TCM clinical diagnosis. The methods used in these studies are introduced, and some interesting results are highlighted. Finally, in a discussion section based on existing KDTCM studies, the current state and main problems of KDTCM work in each subfield are summarized, and the future directions for each subfield are also presented.

The journey of KDTCM in recent years is inspiring, resulting with considerable meaningful discoveries (such as the laboratory-confirmed relationship between CRF gene and *kidney YangXu* syndrome, the high proportion of toxic plants in *Ranunculaceae*, the association between M-cholinoceptor blocking drug and *Solanaceae*, etc.). However, it should be noticed that the KDTCM achievement currently is preliminary. For knowledge discovery, the TCM field is still nearly a piece of virgin soil with copious amounts of hidden gold. Here, the questions arise: where is the gold, what kind of gold is hidden, and how we can mine for the gold? This paper aims at answering these questions based on a review and analysis of existing KDTCM researches, as well as a discussion of future directions. As is indicated by Roddick *et al.* [11], mining over medical, health or clinical data is arguably the most difficult domain for the KDD field. As a huge non-linear complicated system, human body always involves a large amount of mutual influence and dynamic balance among complex factors, which makes it extremely difficult to fully unravel the inner mystery of life phenomenon. The advantage of TCM lies largely in the holistic thinking pattern and its preference for multiple-component therapy based on natural products. However, this also increases the complexity for KDTCM. Besides, currently the data of TCM still suffer from high individuality, ambiguity and incompleteness. All these bring new problems and challenges when traditional KDD methods are applied to TCM field. These problems are partly solved by the studies reviewed in this paper. However, much more work needs to be done. Considering the ever-increasing volume of TCM data and the pressing demand to extract knowledge from these resources, we believe that the usage and development of KDTCM in the future will substantially contribute to the TCM community, as well as modern life science.

Acknowledgements

We gratefully acknowledge all the researchers from the Institute of Information on Traditional Chinese Medicine, China Academy of Traditional Chinese Medicine for the TCM databases and discussion of TCM topics. This research is partly supported by National Basic Research Priorities Programme of China Ministry of Science and Technology (No. 2005DKA32400), subprogram of China 973 project (No. 2003CB317006), National Science Fund for Distinguished Young Scholars of China NSF program (No. NSFC60533040), and also a grant from Program for New Century Excellent Talents in University of Ministry of Education of China (No. NCET-04-0545).

References

[1] Aderem A. Systems biology: its practice and challenges. Cell 2005,121(4):511-513.

[2] Eisenberg DM, Kessler RC, Foster C, Norlock FE, Calkins DR, Delbanco TL. Unconventional medicine in the United States: prevalence, costs, and patterns of use. New Engl J Med 1993,328(4):246-242.

[3] Eisenberg DM, Davis RB, Ettner SL, Appel S, Wilkey S, Van Rompay M, *et al*. Trends in alternative medicine use in the United States 1097: results of a follow-up national survey. J Am Med Assoc 1998,280(18):1569-1575.

[4] Honda K, Jacobson JS. Use of complementary and alternative medicine among United States adults: the influences of personality, coping strategies, and social support. Preventive Med 2005,40(1):46-53.

[5] Thomas KJ, Nicholl JP, Coleman P. Use and expenditure on complementary medicine in England: a population based survey. Comp Ther Med 2001,9:2-11.

[6] Yamashita H, Tsukayama H, Sugishita C. Popularity of complementary and alternative medicine in Japan: a telephone survey. Comp Ther Med 2002,10:84-93.

[7] Fayyad U, Piatetsky-Shapiro G, Smyth P. From data mining to knowledge discovery in databases. AI Mag 1996,17

(3):37-54.

[8] Han J, Kamber M. Data mining: concepts and techniques San Fransisco, CA: Morgan Kaufmann Publishers, 2000.

[9] Bath PA. Data mining in health and medical information. Annu Rev Inform Sci Technol 2004,38(1):331-369.

[10] Altman RB. AI in medicine: the spectrum of challenges from managed care to molecular medicine. AI Mag 1999, 20(3):67-77.

[11] Roddick JF, Fule P, Graco WJ. Exploratory medical knowledge discovery: experiences and issues. SIGKDD Explor 2003,5(1):94-99.

[12] Cios KJ, Moore GW. Uniqueness of medical data mining. Artif Intell Med 2002,26(1-2):1-24.

[13] Zupan B, Lavrac N, Keravnou E. Data mining techniques and applications in medicine. Artif Intell Med 1999, 16 (1):1-2.

[14] Lavrac N. Selected techniques for data mining in medicine. Artif Intell Med 1999,16(1):3-23.

[15] Cios KJ, editor. Medical data mining and knowledge discovery. Heidelberg: Springer-Verlag, 2000.

[16] Kononenko I. Machine learning for medical diagnosis: history, state of the art and perspective. Artif Intell Med 2001,23(1):89-109.

[17] Fan KW. Online research databases and journals of Chinese medicine. J Altern Complement Med 2004,10(6): 1123-1128.

[18] Liu Y, Sun Y. China traditional Chinese medicine (TCM) patent database. World Patent Information 2004,26:91-96.

[19] http://www.tradimed.com (Accessed: 17 May 2006).

[20] Zhou JJ, Xie GG, Yan XJ. Traditional Chinese medicines: molecular structures natural sources and applications Burlington, VT: ASHGATE, 2003.

[21] http://www.cintcm.com (Accessed: 17 May 2006).

[22] Zhou XZ, Wu ZH, Lu W. TCMMDB: a distributed multi-database query system and its key technique implementation. In: Proceedings of IEEE SMC 2001, IEEE computer society, 2001:1095-1100.

[23] Chen HJ, Wu ZH, Huang C, Xu JF. TCM-Grid: weaving a medical grid for traditional Chinese medicine. In: Goos G, Hartmanis J, van Leuwen J, editors. Proceedings of international conference on computational science 2003, lecture notes in computer science 2659. Berlin: Springer-Verlag, 2003:1143-1152.

[24] Zhou XZ, Wu ZH, Yin AN, Wu LC, Fan WY, Zhang RE. Ontology development for unified traditional Chinese medical language system. Artif Intell Med 2004,32(1):15-27.

[25] Fan WY. The traditional Chinese medical literature analysis and retrieval system (TCMLARS) and its application. Int J Spec Libr 2001,35(3):147-156.

[26] McCulloch M, Broffman M, Gao JM. Chinese herbal medicine and interferon in the treatment of chronic hepatitis B: a meta-analysis of randomized, controlled trials. Am J Public Health 2002,92(10):1619-1627.

[27] Yao MC, Ai L, Yuan YM, Qiao YJ. Analysis of the association rule in the composition of the TCM formulas for diabetes. J Beijing Univ Tradit Chin Med 2002,25(6):48-50 (in Chinese).

[28] Jiang YG, Li RS, Li L, Li HQ, Chen B. Experiment on data mining in compatibility law of spleen-stomach prescriptions in TCM. World Sci Technol-Modern Tradit Chin Med Mater Med 2003,5(2):33-37(in Chinese).

[29] Li C, Tang CJ, Peng J, Hu JJ. NNF: an effective approach in medicine paring analysis of traditional Chinese medicine prescriptions. In: Zhou LZ, Ooi BC, Meng XF, editors. Proceedings of DASFAA 2005, lecture notes in computer science 3453. Berlin: Springer-Verlag, 2005:576-581.

[30] Li C, Tang CJ, Peng J, Hu JJ, Zeng LM, Yin XX, et al. TCMiner: a high performance data mining system for multi-dimensional data analysis of traditional Chinese medicine prescriptions. In: Wang S, Yang DQ, Tanaka K,

Grandi F, Zhou SG, Mangina EE, *et al*., editors. Proceedings of ER workshops 2004, lecture notes in computer science 3289. Berlin: Springer-Verlag, 2004:246-247.

[31] He QF, Cui M, Wu ZH, Zhou XZ, Zhou ZM. Compatibility knowledge discovery in Chinese medical formulae. Chin J Inf Tradit Chin Med 2004,11(7):655-658(in Chinese).

[32] Zeng LM, Tang CJ, Yin XX, Jiang YG, Liu J, Liao Y. Mining compatibility of traditional Chinese medicine based on bit- map matrix and bi-support. J Sichuan Univ (Nat Sci Ed) 2005,42(1):57-62(in Chinese).

[33] Zeng LM, Tang CJ, Yin XX, Li C, Hu JJ, Jiang YG. Analysis of correlation based on bidirectional association rules. Comput Eng Des 2005,26(10):2585-2588 (in Chinese).

[34] Zhou ZM, Wu ZH, Wang CS, Feng Y. Mining both associated and correlated patterns. In: Alexandrov VN, van Albada GD, Sloot PM, Dongarra J, editors. Proceedings of ICCS 2006, lecture notes in computer science 3994. Berlin: Springer-Verlag, 2006:468-475.

[35] Zhou XZ, Liu BY, Wu ZH. Text mining for clinical Chinese herbal medical knowledge discovery. In: Hoffmann AG, Motoda H, Scheffer T, editors. Proceedings of DS 2005, lecture notes in computer science 3735. Berlin: Springer-Verlag, 2005:395-397.

[36] Deng K, Liu DL, Gao S, Geng Z. Structural learning of graphical models and its applications to traditional Chinese medicine. In: Wang LP, Jin YC, editors. Proceedings of FSKD 2005, lecture notes in computer science 3614. Berlin: Springer-Verlag, 2005:362-367.

[37] Xiang ZG. A 3-stage voting algorithm for mining optimal ingredient pattern of traditional Chinese medicine. J Software 2003,14(11):1882-1890.

[38] Cao CG, Wang HT, Sui YF. Knowledge modeling and acquisition of traditional Chinese herbal drugs and formulae from text. Artif Intell Med 2004,32(1):3-13.

[39] Wu ZH, Zhou XZ, Liu BY, Chen JL. Text mining for finding functional community of related genes using TCM knowledge. In: Boulicaut JF, Esposito F, Giannotti F, Pedreschi D, editors. Proceedings of the 8th European conference on principles and practice of knowledge discovery in databases. Berlin: Springer-Verlag, 2004:459-470.

[40] Chen XL, Gui XM. Quantitative analysis with multifactor for Chinese herbal medicine: relevant factors of toxicity. J Fujian Coll Tradit Chin Med 1995,5(1):27-30(in Chinese).

[41] Yang GY. Analysis of the properties of 101 blood pressure-reducing plants. J Henan Univ Chin Med 2005, 20 (118):22-27 (in Chinese).

[42] Yao MC, Zhang YL, Yuan YM, Ai L, Qiao YJ. Study on the prediction of the effect attribution of the deficiency-nourishing drugs based on the quantification of TCM drug properties. J Beijing Univ Tradit Chin Med 2004, 27(4): 7-9(in Chinese).

[43] Zhou L, Tang XY, Fu C, Peng SH. Fuzzy clustering analysis of Chinese herbs for relieving exterior syndrome. West China J Pharm Sci 2004,19(5):339-341(in Chinese).

[44] He QF, Zhou XZ, Zhou ZM, Cui M, Wu ZH. Efficacy-based clustering analysis of traditional Chinese medicinal herbs. Chin J Inf Tradit Chin Med 2004,11(7):561-562(in Chinese).

[45] Qi JS, Xu HB, Zhou JY, Lu XH, Yang XL, Guan JH. Factor analysis and cluster analysis of trace elements in some Chinese medicinal herbs. Chin J Anal Chem 1998,26(11):1309-1314(in Chinese).

[46] Qi JS, Xu HB, Zhou JY, Lu XH, Guan JH. Studies on the amount of trace elements and efficacy in Chinese medicinal herbs for treating exterior syndromes. Comput Appl Chem 2003,20(4):449-452 (in Chinese).

[47] Feng XS, Dong HY. Data mining in establishing fingerprint spectrum of Chinese traditional medicines. Prog Pharm Sci 2002, 26(4):194-201 (in Chinese).

[48] Zhang LX, Zhao YN, Yang ZH, Wang JX, Cai SQ, Liu HY. Classifier for Chinese traditional medicine with high-dimensional and small samplesize data. In: Proceedings of WCICA 2004, IEEE computer society, 2004:330-334.

[49] Lu AJ, Liu B, Liu HB, Zhou JJ. Mining association rule in traditional Chinese medicine chemical database. Comput Appl Chem 2005,22(2):108-112 (in Chinese).

[50] Shen ZY. The continuation of kidney study Shanghai: Shanghai Scientific & Technical Publishers, 1990:3-31.

[51] Jenssen TK, Laegreid A, Komorowski J, Hovig E. A literature network of human genes for high-throughput analysis of gene expression. Nat Gen 2001,28(1):21-28.

[52] Yue XQ, Liu Q. Analysis of studies on pattern recognition of tongue image in traditional Chinese medicine by computer technology. J Chin Int Med 2004,2(5):326-329 (in Chinese).

[53] Pang B, Zhang D, Li N, Wang K. Computerized tongue diagnosis based on Bayesian networks. IEEE Trans Biomed Eng 2004,51(10):1803-1810.

[54] Ying J, Li ZX, Li S, Ji L, Liu DL, Ma WY. Collection and analysis of characteristics of tongue manifestations in patients with cerebrovascular diseases. J Beijing Univ Tradit Chin Med 2005,28(4):62-66 (in Chinese).

[55] Lu AP, Zhang SS, Zha QL, Ju DH, Wu H, Jia HW, et al. Correlation between CD4, CD8 cell infiltration in gastric mucosa *Helicobacter pylori* infection and symptoms in patients with chronic gastritis. World J Gastroenterol 2005,11(16):2486-2490.

[56] Deng ZZ, He YT, Yu YM. Comparison between two diagnostic methods of computer's mathematic model and clinical diagnosis on TCM syndromes of rheumatoid arthritis. Chin J Int Tradit West Med 1996,16(12):727-729.

[57] Li S, Lu AP, Zhang L, Li YD. Anti-Helicobacter pylori immunoglobulin G (IgG) and IgA antibody responses and the value of clinical presentations in diagnosis of H. pylori infection in patients with precancerous lesions. World J Gastroenterol 2003,9(4):755-758.

[58] Zhang Q, Zhang WT, Wei JJ, Wang XB, Liu P. Combined use of factor analysis and cluster analysis in classification of traditional Chinese medical syndromes in patients with posthepatitic cirrhosis. J Chin Int Med 2005,3(1):14-18 (in Chinese).

[59] Qin ZG, Mao ZY, Deng ZZ. The application of rough set in the Chinese medicine rheumatic arthritis diagnosis. Chin J Biomed Eng 2001,20(4):357-363 (in Chinese).

[60] Wang XW, Qu HB, Liu P, Cheng YY. A self-learning expert system for diagnosis in traditional Chinese medicine. Expert Sys Appl 2004,26(4):557-566.

[61] Zhang NL, Yuan SH, Latent structure models and diagnosis in traditional Chinese medicine. Technical report HKUST-CS04-12. Department of Computer Science: The Hong Kong University of Science & Technology, 2006 (in Chinese).

[62] Zhang NL, Nielsen TD, Jensen FV. Latent variable discovery in classification models. Artif Intell Med 2004, 30(3):283-299.

[63] Zhang NL. Hierarchical latent class models for cluster analysis. J Machine Learn Res 2004,5(6):697-723.

[64] Zhang NL, Kocka T. Efficient learning of hierarchical latent class models. In: Proceedings of ICTAI 2004, Los Alamitos, 2004:585-593.

[65] Pradhan M, Henrion M, Provan GM, Del Favero B, Huang K. The sensitivity of belief networks to imprecise probabilities: an experimental investigation. Artif Intell 1996,85(1-2):363-397.

3.2 学位论文摘要

本节摘录了中医药数据挖掘与知识发现方向 2000—2018 年共 16 份学位论文资料信息(其中博士学位论文 4 份,硕士学位论文 12 份)。

3.2.1 基于粗集理论的数据挖掘方法的研究

陆伟(指导教师:吴朝晖)
2000 年硕士学位论文

在数据库中挖掘知识(Knowledge Discovery in Database,KDD)是近年来兴起的研究领域之一,其目的是自动地从海量的原始数据中发现隐藏在数据中有价值的知识,并且以用户可以理解的形式表现出来。KDD 对金融、商业、科研等领域有着非常重要的意义。

粗集理论(Rough Set)是近年来新兴的用于分析与表达不完整数据、表达和学习不精确知识的理论与方法。它与传统的处理不确定的理论方法如统计分析、证据理论、模糊集理论等的最大区别在于:它只依赖于知识相关的数据,采用数据之间的近似来表示知识的不确定性,而不需要依赖先验知识对不确定性做定量描述。由于粗集方法具有很好的理论基础和实用前景,因此基于粗集理论的数据挖掘方法正在被广泛地应用于 KDD 系统中,并逐渐成为 KDD 的主流方法之一。

本文的研究工作来源于上述背景。我们的研究目的是对粗集理论在 KDD 中的具体应用进行深入的研究,探讨其具体的实现方法,并且结合其他 KDD 方法构建一个完整的 KDD 系统原型。RoughMiner 是一个由我们自主设计开发的、基于粗集理论框架的通用 KDD 系统原型,它能够实现粗集理论中的基本概念和方法,并在此基础上提供一个完整的 KDD 处理流程。它包括数据准备、数据挖掘、知识检验和评估、结果的表现等步骤。RoughMiner 支持分类、聚类、总结描述、属性相关分析、不确定性分析等多种 KDD 任务。与其他 KDD 系统相比,RoughMiner 具有明显特点:①基于粗集理论的系统框架;②支持 KDD 多阶段处理过程;③支持多种 KDD 任务;④提供多策略选择;⑤基于最小公共交集理论的内核结构;⑥提供有效的知识评估体系;⑦良好的体系结构和系统性能等。

3.2.2 数据挖掘技术及其在中药配伍系统中的应用研究

蔡越君(指导教师:吴朝晖)
2003 年硕士学位论文

中医药是中华民族具有几千年传统的医药学,中华民族繁衍生息到现在,充分证明了中医顽强的生命力及其实用价值。近几年来,中医药科学问题的现代研究不仅是中医药本身的研究重点,而且成为其他学科如化学、药物学研究的重点。随着信息化的深入,中医药信息越来越多,对其整理和归纳的工作也越来越复杂。如何从中找到有用的中医药知识,如何利用以前的临床案例来进行中医证候的诊断,如何利用巨大的方剂知识为中医专家有效地提供新的方剂配伍,是三个急需解决的问题。

数据挖掘技术是为解决机器学习、模式识别、数据库技术等各种领域中的大型实际应用问题而提出的一些工程性方法的集合,主要是为了从大型数据库中高效地发现隐含在其中的知识或规律,并为人类专家的决策提供支持。高频集发现和贝叶斯分类是两种重要的数据挖掘技术。

中药知识发现集中在发现常用的单味药合用模式,在中医术语中称为药对,这可以用高频集发现来解决;中医症候诊断可以看成是在大量临床案例库上的贝叶斯训练器和分类器;解决方剂配伍问题的关键是建立起一个合适的配伍计算机模型。本文在这三个方面做了下面一些工作。

(1)分析高频集发现算法在中药知识发现中的模型,建立起合理的数据结构,并对 Apriori 算法做了一些改进,提出了一个新的参数——有效支持度,以便使找到的药对真正满足中医专家的兴趣,并在几十条中医数据基础上做了一些测试工作。

(2)分析了贝叶斯算法的工作原理,并建立起中医证候诊断的模型,建立起以症状为维度的特征空间、以证候为分类目标的空间,初步建立起一个中医证候诊断的原型演示系统。

(3)研究了中医方剂组方的过程,提出了方剂配方的计算机模型,设计了一个计算机方剂配方系统,给出了计算机方剂组方的具体步骤,探讨了这种模型的可行性和有效性。

(4)开发了一个计算机系统 Formula,它集成了中药药对发现功能、中医证候诊断功能以及在中医专家的支持下的计算机辅助组方功能。

3.2.3　文本挖掘在中医药中的若干应用研究

周雪忠(指导教师:吴朝晖)
2004 年博士学位论文

文本挖掘是人工智能、机器学习、自然语言处理、数据挖掘及相关自动文本处理如信息抽取、信息检索、文本分类等理论和技术相结合的产物,它得到了越来越多研究人员的关注。文本挖掘是数据挖掘研究面向文本数据的自然延伸,其研究仍处于婴儿期,在方法和应用方面均未成熟。中医药学作为生命科学具备中国特色的传统医学组成部分,在疾病诊治和方药使用等方面具有特色和显著的临床疗效,并包含着丰富的知识,几千年的医学实践积累获得了大量的数据。在中医药学信息化建设的基础上进行 KDD 研究具有重要意义。中医药领域未存在文本挖掘的相关研究,本文在多个方面如文献临床复方药物组成和科属配伍知识发现、中医术语及关系抽取和中医证候基因关系知识发现等进行了研究。本文研究内容包括如下四个方面。

(1)进行基于字特征的中文文本分类研究,实验表明字特征是中文文本分类的高效特征表示方法。提出了分布字聚类方法,该方法无须分词,具有低达 10^2 数量级的特征维数和高性能的特点,其与 NB 结合的性能接近基于词特征的 SVM 分类器,微平均准确率达到86%。

(2)进行中医药文献信息抽取研究,提出了 Bubble-bootstrapping 和 ATP 方法。该方法无须任何浅层中文自然语言处理、专业词库和已标注的训练语料,是一种接近无导师的可缩放性、可移植性信息抽取方法。在近 40 万篇文献题录的复方名称和疾病名称抽取实验中,取得了平均准确率达99%、F1 值达 65% 左右的结果。应用于中医药文献自动标引的副主题词抽取,达到 80% 的 F1 值。ATP 是一种 semi-hard 的模式方法,是未来信息抽取研究的技术方向之一。

(3)进行文献临床复方药物组成文本挖掘研究,提出了复方科属配伍的概念,并进行了临床复方科属配伍知识发现研究,实现了 MeDisco/3T 文本挖掘系统。MeDisco/3T 实验表明,复方文本挖掘研究具有较高的质量和实际应用价值,复方用药中存在科属配伍的规律,并能进行挖掘发现。

（4）整合利用中医药文献库和生物医学文献库（MEDLINE）进行中医证候和基因相关关系知识发现研究,实现了原型系统 MeDisco/3S,并进行了初步实验和分析。结果表明,MeDisco/3S 能为辅助中西医结合研究和生命科学交叉研究提供智能化的知识发现平台,是进行生物医学文本挖掘和多学科信息整合研究的典型范例。

3.2.4　中医方剂数据挖掘平台研发

何前锋（指导教师：吴朝晖）

2005 年硕士学位论文

方剂配伍规律的研究是中医药信息化重大课题之一,是当前方证相关研究的关键点。方剂配伍的研究在中医药理论体系的整理完善、处方专家系统研发、物质有效成分配比的研究等多方面展开。随着中医药的信息化,方剂数据得到逐步积累,从而形成了几大方剂数据库。数据挖掘研究成果以及相关技术分析方剂数据库,为方剂配伍规律研究提供了又一有效的途径。本文使用数据挖掘相关技术做了以下几个方面的研究开发工作：

（1）提出了使用方剂挖掘平台研究方剂配伍的方法,并描绘了平台可能获得的应用；

（2）整理总结了方剂数据的特点并针对特点提出相应的数据预处理方案；

（3）分析了方剂数据挖掘平台的主体功能,设计了平台的整体框架；

（4）完成了方剂数据挖掘平台挖掘分析模块的原型开发；

（5）使用方剂数据挖掘平台对方剂数据库进行了一些典型的应用分析；

（6）实现了高频分析算法在网格环境下的应用。

3.2.5　文本分类技术及其在中医药文献中的应用

陈君利（指导教师：吴朝晖）

2005 年硕士学位论文

文本自动分类是文本挖掘最重要的研究方向之一,解决的是根据文本的内容自动确定其类别的问题。文本可以关联到预定义的一个或者多个类别,对应于单标签（single-label）和多标签（multi-label）分类问题。对于单标签英文文本分类技术的研究已经较为成熟,但是很少有研究系统地、专门地处理多标签数据,特别是多标签中文文本数据。本文实现了一种多标签中文文本自动分类系统,并将其应用于中医药文献主题自动标引,即根据文献内容自动确定文献副主题词类别,相当有效地解决了自动标引中的难点：副主题词的标注问题。此外,我们还开发了一个证候分子生物学在线挖掘原型系统,应用文本挖掘方法将中医学和分子生物学联系起来。本文主要做了以下几个方面的工作。

（1）基于 CMU 的 Bow 系统,开发了多标签中文文本自动分类系统 Bow_TCM。多标签文本分类是一个非常重要的研究方向,同时也是一个难以解决的问题,尤其是多标签中文文本分类,据我们所知仍然没有令人满意的系统。并且由于缺少统一的语料库以及中文语言自身的问题,很难对中文分类系统及分类方法的优劣做出严格的比较。Bow_TCM 系统基于 Boosting 算法和字特征表示,能够接受多种格式的训练文本,训练后进行分类和系统性能评估,很大程度上解决了现存的一些问题。

(2)研究了中医药文献主题自动标引的现状,应用多标签中文文本自动分类方法进行医学文献自动标引,即根据文献内容自动确定文献副主题词类别。在中医药学语料库 TCM-MED 和英文标准语料库 Reuters21578 中应用三种方法进行对比试验,取得了比较好的实验结果。实验结果表明,系统具有一定的实用性。TCM-MED 训练集由中国中医界的权威机构、专业人员编辑而成,它的标准性可以和 OHSUMED 相比较,我们推荐 TCM-MED 作为标准中文语料库。

(3)开发了中医证候分子生物学在线挖掘系统原型,旨在通过 MEDLINE 信息和中医药学证病数据找出中医证候和基因蛋白质可能的关联。目前基因组学的研究从结构基因组学转向了功能基因组学,探究基因的生物功能和揭示基因之间的相互关系是生物学领域的研究热点。我们从中医证候整体论的角度来观察基因功能组,通过证候找出其对应的基因网络,并通过证候疾病、疾病基因关系分割基因网络,有望将中医整体观点和西医分子观点结合起来。

3.2.6　中医方剂数据挖掘模式和算法研究

周忠眉(指导教师:吴朝晖)

2006 年博士学位论文

中医药学是中华民族五千年优秀文化的瑰宝和科学发展的结晶,为人民的健康和生存质量的提高做出了极大贡献。方剂学在中医药学中占有重要位置,方剂是中医药学理、法、方、药的一个重要组成部分,其配伍规律有着深刻的科学内涵。

几千年来,中医药领域的无数临床实践与理论研究积累了海量的中医方剂,这些中医方剂包含在中医药古籍、文献以及当前的临床研究文献中。近年来,浙江大学计算机学院 CCNT 实验室和中国中医科学院合作共建了大量方剂数据库,如何有效地利用这些宝贵的数据库资源就成了发展中医药必须面对的一个问题。而数据挖掘所擅长的正是从海量的数据中发现有意义的模式、知识,这是分析中医药海量中医方剂所需要的技术。本文利用数据挖掘技术从大量方剂中抽取有意义的药物组配模式,为方剂理论研究和临床实践研究提供现代技术手段。

本文的主要工作是提出一系列适合方剂数据挖掘的挖掘模式和算法,并将各算法集成研发方剂数据挖掘系统。

频繁关联模式能反映模式中各项目之间的关联关系。然而,与频繁模式挖掘特点类似的是,当最小关联度界设得太低时,频繁关联模式挖掘会产生大量的频繁关联模式,不利于人工分析,因此本文提出最大频繁关联模式挖掘和挖掘算法。因为所有的频繁关联模式都可以从最大频繁关联模式中导出,所以最大频繁关联模式挖掘对挖掘结果不丢失信息量。实验证明,最大频繁关联模式挖掘既可以减少结果模式的数量,又提高了算法的效率。

关联挖掘和相关挖掘是两种不同的数据挖掘任务。实验证明,大量极其关联的频繁关联模式各项目之间不存在相关关系。本文在数据挖掘过程中将关联兴趣度度量与相关兴趣度度量结合,提出关联且相关频繁模式挖掘和挖掘算法。实验证明,关联且相关频繁模式各项目之间不但关联,而且存在相关关系,这提高了模式的兴趣性。

由于相关模式的定义条件较弱,即只要模式各项目之间存在相关关系,必为相关模式,这致使许多关联且相关频繁模式各项目之间仍然存在大量的独立关系,即关联且相关频繁模式任意两个子集不一定都是相关的。鉴于此,本文提出互为正相关频繁模式挖掘和挖掘算法。互为正相关频繁模式任意两个子模式不但关联,而且正相关。实验证明,互为正相关频繁模式挖掘能有效去除模式中各项目之间有独立关系的那些关联且相关频繁模式。由于互为正相关频繁模式挖掘产生的结果模式数量比关联且相关频繁模式挖掘少,所以互为正相关频繁模式挖掘算法的执行效率比关联且相关频繁模式挖掘高。

实验表明,大量的关联规则两边不具有相关关系,于是本文提出把关联且相关规则的挖掘和挖掘算法作为关联规则挖掘的补充。关联且相关规则两边不但关联而且正相关,所以关联且相关的规则挖掘能提高规则的兴趣度,比关联规则挖掘更有利于有意义规则的发现。

目前几乎所有与度量模式相关的兴趣度度量都不适合挖掘长模式,又没有上下界便于参数输入时的控制。本文利用概率统计中事件的独立性定义,提出新的度量模式相关性的兴趣度度量——相关自信度。该度量建立在概率统计理论上,定义合理,有上下界-1和$+1$,而且此度量还适合挖掘模式中项目个数大于2的长模式。

本文集成了所有的方剂数据挖掘模式和算法,设计研发了方剂药物组配模式分析系统和方剂功效分析系统。通过该系统,不仅可以抽取方剂中有关联和/或相关药物的组配模式,探讨这些模式中药物组配后功效的变化情况,探讨与这些模式配伍的高频药物及这些高频药物的功效情况,还可以通过在模式中添加高频药物,探讨模式药物变化后功效的变化情况及方剂因所含模式的药物变化而发生功效变化的情况。

3.2.7　中医临床数据仓库的设计与构建

于彤(指导教师:吴朝晖)

2006 年硕士学位论文

本文主要讨论一个面向中医临床研究的示范性数据仓库系统的设计与构建。该数据仓库将多个电子病例管理系统中产生的大量临床数据进行集成和结构化存储,并在此基础上建立多种面向中医临床研究的应用,从而快速地向被授权的用户提供全面而准确的中医临床信息和知识。

与商业环境中的传统应用相比,中医临床领域模型的复杂性向数据仓库的数据建模技术提出了新的需求。本文将首先提出中医临床领域模型和电子病例的结构,然后介绍基于 EAV 模型对临床数据进行建模的方法,并通过对多维模型进行扩展来处理临床数据中事实与维度之间的多对多关系、双时效性事实和非正规维度等复杂情况。

临床数据仓库的主要应用是信息检索、OLAP 和数据挖掘等。本文对元数据驱动的临床信息检索工具的设计,选择视图进行物理化的策略,定制查询环境的设计,业务元数据的表示和管理,以及信息共享与安全机制等应用设计问题进行了阐述。

项目中自主研发了一套较为成熟的面向中医临床领域的数据抽取、转换和装载工具,该套工具已将数千份电子病例成功地导入数据仓库中。同时建立了支持关系型 OLAP 的数据集市,并实现了从数据仓库到数据集市的数据模式转换。

项目使用多个业务智能领域优秀的开源项目,以相对低廉的成本在较短的时间内开发出一个基于 Web 的 OLAP 平台。其中分别使用 BIRT 和 Mondrian 作为报表生成和多维分析的实现框架,并增加元数据管理工具、主题浏览和 ad hoc 查询生成界面等外围组件。在此框架基础上,开发人员可以集中精力处理中医临床领域的业务逻辑,使软件更好地满足临床分析人员的特定需要。

3.2.8　中医药知识发现可靠性研究

封毅(指导教师:吴朝晖)
2008 年博士学位论文

知识发现可靠性是知识发现领域中一个重要但容易被忽视的主题。随着知识发现和数据挖掘技术的广泛应用,有一个问题逐渐引起人们的关注:在什么条件下知识发现是可靠的,或者说在什么条件下所发现的知识是可靠的? 近年来在知识发现可靠性方面的研究,大多关注于某一具体数据挖掘模型下的可靠性问题。而对于不同模型间存在的可靠性共同主题,比如数据质量、评估方法等,迄今为止仍没有一项系统性研究。针对知识发现可靠性的共同主题,进行分阶段、系统化的总结和梳理,已成为知识发现可靠性研究的一大迫切需要。

在知识发现技术所应用的各个领域中,有一个领域特别需要知识发现可靠性的研究,即中医药领域。作为中华民族重要文化财富和学术成就的中医药,近年来面临着生存和发展的挑战。如何把这一挑战化为中医药发展的契机,利用知识发现技术促进中医药的跨越式发展,已成为中医药研究人员的一项重要课题。近年来中医药信息化工作已为知识发现创造了有利条件。然而,由于中医药数据自然语言性强,数据表达含义丰富,表达方式多样化,而且在数据质量上还面临较大问题,在具备这些特征的数据上所进行的知识发现,相比其他领域来讲,就更加需要关注和研究其可靠性问题。

在这一背景下,本文围绕中医药知识发现可靠性这一主题,从知识发现整个生命周期的各个阶段对可靠性因素进行探讨,提出了知识发现可靠性框架 PBRF-KD。针对中医药知识发现中比较突出的可靠性问题,重点探讨中医药知识发现中的结构性因素、表达性因素和信任性因素三大问题。本文的研究工作与贡献包括如下几个方面。

(1)提出了基于过程的知识发现可靠性框架。针对与现有知识发现可靠性研究模型相关的特点,提出了一个与模型/应用无关的知识发现可靠性框架 PBRF-KD,该框架采用基于过程的思路对知识发现整个流程中的各个阶段和可靠性因素进行了梳理,归纳出 7 种可靠性相关因素。该框架为知识发现项目设立了整套与可靠性相关的蓝本。

(2)提出了与结构相关的可靠性因素的优化方法。分析了中医药知识发现中与结构相关的可靠性因素,主要指数据完整性。针对文本型字段的完整性问题,提出了基于顺序半相关度量的中医药文本缺失字段填补方法。针对中医药文献类别标签缺失的问题,提出了基于 M-Similarity 的多标签文本分类方法。

(3)提出了与表达相关的可靠性因素的优化方法。分析了中医药知识发现中与表达相关的可靠性因素,主要指表达粒度和表达一致性。针对表达粒度,提出了基于规则的表达粒度细分方法。针对表达一致性,提出了基于本体的表达一致化方法。该套方法有助于提高中医药与表达相关的可靠性。

(4)提出了与信任相关的可靠性因素的优化方法。分析了中医药知识发现中与信任相关的可靠性因素,主要指数据可信度。针对中医药特有的数据可信度问题,提出了基于历史文献认可度的数据可信度衡量方法,以及基于互联网知名度的数据可信度衡量方法。此外,基于这两种可信度衡量方法,提出了基于数据可信度的加权频繁模式挖掘算法,并在消渴方和脾胃方数据集上获得了有意义的结果。该套方法有助于提高中医药与信任相关的可靠性。

3.2.9 DartSpora 数据挖掘平台的构建及其在中医方剂领域的应用

吴毅挺(指导教师:陈华钧)

2008 年硕士学位论文

在信息时代,随着互联网的发展,人类积累了海量数据。激增的数据背后隐藏着许多重要的信息,人们希望能够对其进行更高层次的分析,以便更好地利用这些数据,因而数据挖掘显得越来越重要。数据挖掘是一个复杂而又需求庞大的任务。虽然已经建立了很多方法来处理层出不穷的问题,但依然还需要面临许多挑战。数据挖掘需求的快速变化,要求平台和工具能够支持对已有方法的最大程度重用和创新组合,同时能够简单快速地集成新的方法。

随着中医药的信息化进程的推进,数据挖掘也越来越广泛地被应用到中医药领域。方剂数据经过中医学界及相关领域广大工作者的不懈努力,被整理形成几大方剂数据库。复方数量达十几万首,其中中医古方剂库就包含了 8 万方剂,为研究方剂配伍规律打下了坚实的基础。

在本文中,我们设计并开发了 DartSpora 数据挖掘平台,与中国中医科学院合作,将 DartSpora 平台应用到中医方剂领域,研究方剂配伍规律。本文的主要研究内容如下。

(1)应用 AJAX 技术通过 Google Web Toolkits、GWT-EXT 开源框架和 Rapid Miner 开源项目设计与实现 DartSpora 数据挖掘平台。包括实验管理模块、DartGrid 模块、数据库连接管理模块、用户管理模块等。

(2)整合 DartSpora 与 DartGrid,以提供基于语义集成的分布式数据库访问。用户在不需要了解基于语义集成的分布式数据库结构的情况下,凭借自身的领域知识就能获取需要的数据,并进行数据挖掘。

(3)针对中医方剂数据的特点,设计基于规则的替换与拆分预处理方法,提高了中医方剂数据处理的效率和可配置性。

(4)改进传统经典 Apriori 算法,引入数据权值,开发 WApriori 算法;分别以互联网知名度和历史文献认可度为权值,对脾胃方剂进行挖掘。将实验室已开发的各种算法移植到 DartSpora 平台。

(5)DartSpora 平台在中医方剂领域的应用案例。主要包括基于规则的替换与拆分进行中医方剂预处理、病毒性心肌炎方剂最大高频模式挖掘、脾胃方基于数据可信度的加权频繁模式挖掘。

3.2.10 中医药数据挖掘平台与服务

秘中凯(指导教师:姜晓红、陈华钧)

2010 年硕士学位论文

数据挖掘技术历经近二十年发展,逐步趋于成熟,在商业数据处理和互联网数据分析等应用中获得了巨大的成功,并逐步向更广阔的领域拓展其应用。而中国传统医药学以上千年的积累汇聚了种类繁多、内容丰富的医学典籍与记录,这些资源中蕴含了大量未知的知识与规律,而这些知识将对现代中医学的发展发挥重要作用。近十年,浙江大学 CCNT 实验室与中国中医科学院中医药信息研究所致力于中医药数据的信息化,建成了多个具有相当规模的中医数据库,为该领域的数据挖掘工作打下了良好的基础。但是,在研究和应用中还是面临着不少实际问题:没有明确的方案规划标准;各种挖掘应用平台功能相对单一,无法有效便利分享和重用资源;无法有效处理大规模数据挖掘任务。

面对中医药领域数据挖掘发展中的实际需求,浙江大学 CCNT 实验室数据挖掘组设计开发了在线数据挖掘服务平台 DartSpora。该平台借鉴和使用了开源数据挖掘软件的设计理念与资源,并以 Web 服务的方式为中医药领域的研究人员提供丰富的领域相关挖掘服务。笔者在该项目中负责 DartSpora 服务平台 2.0 版本的系统设计和大部分模块开发工作,并参与了分布式并行数据挖掘算法库的设计和开发。在 2.0 版本的挖掘平台基础上,笔者与数据挖掘组的其他同事和中国中医科学院的工作人员合作制定了一系列中医领域研究应用的挖掘方案实例,用于相关领域问题的解决和平台使用的参考。

3.2.11　基于 MapReduce 的中医药并行数据挖掘服务

刘洋(指导教师:陈华钧、姜晓红)
2010 年硕士学位论文

随着中医药信息化的进一步深入,更广泛的中医药临床数据被规范化整理,形成了大量标准的中医药数据库,使得中医药信息的数据进一步膨胀,而原有的单机版 DartSpora 数据挖掘软件无法满足这种对海量数据进行挖掘的要求。针对这种新的需要,我提出了基于 MapReduce 的中医药并行数据挖掘服务框架,以满足中医药研究对更高性能计算能力的要求。这种方法可以充分利用已有的高性能集群的计算能力,为 DartSpora 平台提供更强大的后台支撑。同时,这种服务方式又具有一定的通用性,可以为一些非领域内的挖掘要求服务。

在这个针对中医药研究的并行服务框架中,我具体实现了以下内容。

(1)设计并实现了可视化交互平台,以及可编程的 Web Service 服务。

(2)在并行框架集成的算法库中,具体开发了:①针对单图的频繁模式发现算法,并应用到中医方剂组成配伍的研究中;②实现了简化点式互信息算法,并把其应用于中医临床数据。

3.2.12　超数据集成挖掘方法与技术研究

周春英(指导教师:吴朝晖、陈华钧)
2012 年博士学位论文

超数据(Hyperdata)是被连接到其他数据对象的数据对象。超数据经过语义关系连接形成了数据网络(Data Web)。超数据可以为集成挖掘提供丰富的、相互关联的数据。然而,超数据具有的高关联性、分布性和海量性也给超数据集成挖掘带来一系列困难。从目前超数据的研究现状来看,还缺乏比较有效的、系统性的研究来解决这些困难以支持超数据集成挖掘。

基于上述背景,本文围绕超数据集成挖掘,从超数据准备、超数据集成挖掘方法和大规模超数集成挖掘原型系统三个方面入手,针对超数据的分布性、高关联性和海量性带来的问题提出相应的解决方法。本文的主要研究内容和贡献可以概括为以下几个方面。

- **超数据准备**(包括超数据获取和集成两部分工作)

(1)超数据获取:一种基于领域本体的文本自动获取超数据图的方法

为了实现文本向超数据的转化,提出一种基于领域本体的从文本自动获取超数据图的方法。超数据图由多个超数据节点和它们之间多维的、复杂的语义关系构成。句子是文本的基本组成单元。一个句子可能含有多个超数据节点,并且它们之间可能存在多种不同类型的语义关系。该方法将超数据图作为句子的超数据信息的表达单元,然后利用自然语言处理、数据挖掘、概率统计技术实现从一个句子自动提取超数据图,从而实现文本自动向超数据的转化。

(2)超数据集成:一种基于语义的多个超数据源的糅合方法

数据质量越高,数据挖掘的性能往往也越高。超数据的分布性带来了数据模式和数据内容两方面的异质异构。为了解决数据不一致和冗余的问题,本文提出了一种基于语义的多个超数据源的糅合方法。针对数据模式的异质异构,利用语义映射把多个具有不同数据模式的超数据源映射到一个统一的本体模式,从而解决数据模式的差异;针对数据内容的异质异构,提出一个综合了语义推理和文本挖掘技术的超数据实体识别方法,从而识别不同超数据节点指向同一个现实世界实体的情况。

- **超数据挖掘方法**(包括概念描述和挖掘方法)

(3)超数据的概念描述:一种基于语义图模板的概念描述方法

超数据以 RDF 格式存在,是高度结构化数据,并不能直接运用传统数据挖掘方法。概念描述的目的是针对数据的模式、挖掘方法,产生数据的特征和比较描述。本文针对超数据的数据模式,提出一种基于语义(RDF)图模板的概念描述方法,其中语义图模板可以描述 RDF 数据模型所携带的三种信息源,包括描述性属性、语义关系和语义图结构,可以用来实现超数据的概念描述,从而为后面的挖掘方法提供数据。

(4)超数据的挖掘方法:概率语义学习模型

超数据源以 RDF 形式存贮数据,并提供标准的 SPARQL 语言作为查询接口。与其他数据类型不同,超数据具有高关联性和分布性。针对分布式的 RDF 数据源,利用语义图模板的概念来描述超数据所携带的属性特征,以解决超数据的高关联性、分布性给集成挖掘带来的问题。在此之上,提出了扩展了传统贝叶斯网络的概率语义学习模型,以实现多个超数据源的集成挖掘。另外,为了提高机器学习模型在训练数据不准确或不足的情况下的性能,提出了一种综合利用标记数据和未标记数据的半监督学习方法以提高性能。

- **挖掘方法的可规模性**

(5)一种基于云计算框架的大规模超数据集成挖掘原型系统

针对大规模超数据的集成挖掘,本文提出了一个基于云计算框架(MapReduce 和 Hadoop)的大规模超数据集成挖掘原型系统。该系统支持大规模超数据的存贮、语义查询和基于概率语义学习模型的集成挖掘。本文围绕超数据集成挖掘,从超数据准备、超数据集成挖掘和基于云计算框架的大规模超数据集成挖掘原型系统三个方面入手,针对超数据的高关联性、分布性和海量性给超数据集成挖掘带来的困难,分别提出了以下方法。①超数据获取:一种基于领域本体的从文本自动获取超数据图的方法,用来实现文本向超数据的转化。②超数据集成:一种基于语义的多个超数据源糅合方法,用来解决超数据的分布性带来的数据模式和数据内容的异质异构问题。③超数据概念描述:一种基于语义图模板的超数据概念描述方法,用来描述超数据(RDF)所携带的三种信息源(描述性属性、语义关系和语义图结构),从而为挖掘方法提供特征和比较描述。④超数据挖掘:一种扩展了传统贝叶斯网络学习的概率语义学习模型,它通过利用语义图模板描述的特征变量代替传统的属性变量实现扩展;一种半监督学习方法,用来改善概率语义学习在训练数据不准确或不足情况下的性能。⑤针对超数据的海量性,提出并开发了一个基于云计算框架(Hadoop 和 MapReduce)的大规模超数据集成挖掘原型系统,从而提高超数据挖掘方法的可规模性。

本文提出了超数据集成挖掘的相关方法和原型系统,试图解决超数据的高关联性、分布性和海量性给集成数据挖掘的超数据获取、集成、概念描述和挖掘方法等过程带来的问题,并且开发了一个基于云计算框架的大规模超数据集成挖掘原型系统以提高挖掘方法的可规模性,从而为今后的超数据集成挖掘研究和应用提供理论与技术基础。

3.2.13　几种机器学习算法的改进及其在中药成分分析中的应用

刘明魁(指导教师:姜晓红、陈华钧)
2012 年硕士学位论文

机器学习算法在中药成分分析、成分与疾病关系的研究中一直起着重要的作用。利用机器学习技术对中药成分进行发掘是中药现代化的重要方法。本文主要研究几种机器学习算法的改进,并分析它们在中药成分分析、成分与证候的关系中的应用。

本文提出了根据疾病的历史记录提取成分对应的疾病集合和频次以及 TF-IDF 权重的计算方法。接着本文提出了中药成分之间的相似度计算方法。并改进了 K-medoids 算法,然后分析了改进的 K-medoids 算法在中药成分聚类分析中的效果,最后给出了聚类分析的评价方法。

本文提出了一种基于中药成分 IDF 值的黑名单算法,并介绍了基于中药成分 IDF 的黑名单算法在中药成分分析研究中的应用。此算法在提高黑名单的自动化、可解释性以及降低数据量和减少冗余信息方面取得了一定成果。

协同过滤(CF)是最成功的推荐系统的方法之一。本文提出了一种改进的概率矩阵分解的模型;接着分析了改进的非负概率分解,以及这些模型在 MovieLens 数据集中的实验结果,并比较几种算法之间的优劣;最后提出了可行的改进的概率矩阵分解模型在中药成分和证候的关系预测和分析中应用的设想。

3.2.14　基于主题模型的中医药隐含语义信息挖掘

商任翔(指导教师:姜晓红、陈华钧)
2013 年硕士学位论文

信息检索领域很多应用都需要挖掘隐含在字、词(中医药处方里面的药剂、化学成分)背后的含义,通过运用统计规律对样本进行学习,可以挖掘出这些词的潜在语义,进而克服单个字词精确匹配带来的一词多义的问题。“取象比类”是贯穿中医药知识体系的思维模式,它本身包含了利用统计规律来刻画中医药方剂的作用机制。

LDA 主题模型是一个文档-主题-词汇三层贝叶斯模型,它能够很好地挖掘词语的潜在语义,将统计学习挖掘的方法应用在中医药知识发现的领域中。文档即中医处方。词汇对应于处方中的方剂、药品。通过运用主题模型对大量中医处方的数据挖掘,可以建立处方、主题、药剂之间的关系模型,并融合到已有的中医药语义 Web 的知识网络中,这对中医药知识完整描述和新知识的发现意义重大。

本文主要研究主题模型在中医药信息挖掘领域的应用,主要贡献如下。

(1)改进 Gibbs-LDA(Gibbs-Latent Dirichlet Allocation)算法,构建主题模型对中医药处方数据进行分析。

(2)使用 RDF 对主题模型训练出来的知识进行描述,并融合到中医药语义知识网络之中,设计并实现其语义网络图的可视化算法,为中医药之间的相互作用机理提供统计意义上的支持和形象的展示。

(3)在中医药数据挖掘平台 Spora 上增加基于主题模型的数据挖掘算子,使得普通用户能够共享主题模型并进行中医药数据挖掘方法的实践应用。

(4)设计并实现用户对海量资源访问控制的管理系统——IAM(Identify and Access Management)。

3.2.15　基于文本语义分块的中医病情分类问题研究

付钊(指导教师:姜晓红)
2018 年硕士学位论文

中医智能医疗研究对于解决我国中医传承难、中医资源匮乏、中医"看病难"等一系列问题具有十分重要的意义。其中,智能辨证是中医智能医疗中最基本而又最关键的一步。本文通过将智能辨证问题抽象为一个病情文本分类问题,首先提出基于分块向量的病情文本相似性计算方法,将病情文本按照所描述的病位划分为块,并赋予各个病位块不同的权重来区分主次症状,通过计算块向量的余弦夹角找出两段病情文本的相似症状。然后,结合自然语言处理和数据挖掘相关技术,给出了中医病情文本分类模型。最后,以中医肾病综合征七种分型患者的病程数据为基础,通过实验将基于文本块向量相似性的病情分类模型与传统的文本分类模型进行对比。实验结果表明,本文提出的基于文本块向量相似的病情分类模型具有更高的准确性。论文主要贡献如下。

(1)研究传统的文本表示、文本相似性计算方法,并分析各个方法的优缺点,实现基于 TF-IDF 特征的随机森林病情分类模型和 SVM 病情分类模型,两种模型的 F1 值分别为 75.38% 和 75.20%。

(2)针对中医病情文本,提出了一种基于分块向量的病情文本特征表示方法,更准确地表达了文本语义;以病位词的文档频率为块权值,区分主次症状。

(3)在基于分块向量的病情文本特征表示方法的基础上,提出了一种基于文本分块向量的相似性计算方法(Similarity Based On Block Vector,SBBV),并与现有的文本相似性计算方法做实验对比,证明该方法的准确率明显高于现有方法。

(4)在基于文本块向量特征的文本相似性计算方法的基础上,进一步提出了相应的中医病情文本分类模型,综合 F1 值达到 90.81%。最后,融合病情的非文本特征,提出了多维度的中医病情分类方法,综合 F1 值较文本分类模型提升近 1%。

3.2.16　中药生产工艺的智能优化研究

李金昌(指导教师:姜晓红)
2018 年硕士学位论文

随着智能制造技术在世界范围内兴起,中药生产也从数字化走向智能化。在中药生产智能化进程中,为了逐步提升产品质量指标,不断优化生产工艺。本文通过深入研究工业上工艺优化的相关工作,提出一种中药生产工艺智能优化方案。该方案共包括工艺参数离线优化与工艺参数在线反馈两个模块,其中工艺参数离线优化模块又包括关键工艺参数筛选、质量指标预测、工艺参数优选三方面工作,本文的主要工作和贡献概括如下。

(1)调研关键工艺参数筛选相关算法,提出了 BCA(Bidirectional Clustering Analysis)双向聚类关键工艺参数筛选法。通过与皮尔逊参数法和逐步回归系数方法相比较,本文提出的算法在关键工艺参数筛选准确度上具有明显的优势,准确率在 98% 以上。

(2)调研质量指标预测相关算法,提出了利用 GA 遗传算法优化 BP 神经网络建立质量指标预测模型。通过与回归预测算法、贝叶斯预测算法、BP 神经网络算法相比,在预测精准度上有明显的优势,总体相对误差控制在 4‰ 以内。

(3)调研工艺参数优选相关算法,针对 NSGA-Ⅱ 算法波动大、不收敛的不足,提出了 INSGA 算法。通过实验对比,INSGA 算法的稳定性和收敛效果有明显提升,同时利用该算法优化后的工艺参数,对应的产品质量指标提升 23%。

(4)调研工艺在线反馈相关算法和技术难点,提出了基于最优工艺响应面的 PIA(Process Intelligent Adjustment)智能反馈方法。在生产过程中,当质量指标偏离预期阈值时,通过该方法快速调节工艺参数,使得最终质量参数达到预期阈值,实现工艺参数智能调节,进而提升产品质量指标。

(5)实现了中药生产过程知识系统 PKS(Process Knowledge System)。该系统利用生产中的数据,通过数据挖掘、统计分析等手段,实现中药生产中实时监控、工艺智能优化等相关功能,保证了中药生产的可靠性和产品的稳定性。

3.3　学术论文摘要

本节摘录了中医药数据挖掘与知识发现方向 2001—2016 年共 26 篇主要学术论文(分别发表在 *Briefings In Bioinformatics*、*Artificial Intelligence in Medicine*、《浙江大学学报》、*PKDD*、*APPT*、*WWW* 等国内外期刊和会议论文集上)。

3.3.1　中药复方组成规律的关联规则发现系统

陆伟,王雁峰,吴朝晖
首发于《浙江大学学报(工学版)》,2001,35(4):370-373

本文主要讨论如何将知识挖掘中的关联规则发现算法应用于传统中药复方数据库,以求发现中药单方之间的配伍规律。为了实现高效的关联规则发现以及提高系统的灵活性,系统采用了基于数据立方体的关联规则发现方法,其目标数据是包含了 2500 条中药复方信息的数据库。系统能够根据用户的设定,从数据库中发现治疗某一特定疾病的所有复方中不同单方之间的关联规则。

3.3.2　基于文本挖掘的中医学文献主题自动标引

周雪忠,崔蒙,吴朝晖
首发于《中国中医药信息杂志》,2003,10(1):71-74

　　由于计算机、数据仓库及网格技术的发展,大量数字化科技文献的 Internet 共享和知识挖掘需求越来越迫切。如何采用计算机技术自动或半自动地完成文献的编辑(包括文摘标引关键字的提取等),以减少在文献编辑中人为的不确定性和错误,同时降低人力物力的需求,从而提高文献分类、检索的效率和质量,已经是异常突出和重要的问题。在中医领域,由于文献资源具有很高的临床价值和理论价值,大量人员从事文献的原始的手工编辑任务。而在实际使用中的《中医药学主题词表》《英汉对照医学主题词标引树状结构表》《医学主题词标引》等词库和规则知识为中医文献自动标引提供了基础资源条件,同时中医学语言是一种次语言(sublanguage),基于次语言的语言处理技术能对中医文本进行相当深度的理解式分析和知识抽取。本文将根据文献标引人员的实践经验,面向文献的题名和文摘(文摘可自动生成,考虑到准确性,本文的系统目前仍基于手工编辑的文摘),采用基于机器学习的信息抽取及文本分类等文本挖掘方法研究中医文献主题词的自动标引,并简单介绍我们正在研究的中医文献主题自动标引系统框架。本文的第二节介绍文本处理技术如信息抽取、文本挖掘及文献主题标引等内容;第三节分析本文采用的机器学习方法;第四节介绍主题标引的难点、解决方法、模糊词识别和概念语义组配等;第五节提供本文的 IE-based 主题标引系统结构及其各部分功能的简要分析;第六节是结论。

3.3.3　文本知识发现:基于信息抽取的文本挖掘

周雪忠,吴朝晖
首发于《计算机科学》,2003,30(1):63-66

In the general context of Knowledge Discovery, Knowledge Discovery in Text (KDT), which uses Text Mining techniques to extract and induce hidden knowledge from unstructured text data, surges in the data and natural language processing research. KDT is a multi-discipline of Artificial Intelligence, Machine learning, Natural Language Processing and Information Extraction & Information Retrieval. This paper presents an overview of Text Mining with a stressing on its IE (Information Extraction)-based induction and specific sublanguage fields oriented practices.

3.3.4　Mining Frequent Maximum Patterns with Constraint

Zhongmei Zhou, Zhaohui Wu
首发于 *Journal of Fudan University* (*Nature Science*),2004,43(5):746-749

Frequent pattern mining often generates a very large number of patterns and rules, which reduces not only the efficiency but also the effectiveness of mining. Recent work has highlighted the importance of the paradigm of constraint-based frequent maximum pattern mining. It gives the definition of the frequent maximum pattern with constraint and develops an algorithm for mining frequent maximum patterns with convertible anti-monotone constraints.

3.3.5　古代方剂与新药方剂高频药组配情况分析

周忠眉,林宝德,肖青

首发于《漳州师范学院学报(自然科学版)》,2004,17(1):19-21

数据挖掘是从海量数据中获取知识的一种重要手段,高频集挖掘是数据挖掘的一种重要方法。本文通过挖掘古代方剂与新药方剂的高频药对,探讨古代方剂与新药方剂高频药组配异同情况。

3.3.6　数据挖掘在方剂配伍规律研究应用的探讨

周忠眉

首发于《漳州师范学院学报(自然科学版)》,2003,16(4):31-35

中医药学以其独特的强大优势,成为中华民族优秀文化及世界传统医学的重要组成部分。世界卫生组织已经把中医药纳入其管理体系,今年五月在日内瓦举行的世界卫生组织大会,也将传统医药的发展战略列入了议题。从国家层面上整体推动我国传统医学发展,已成为国家发展的主体战略目标之一。

中医药是中华民族的瑰宝,进行中医药的数据挖掘是中医药现代化研究的重要组成部分,是对中医药几千年沉淀的宝贵历史数据进行去伪存真、去粗取精的过程,也是更好地推进中医药的发展,保持其优势与特色的重要方法。中药配伍规律及方剂学是历代医学于临床遣药组方中经过千锤百炼的经验凝结,并升华为中医理论。中药复方的配伍规律是中医药的脊梁与灵魂。中药复方的配伍规律所研究的内容丰富多彩,包括药与药之间有相须、相使、相杀、相恶等关系,药物之间的十八反、十九畏内涵,药物在配伍中的地位——君臣佐使等内容。但是中药复方的配伍规律不能仅停留于传统的经验及理论,应该借用数据挖掘等高科技手段揭示其科学的内涵。

3.3.7　A Multi-Label Chinese Text Categorization System Based on Boosting Algorithm

Junli Chen, Xuezhong Zhou, Zhaohui Wu

首发于 *CIT*,2004:1153-1158

This paper presents a multi-label Chinese text categorization system based on Chinese character features and the boosting algorithm. This system has been successfully evaluated on the TCM-MED dataset provided by China Academy of Traditional Chinese Medicine (TCM) and the Reuters-21578 benchmark. We suggest that the TCM-MED dataset should be used as a standard corpus for the Chinese text categorization tasks. We have also carried out experiments to compare the performance of the boosting algorithm with two other traditional algorithms on the same datasets. The results indicate that for the design of a multi-label Chinese text categorization system, the boosting algorithm has a high performance and outperforms the other two algorithms.

3.3.8　方剂中配伍知识的发现

何前锋,崔蒙,吴朝晖,周雪忠,周忠眉

首发于《中国中医药信息杂志》,2004,11(7):655-658

　　数据挖掘是计算机处理大量数据、发掘有效知识的方法。高频集挖掘是数据挖掘中最基本的手段,在关联规则挖掘、相关关系挖掘、因果关系挖掘和多维模式挖掘中都起着重要的作用。笔者尝试利用高频集挖掘的方法,对中国方剂数据库、中药新药品种数据库、中药成方制剂标准数据库中各方剂药物组成数据进行了分析,并使用中国中药药对数据库中的药对组成与各方剂数据库中所得到的高频用药组合之间的数据进行了比较分析。

3.3.9　基于中药功效的聚类分析

何前锋,周雪忠,周忠眉,崔蒙,吴朝晖

首发于《中国中医药信息杂志》,2004,11(6):561-562

　　笔者使用数理统计的方法,采用较新的数据挖掘技术,对中药库中大量数据进行分析,研究的焦点转向组成方剂的单味药,从对单味药按照功效进行分类入手,逐步由简到繁探索方剂的配伍规律。

3.3.10　Distributional Character Clustering for Chinese Text Categorization

Xuezhong Zhou, Zhaohui Wu

首发于 *PRICAI*,2004,*LNAI* 3157:575-584

　　A novel feature generation method-distributional character clustering for Chinese text categorization, which avoids word segmentation, is presented and experimentally evaluated. We propose a hybrid clustering criterion function and bisecting divisive clustering algorithm to improve the quality of clusters. The experimental results show that distributional character clustering is an effective dimensionality reduction method, which reduces the feature space to very low dimensionality (e.g. 500 features) while maintaining high performance. The performance is much better than information gain. Moreover, Naïve Bayes classifier with distributional character clustering has state-of-the-art performance in Chinese text classification.

3.3.11　Text Mining for Finding Functional Community of Related Genes Using TCM Knowledge

Zhaohui Wu, Xuezhong Zhou, Baoyan Liu, Junli Chen

首发于 *PKDD*,2004,*LNAI* 3202:459-470

　　We present a novel text mining approach to uncovering the functional gene relationships, maybe, temporal and spatial functional modular interaction networks, from MEDLINE in large scale. Other than the regular approaches, which only consider the reductionistic molecular biological knowledge in MEDLINE, we use TCM knowledge (e.g. Symptom Complex) and the 50000 TCM bibliographic records to automatically congregate the related genes. A simple but efficient bootstrapping technique is used to extract the clinical disease names from TCM literature, and term co-occurrence is used to identify the disease-gene relationships in MEDLINE abstracts and titles. The underlying hypothesis is that the relevant genes of the same Symptom Complex will have some biological interactions. It is also a probing research to study the connection of TCM with modern biomedical and post-genomics studies by text mining. The preliminary results show that Symptom Complex gives a novel top-down view of functional genomics research, and it is a promising research field while connecting TCM with modern life science using text mining.

3.3.12　生物医学文献知识发现研究探讨及展望

周雪忠,吴朝晖,刘保延

首发于《复杂系统与复杂性科学》,2004,1(3):45-55

采用文本挖掘技术处理海量生物医学科技文献和文本注释型数据库,从而发现创新知识如基因、蛋白质、疾病、药物及其相互关系的研究是当前人工智能和数据挖掘领域研究的热点。本文对生物医学文献知识发现的研究内容、研究成果以及基于文本挖掘的关键技术诸方面进行了系统的分析和阐述。通过分析中医药学数据的特点,提出了基于文本挖掘的中医证候分子生物学知识发现研究。该方法的特点是综合利用中医药学文献和 MEDLINE,获得创新的证候与基因相关知识。初步实验表明,文本挖掘技术有望为证候的分子水平研究提供辅助和支撑手段。

3.3.13　Text Mining for Clinical Chinese Herbal Medical Knowledge Discovery

Xuezhong Zhou, Baoyan Liu, Zhaohui Wu

首发于 DS,2005,LNAI 3735:396-398

Chinese herbal medicine has been an effective therapy for healthcare and disease treatment. Large amount of TCM literature data has been curated in the last ten years, most of which is about the TCM clinical researches with herbal medicine. This paper develops text mining system named MeDisco/3T to extract the clinical Chinese medical formula data from literature, and discover the combination knowledge of herbal medicine by frequent itemset analysis. Over 18000 clinical Chinese medical formula are acquired, furthermore, significant frequent herbal medicine pairs and the family combination rule of herbal medicine have primarily been studied.

3.3.14　Multi-Label Text Categorization Using k-Nearest Neighbor Approach with M-Similarity

Yi Feng, Zhaohui Wu, Zhongmei Zhou

首发于 SPIRE,2005,LNCS 3772:155-160

Due to the ubiquity of textual information nowadays and the multitopic nature of text, it is of great necessity to explore multi-label text categorization problem. Traditional methods based on vector-space-model text representation suffer the losing of word order information. In this paper, texts are considered as symbol sequences. A multi-label lazy learning approach named kNN-M is proposed, which is derived from traditional k-nearest neighbor (kNN) method. The flexible order-semisensitive measure, M-Similarity, which enables the usage of sequence information in text by swap-allowed dynamic block matching, is applied to evaluate the closeness of texts on finding knearest neighbors in kNN-M. Experiments on real-world OHSUMED datasets illustrate that our approach outperforms existing ones considerably, showing the power of considering both term co-occurrence and order on text categorization tasks.

3.3.15 Efficiently Mining Both Association and Correlation Rules

Zhongmei Zhou, Zhaohui Wu, Chunshan Wang, Yi Feng

首发于 *FSKD*,2006,*LNAI* **4223**:369-372

Associated and correlated patterns cannot fully reflect association and correlation relationships between items like both association and correlation rules. Moreover, both association and correlation rule mining can find such type of rules,"the conditional probability that a customer purchasing A is likely to also purchase B is not only greater than the given threshold, but also significantly greater than the probability that a customer purchases only B. In other words, the sale of A can increase the likelihood of the sale of B." Therefore, in this paper, we combine association with correlation in the mining process to discover both association and correlation rules. A new notion of a both association and correlation rule is given and an algorithm is developed for discovering all both association and correlation rules. Our experimental results show that the mining combined association with correlation is quite a good approach to discovering both association and correlation rules.

3.3.16 Efficiently Mining Maximal Frequent Mutually Associated Patterns

Zhongmei Zhou, Zhaohui Wu, Chunshan Wang, Yi Feng

首发于 *ADMA*,2006,*LNAI* **4093**:110-117

Mutually associated pattern mining can find such type of patterns whose any two sub-patterns are associated. However, like frequent pattern mining, when the minimum association threshold is set to be low, it still generates a large number of mutually associated patterns. The huge number of patterns produced not only reduces the mining efficiency, but also makes it very difficult for a human user to analyze in order to identify interesting/useful ones. In this paper, a new task of maximal frequent mutually associated pattern mining is proposed, which can dramatically decrease the number of patterns produced without information loss due to the downward closure property of the association measure and meanwhile improve the mining efficiency. Experimental results show that maximal frequent mutually associated pattern mining is quite a necessary approach to lessening the number of results and increasing the performance of the algorithm. Also, experimental results show that the techniques developed are much effective especially for very large and dense datasets.

3.3.17 Efficiently Mining Mutually and Positively Correlated Patterns

Zhongmei Zhou, Zhaohui Wu, Chunshan Wang, Yi Feng

首发于 *ADMA*,2006,*LNAI* **4093**:118-125

Positive correlation mining can find such type of patterns,"the conditional probability that a customer purchasing A is likely to also purchase B is not only great enough, but also significantly greater than the probability that a customer purchases only B."However, there often exist many independence relationships between items in a correlated pattern due to the definition of a correlated pattern. Therefore, we mine mutually and positively correlated patterns, whose any two sub-patterns are both associated and positively correlated. A new correlation interestingness measure is proposed for rationally evaluating the correlation degree. In order to improve the mining efficiency, we combine association with correlation and use not only the correlation measure but also the association measure in the mining process. Our experimental results show that mutually and positively correlated pattern mining is a good approach to discovering patterns which can reflect both association and positive correlation relationships between items at the same time. Meanwhile, our experimental results show that the mining combined association with correlation is quite a valid method to decrease the execution time.

3.3.18　Mining Both Associated and Correlated Patterns

Zhongmei Zhou, Zhaohui Wu, Chunshan Wang, Yi Feng

首发于 *ICCS*, 2006, *LNCS* 3994:468-475

Association mining cannot find such type of patterns, "the conditional probability that a customer purchasing *A* is likely to also purchase *B* is not only greater than the given threshold, but also much greater than the probability that a customer purchases only *B*. In other words, the sale of *A* can increase the likelihood of the sale of *B*." Such kind of patterns are both associated and correlated. Therefore, in this paper, we combine association with correlation in the mining process to discover both associated and correlated patterns. A new interesting measure corr-confidence is proposed for rationally evaluating the correlation relationships. This measure not only has proper bounds for effectively evaluating the correlation degree of patterns, but also is suitable for mining long patterns. Our experimental results show that the mining combined association with correlation is quite a valid approach to discovering both associated and correlated patterns.

3.3.19　Complex Network Analysis on TCMLS Sub-Ontologies

Jun Ma, Huajun Chen

首发于 *SKG*, 2007:551-553

TCMLS is the largest Traditional Chinese Medicine ontology all over the world. This paper surveys the topology of TCMLS sub-ontologies in complex networks way. The result indicates that the network, composed of concepts and instances, displays both patterns of small-world and scale-free.

3.3.20　Integrative Mining of Traditional Chinese Medicine Literature and MEDLINE for Functional Gene Networks

Xuezhong Zhou, Baoyan Liu, Zhaohui Wu, Yi Feng

首发于 *Artificial Intelligence in Medicine*, 2007, 41(2):87-104

Objective: The amount of biomedical data indifferent disciplines is growing at an exponential rate. Integrating these significant knowledge sources to generate novel hypotheses for systems biology research is difficult. Traditional Chinese medicine (TCM) is a completely different discipline, and is a complementary knowledge system to modern biomedical science. This paper uses a significant TCM bibliographic literature database in China, together with MEDLINE, to help discover novel gene functional knowledge.

Materials and methods: We present an integrative mining approach to uncover the functional gene relationships from MEDLINE and TCM bibliographic literature. This paper introduces TCM literature (about 50000 records) as one knowledge source for constructing literature-based gene networks. We use the TCM diagnosis, TCM syndrome, to automatically congregate the related genes. The syndrome-gene relationships are discovered based on the syndrome-disease relationships extracted from TCM literature and the disease-gene relationships in MEDLINE. Based on the bubble bootstrapping and relation weight computing methods, we have developed a prototype system called MeDisco/3S, which has name entity and relation extraction, and online analytical processing (OLAP) capabilities, to perform the integrative mining process.

Results: We have got about 200000 syndrome-gene relations, which could help generate syndrome-based gene networks, and help analyze the functional knowledge of genes from syndrome perspective. We take the gene network of Kidney-Yang Deficiency syndrome (KYD syndrome) and the functional analysis of some genes, such as CRH (corticotropin releasing hormone), PTH (parathyroid hormone), PRL (prolactin), BRCA1 (breast cancer 1, early onset) and BRCA (breast cancer 2, early onset), to demonstrate the preliminary results. The underlying hypothesis is that the related genes of the same syndrome will have some biological functional relationships, and will constitute a functional network.

Conclusion: This paper presents an approach to integrating TCM literature and modern biomedical data to discover novel gene networks and functional knowledge of genes. The preliminary results show that the novel gene functional knowledge and gene networks, which are worthy of further investigation, could be generated by integrating the two complementary biomedical data sources. It will be a promising research field through integrative mining of TCM and modern life science literature.

3.3.21 Information Retrieval and Knowledge Discovery on the Semantic Web of Traditional Chinese Medicine

Zhaohui Wu, Tong Yu, Huajun Chen
首发于 *WWW*, 2008: 1085-1086

We conduct the first systematical adoption of the Semantic Web solution in the integration, management, and utilization of TCM information and knowledge resources. As the results, the largest TCM Semantic Web ontology is engineered as the uniform knowledge representation mechanism; the ontology-based query and search engine is deployed, mapping legacy and heterogeneous relational databases to the Semantic Web layer for query and search across database boundaries; the first global herb-drug interaction network is mapped through semantic integration, and the semantic graph mining methodology is implemented for discovering and interpreting interesting patterns from this network. The platform and underlying methodology are proved effective in TCM-related drug usage, discovery, and safety analysis.

3.3.22 Semantic Web for Integrated Network Analysis in Biomedicine

Huajun Chen, Li Ding, Zhaohui Wu, Tong Yu, Lavanya Dhanapalan, Jake Y. Chen
首发于 *Briefings In Bioinformatics*, 2009, 10(2): 177-192

The Semantic Web technology enables integration of heterogeneous data on the World Wide Web by making the semantics of data explicit through formal ontologies. In this article, we survey the feasibility and state of the art of utilizing the Semantic Web technology to represent, integrate and analyze the knowledge in various biomedical networks. We introduce a new conceptual framework, semantic graph mining, to enable researchers to integrate graph mining with ontology reasoning in network data analysis. Through four case studies, we demonstrate how semantic graph mining can be applied to the analysis of disease-causal genes, Gene Ontology category cross-talks, drug efficacy analysis and herb-drug interactions analysis.

3.3.23　MapReduce-Based Pattern Finding Algorithm Applied in Motif Detection for Prescription Compatibility Network

Yang Liu, Xiaohong Jiang, Huajun Chen, Jun Ma, Xiangyu Zhang
首发于 *APPT*,2009,*LNCS* 5737:341-355

Network motifs are basic building blocks in complex networks. Motif detection has recently attracted much attention as a topic to uncover structural design principles of complex networks. Pattern finding is the most computationally expensive step in the process of motif detection. In this paper, we design a pattern finding algorithm based on Google MapReduce to improve the efficiency. Performance evaluation shows that our algorithm can facilitate the detection of larger motifs in large-size networks and has good scalability. We apply it in the prescription network and find some commonly used prescription network motifs that provide the possibility to further discover the law of prescription compatibility.

3.3.24　Collaborative Semantic Association Discovery from Linked Data

Qingzhao Zheng, Huajun Chen, Tong Yu, Gang Pan
首发于 *IRI*,2009:394-399

The efforts of publishing and interlinking structured data on the Semantic Web will result in a global network of databases, or the Linked Data, which provides huge potential for discovering hidden relationships. We present a multi-agent framework for Semantic Associations Discovery (SAD) from distributed linked data on the Semantic Web. Here, agents collaborate in SAD by publishing inter-dependent hypotheses and evidences, giving rise to an evidentiary network that connects and ranks diverse knowledge elements. We evaluate this framework through simulation, and the results show that the framework is suitable in cross-domain relationship discovery tasks.

3.3.25　一种稳定的并行分布式频繁集挖掘算法及其应用

秘中凯,姜晓红,雷蕾
首发于《计算机应用与软件》,2011,28(3):83-85,124

为解决大规模医药数据分析中的频繁集挖掘问题,提出一种稳定且具有良好扩展性的并行分布式算法 P-FIM。该算法将挖掘任务分割成无相互依赖关系的同构子任务,实现有效的并行计算;并且充分利用 Map/Reduce 框架和集群环境的优势,提高自身的鲁棒性和负载均衡能力。采用最大规模 512 万条记录的中医药方剂数据进行算法性能分析实验,其结果表明,该算法在分布式集群环境中表现稳定,随着集群规模的增加,其加速比接近线性。以 P-FIM 算法为基础设计实现的中医药数据相关性分析方案,可有效地从大规模临床数据中获得全面、可靠的病、症、药间相关性的信息。

3.3.26 An Intelligent Medicine Recommender System Framework

Youjun Bao, Xiaohong Jiang

首发于 *ICIEA*,2016:1383-1388

More and more people are caring about the health and medical diagnosis problems. However, according to the administration's report, more than 200 thousand people in China, even 100 thousand in USA, die each year due to medication errors. More than 42% medication errors are caused by doctors because experts write the prescription according to their experience which is quite limited. Technologies as data mining and recommender technologies provide possibilities to explore potential knowledge from diagnosis history records and help doctors to prescribe medication correctly to decrease medication errors effectively. In this paper, we design and implement a universal medicine recommender system framework that applies data mining technologies to the recommendation system. The medicine recommender system consists of database system module, data preparation module, recommendation model module, model evaluation, and data visualization module. We investigate the medicine recommendation algorithms of the SVM (Support Vector Machine), BP neural network algorithm and ID3 decision tree algorithm based on the diagnosis data. Experiments are done to tune the parameters for each algorithm to get better performance. Finally, in the given open dataset, SVM recommendation model is selected for the medicine recommendation module to obtain a good trade-off among model accuracy, model efficiency, and model scalability. We also propose a mistake-check mechanism to ensure the diagnosis accuracy and service quality. Experimental results show our system can give medication recommendation with excellent efficiency, accuracy and scalability.

3.4 学术著作

本节主要介绍了中医药数据挖掘与知识发现方向 2 部相关著作(为同一内容的中英文两个版本),即 2008 年由 Springer 和浙江大学出版社联合出版的 *Semantic Grid:Model,Methodology, and Applications*,以及 2008 年由浙江大学出版社出版的《语义网格:模型、方法与应用》,摘录了其前言和一级目录信息。

3.4.1 Semantic Grid:Model,Methodology,and Applications

Zhaohui Wu,Huajun Chen

首发于 **Springer 和浙江大学出版社,2008**

Preface

The Internet has been an indispensable means of communication in our daily life. We rely upon it to communicate with others, search information to procure a solution to a knotty problem, book tickets to arrange our trips, look for business opportunities, entertain ourselves, and so forth. Without the Internet our life would have been a largely different one. However, has the Internet reached its full potential?Can it change our life more than we have seen?What will the Internet and the Web look like 20 years later?

A plurality of researchers from different areas have been working on these issues for a long time. At the fore, two distinguished and influential ones are Grid Computing and the Semantic Web.

The term the Grid was first used around 1990 as a metaphor for making the use of computer power as easy as the electric power Grid. It was originally coined as a new paradigm for solving computation-intensive problems by taking advantage of the computation power of idling computers, which could be a super computer or just a desktop computer. Grids were then described as well-organized virtual systems that may span across many organizational boundaries. Grid applications feature in the capability of the dynamic formation of cross-institutional Virtual Organizations in an *ad hoc* way to enable coordinated resource sharing and problem-solving across multiple administrative domains on the Internet.

The term Semantic Web was coined around 1998 by the web inventor Tim Berners Lee. It aims at leading the Web to its full potential by making its content machine-understandable. It draws on the standardization effort of a formal representation framework and advanced web languages such as RDF/OWL that can be used to enrich web resources with semantic descriptions and describe complex semantic relations among them. The semantic theory underlying this formal representation framework provides a formal account of meaning in which the logical relationship of web resources, which can be a webpage, a database record, a program, a web service, and so forth, can be explicitly described and specified without loss of the original meaning. This makes the web smarter and more intelligent, thereby enabling more sensible searches, far more accurate information retrieval, and seamless information integration.

Basically, Grids are concerned with the design and development of the architecture of the future Internet. Their ultimate goal is to provide a flexible, adaptive, manageable, service-oriented architecture for future Internet-based applications. Meanwhile, the Semantic Web looks at the semantic heterogeneity issue that has hindered almost all integration systems in the perspective of information representation. Although these two technologies offer different solutions, they actually complement each other. The concept of the Semantic Grid was then brought up by many researchers with the intention of combining them together to address many difficult problems that cannot be resolved by only one of them.

Commonly, the *Semantic Grid* refers to a branch subject under the umbrella of *Grid Computing* in which computing resources and services are described in a meaningful way that can be discovered, aggregated, joined up more readily and automatically. The description typically draws upon the technology of the Semantic Web, such as the Resource Description Framework (RDF) and Web Ontology Language (OWL). It is stated that the semantic grid, as a combination of the technologies from both grid computing and the semantic web, would provide a promising alternative for developing a future interconnection environment, particularly geared to enable highly selective resource sharing, very sensible knowledge discovery and collective intelligence.

As a synthesis of many different technologies, the Semantic Grid has a broad spectrum of topics. The book attempts to give a comprehensive introduction of these topics, including knowledge representation and semantic description for semantic grid applications, semantic-based data integration, grid service management and process orchestration, trust management in grids, ontology management for problem solving in the semantic grid, and integrative knowledge discovery based on the integration capability of the semantic grid.

How to use this book. This book can be a reference book for researchers in Internet-related technologies. Generally, the topics in Chapters 2—4 are introduced in a fundamental way, while the ones in Chapters 5—8 are presented from an applied perspective. Moreover, Chapters 9, 10 are devoted to the experience of applying specific semantic grid technology to two typical application domains: the life science domain and an intelligent transportation system. Specifically, this book is organized in the following structure:

- Chapter 2 describes the relationship between knowledge representation and the semantic grid. The semantic web languages largely draw upon the fruits of the long-standing research on knowledge representation in the area of artificial intelligence. A good information representational framework is vital for a smarter and more intelligent grid system. For example, grid resource discovery relies upon a better description of the resources and the relationships between them. Rules are useful for specifying mappings, coordination policy, security settings, transaction configurations, and trust dependencies for grid applications.

- Chapter 3 describes typical issues such as sub-ontology management for a problem solving in the Semantic Grid. With the Semantic Grid as the problem solving environment, we will face many unexpected problems as in traditional problem solving. The problems to be solved are often complex and refer to large-scale domain knowledge from crossover disciplines. This chapter focuses on how to manage and reuse ontology that embodies domain knowledge based on the infrastructure of the Semantic Grid.

- Chapter 4 mentions an important issue: trust management in the Semantic Grid. Enabling trust to ensure more effective and efficient interaction is at the heart of the Semantic Grid vision. This chapter presents an integrated computational trust model based on statistical decision theory and Bayesian sequential analysis. The model helps users to select an appropriate service provider within the Semantic Grid environment.

- Chapter 5 introduces specific technology that can be used for semantic data integration in the Semantic Grid, with particular emphasis on integrating relational databases with semantic web ontologies. Integrating legacy relational databases is important for both Grid and Semantic Web applications. However, experience in building such applications has revealed a gap between semantic web languages and the relational data model. This chapter presents an intelligent framework with a formal mapping system to bridge the gap, and studies the problem of reasoning and query answering using the semantic view of the mapping system.

- Chapter 6 provides a comprehensive introduction to service management in the Semantic Grid including service description, service orchestration, service discovery, service composition, and so on. How to collaborate, cooperate and co-experiment conveniently and efficiently in the grid environment has become a hot topic in the research and application of the grid, and service flow management will be the key technology in solving the problem.

- Chapter 7 proposes the general ideas and the preliminary implementation of knowledge discovery in the Semantic Grid, with the emphasis on mining based semantic integration. The Semantic Grid provides a new computational environment, and also a new architecture for data mining. The dynamic extension of the algorithm, the transparent integration of data, and the circular refinement of knowledge, are main characteristics of knowledge discovery using such architecture, as high-level services of the Semantic Grid, data mining and knowledge discovery greatly enhance the effectiveness of the Semantic Grid.

• Chapter 8 presents a semantic grid platform called DartGrid. The Semantic Grid combines many technologies coming from the Grids, the Web Service and the Semantic Web. Organic integration of these technologies that are actually complement each other can result in competent implementation for both Grid and Semantic Web applications. This chapter presents a semantic grid implementation, called DartGrid, which is made up of several components that are intended to support data integration and service management in Grids.

• Chapter 9 introduces the application of the specific technology of the Semantic Grid in building an e-Science environment for the Traditional Chinese Medicine community from the perspectives of knowledge engineering, data integration, and knowledge discovery.

• Chapter 10 introduces the attempted application in an intelligent transportation system, the goal of which is to build an integrated intelligent transportation information and service platform, to integrate traffic data resources and cooperate with existing ITS subsystems and services.

The book is the result of several years of study, research and development of the faculties, PhD candidates and many others affiliated to the CCNT Lab of Zhejiang University. We would like to give particular thanks to Yuxin Mao, Xiaoqing Zheng, Shuiguang Deng, Yi Feng, Yu Zhang, Chunyin Zhou, Tong Yu, Wei Shi, Guozhou Zheng, Jian Wu who have devoted their energy and enthusiasm to the book and relevant projects.

In addition, the work in this book was mainly sponsored by the China 973 project of the Semantic Grid initiative (No. 2003CB317006), the National Science Fund for Distinguished Young Scholars of China NSF Program (No. NSFC60533040), the Program for New Century Excellent Talents in University of the Ministry of Education of China (No. NCET-04-0545). The work was also partially supported by the National Program for Modern Service Industry (2006BAH02401), the Program for Changjiang Scholar (IRT0652) and the NSFC Program under Grant No. NSFC60503018 and NSFC60603025.

The Semantic Grid is still an undergoing area of rapid development. Although this book cannot give a complete account of all issues and topics, we hope it can shed some light on the most important aspects relevant to the future Internet and can be valuable for those who are interested in the future development of the amazing Internet technology.

Contents

3.4.2 语义网格:模型、方法与应用

吴朝晖,陈华钧

首发于浙江大学出版社,2008

前言

随着互联网的发展与普及,以智能分布式的方式协同共享与集成管理海量的网络信息资源,已经成为一个十分突出的难题和亟待解决的问题。语义网格作为网格计算的一个分支,用一种包含语义的方式描述各类网格资源,使之更加易于被发现、聚合和连接。这种资源描述通常是基于语义Web的关键技术如 RDF 和 OWL 来实现的。语义网格将以语义 Web 为代表的语义技术和以网格计算为代表的体系架构技术结合起来,为下一代互联网提供了开放、安全、有序、可扩展的管理体系架构,并支持解决和实现复杂网络环境下跨多个机构的大规模分布式协同计算与信息共享问题。

语义网格作为网格计算和语义 Web 的交叉技术,为未来互联网环境的发展提供了新的思路、技术和方法。本书针对这一发展趋势进行了有益的探讨与探索,并对语义网格所涉及的一些主要问题展开了广泛的讨论。具体而言,重点针对语义网格中的语义表达与知识表示方法、语义网格中的数据集成与管理、基于语义的流程组合与服务拼接、语义网格中的信任管理与问题求解,以及基于语义网格的数据挖掘与知识发现等问题,进行了分析和探讨。最后,综合理论探索和应用研究,探讨了语义网格中的各种技术如何被实际应用到医学信息学和智能交通管理系统。

本书第 1 章介绍了语义网格的概念和发展历程。第 2、3、4 章从理论方法和模型的角度探讨了语义网格相关的核心问题,比如第 2 章从人工智能知识表达领域出发,阐明了知识表达技术是语义网格的核心技术之一,是人工智能技术在互联网领域的重要应用。第 3 章探讨了语义网格环境下的复杂问题求解。第 4 章提出了一个语义网格中的分布式信任计算模型。第 5、6、7、8 章从关键技术的角度对语义网格进行了介绍。第 5、6 章介绍了基于语义的数据库网格技术,即如何在语义网格中整合和管理跨多个机构的数据库资源。其中的一些关键技术包括语义映射技术、语义注册技术、语义查询重写技术等。第 7 章介绍了基于语义的服务流程发现与组合技术,即如何在语义网格中整合跨多个机构的流程服务资源。其中的一些关键技术包括服务流程的语义组合、基于语义的服务发现等。第 8 章介绍了语义网格中的数据挖掘与知识发现。第 9 章从数据管理、流程组合和消息中间件三个方面介绍了一个称为 DartGrid 的语义网格平台系统。第 10、11 章分别介绍了语义网格的中医药应用和在 ITS 智能交通系统中的应用,从应用的角度具体介绍了语义网格的相关关键技术的潜在应用价值。

本书是经过浙江大学 CCNT 实验室的众多科研人员多年学习、研究和工程实践沉淀的成果。参与本书工作的人员包括郑骁庆、毛郁欣、周春英、张宇、邓水光、封毅、于彤、郑国轴、施伟、吴健等。在此对他们表示衷心的感谢。

本书所介绍的工作主要得到了国家自然科学基金杰出青年基金"智能空间的语义模型与行为感知认证"(No. NSFC60533040)、国家"973"计划语义网格专项子项目"语义网格在中医药知识共享与服务中的应用"(No. 2003CB317006)、教育部新世纪人才计划"面向普适计算的嵌入式语义网格及若干关键技术研究"(No. NCET-04-0545)和现代服务业服务基础技术研究(2006BAH02A01)项目的资

助;此外,参与本书相关项目的其他研究人员还得到了长江学者和创新团队发展计划资助(IRT0652)、国家"863"高科技发展计划(No. 2006AA01A122)、国家自然科学基金项目(NSF60503018,NSF60603025)、国防预研(No.060651306030101,No.9140A06060307JW0403,No.A1420060153)等的资助;本书的出版得到"国家科学技术学术著作出版基金"的资助。在此,一并表示感谢。

语义网格是当前处于科学前沿的论题,许多理论和思想还处于探索阶段,由于作者的水平和经验有限,错误和不妥之处在所难免,恳请读者给予批评指正,共同推进下一代互联网技术研究的进步与发展。

目录

3.5　发明专利

本节摘录了中医药数据挖掘与知识发现方向 6 项相关发明专利(于 2010—2020 年得到授权)。

3.5.1　一种基于复杂网络的压缩空间高效搜索方法

吴朝晖,张宇,陈华钧

专利号:ZL200810121364.X;授权公告号:CN101388024B;授权公告日:2010-11-10

本发明涉及一种基于复杂网络的压缩空间高效搜索方法。该方法在复杂网络中挖掘出影响力较大的核心节点作为初始活跃节点,然后根据网络有向边上的影响力权重继续激活网络中的其他节点,从而使得尽可能多的节点被激活。这个问题可以转化为图论中的网络覆盖最大化问题,在数学上已经被证明是 NP 难问题。在复杂网络中,不同的参数度量方法只能考察复杂网络某一方面的特性,因此本发明提出了一种基于启发信息的压缩空间搜索算法,通过普通贪心算法、爬山算法、高入度启发信息算法的预先处理,在全局范围中选出三个有序最优结点集,合并成一个混沌的候选结点集,并补充加入上述三种算法的次优结点集,构成一个在有效时间内可以进行完全枚举的候选结点全集。本发明的搜索算法将一个巨大、松散、带有极大冗余信息的原解空间,压缩成一个计算机可处理的、集中的、带有高启发信息的另一个解空间,从而保证最大可能地找出一组较优解。

3.5.2　用于分析中医方剂药物组配规律的泛化关联规则挖掘方法

吴朝晖,于彤,封毅,姜晓红

专利号:ZL200710156365.3;授权公告号:CN101149751B;授权公告日:2012-06-06

本发明公开了一种用于分析中医方剂药物组配规律的泛化关联规则挖掘方法。该方法实质上是一种结合关联规则挖掘和领域知识表示的泛化关联规则挖掘方法,它将语义万维网技术作为领域知识表示的主要手段。该方法涉及一个知识发现器,该装置利用领域知识库所提供的术语系统和领域规则完成数据挖掘过程,并将挖掘结果以知识提案的形式提交领域知识库,由领域专家进行验证和评价。其中的数据挖掘过程包括:首先,从中医方剂学数据源中提取所需数据;其次,在数据中挖掘有意义的频繁模式并进行语义标注;最后,根据被标注模式进行泛化规则的提取和推理。其中,使用语义万维网技术构建领域知识库,实现信息和知识在该方法所涉及的部件之间的传递。

3.5.3　基于操作流的异步交互式数据挖掘系统及方法

吴朝晖,吴毅挺,秘中凯,付志宏,封毅,姜晓红,陈华钧

专利号:ZL200810060418.6;授权公告号:CN101276371B;授权公告日:2012-12-05

本发明涉及 AJAX 领域和数据挖掘集成技术领域,公开了一种基于操作流的异步交互式数据挖掘系统(包括客户端和服务器端),客户端采用 GWT-EXT 构建 AJAX 用户界面;服务端架设在 Web 容器上,包括以下几个模块:基于语义集成的分布式数据库模块,操作符参数模块,用户管理模块,Rapid Miner 内核模块。本发明具有无须安装软件、使用方便的优点。

3.5.4　基于 LDA 主题模型的中医药数据挖掘方法

姜晓红,严海明,商任翔,吴朝晖,陈英芝

专利号:ZL201310276021.1;授权公告号:CN103365978B;授权公告日:2017-03-29

本发明涉及中医药信息检索领域,公开了一种基于 LDA 主题模型的中医药数据挖掘方法,包括以下具体步骤:①先在 LDA 模型中确定处方-主题和主题-药剂两组先验,处方-主题和主题-药剂分别由超参数 α 和 β 确定,使用 AS 方式对两组先验进行先验假设;②确定 LDA 模型中的主题数目;③采用 Gibbs 采样方法对上述 LDA 模型进行求解;④生成 LDA 模型的语义 RDF 文档,将 LDA 模型的结果映射至四元组,并用语义 RDF 文档进行表示;⑤将药剂和处方进行关联,建立处方-主题-药剂的可视化结构网络。本发明适用于海量中药处方的处理和挖掘,可以得到可视化的结构模型。

3.5.5　一种获取多维数据稳定性的方法和系统

吴朝晖,包友军,姜晓红,毛宇,陈英芝

专利号:ZL201510100623.0;授权公告号:CN104731875B;授权公告日:2018-04-17

本发明适用于数据处理领域,提供了一种获取多维数据稳定性的方法和系统。所述方法包括:获取连续型多维数据;将所述连续型多维数据处理为低维数据;对所述低维数据进行均值分析,获取距离向量;对所述距离向量进行显著性分析,获取超半径 $r1$ 和 $r2$;通过预设的数据稳定性判断模型对所述多维数据进行稳定性评估。计算均值点到各个数据点的欧式距离,欧式距离的计算考虑所有的维度,并根据显著性要求计算出 $r1$ 和 $r2$,使得方法的扩展性很好。当数据集的维度非常高时,可以采用 PCA 降维方法对数据进行降维。

3.5.6 一种中医病情文本相似度的计算方法

姜晓红,付钊,陈广,杜定益,吴朝晖

专利号:ZL201810359667.9;授权公告号:CN108647203B;授权公告日:2020-07-07

本发明公开了一种中医病情文本相似度的计算方法,包括:基于规则和统计的短语识别,得到文本块;文本块划分,得到文本语义分块;计算文本语义分块的权值;计算文本语义分块向量;组合文本语义分块特征,得到病情文档特征;根据病情文档特征,计算文本相似度。本发明以文本语义分块为最小粒度来表示病情文本特征,将病情文本按照所描述的病位划分为文本语义分块,并赋予各个文本语义分块不同的权重来区分主次症状,通过计算文本语义分块向量夹角的余弦值找出两段病情文本的相似症状,最后按照权重进行加权,得出两段病情文本的相似度,克服了传统文本相似度计算方法或丢失语义信息,或不能突出病因主次的缺点。

第4章　中医药云平台与服务计算

云计算是分布式计算、并行计算和网格计算的进一步发展,云平台能够组合大量资源,如各种类型的基础设施、数据资源、平台软件、存储系统等,组成一个可共享的庞大资源池,使上层应用通过这个资源池获取想要的各种服务。云计算为实现大规模计算资源、存储资源、数据资源、软件资源和知识资源的集成共享服务提供了一种理想的解决方案,为中医药信息共享进一步提升为跨域的中医药知识服务提供了技术基础。

中医药产业发展,需要整合基础研究科研院所、临床诊疗医院、中药生产企业、社区健康服务等整个中医药产业链的数据、信息和知识资源,因此建设基于语义云平台的跨行业的中医药知识服务大平台,提供跨界知识服务,对于推进中医药产业发展以及提升中医药监管能力和效率,都具有重要意义。

中医药智能计算研究团队在知识服务平台方面的研究工作也是随着技术的发展而变化的,从最初的数据库网格技术,到数据挖掘和知识发现,最后走向基于云平台的跨域知识服务平台。起初我们主要解决异质异构数据库的集成和共享问题,开发了 DartGrid 原型系统;在此基础上,构建知识库网格,使得在中医药领域的专家、学者、企业可以在集成的 TCM 数据网格上实现知识发现和共享;随着语义网技术的兴起,我们又开发了基于 Web 的语义本体的协同加工平台,支持中国中医科学院中医药信息研究所进行中医药领域的本体建设;之后又建设了基于语义网格的中医药科学数据平台。

在中医药云平台与服务计算研究中,我们着重从以下几个方面进行了研究。

(1)语义网格关键技术

研究了语义网格的关键技术,提出了知识服务平台的体系架构,包括资源的一体化平台、信息服务、知识服务引擎,支持上层包括的中医药知识服务应用。早在 2003 年就开始研究基于语义网的知识库系统,提出了通用的知识库网格架构[1]和知识库网格模型[2]。同时研究了数据库网格安全架构、基于语义的消息通信机制、语义网的可信任问题以及跨域协同和网络监控问题[3-8]。

[1] Wu Z, Chen H, Xu J. Knowledge base grid: A generic grid architecture for semantic web[J]. Journal of Computer Science and Technology,2003,18(4):462-473.

主要研究了基于语义网构建大规模知识库系统的技术。提出了一种通用的知识库网格(KB-Grid)架构来组织、发现、利用、管理 Web 上的知识库资源。KB-Grid 由四个主要部分构成:语义浏览器可以搜索浏览语义信息,知识服务器起到 Web 知识容器的作用,本体服务器用于管理 Web 本体,知识库目录服务器用于知识库的注册和分类。同时为实现知识库网格上的语义通信定义了知识服务的参考模型。为验证此架构,实现了一个中医药知识库网格。

[2] 徐杰锋.知识库网格模型的研究[D].杭州:浙江大学,2004.

主要研究了知识库网格的核心关键技术。定义了知识库网格 DartGrid/KG 的抽象服务模型和核心协议。抽象模型包括语义浏览器、知识服务器、本体论服务器和知识库目录服务器。核心协议则包括语义注册协议、本体论查询协议、本体论验证协议和融合协议。

[3] 王闰.基于 GSI 的数据库网格安全基础架构[D].杭州:浙江大学,2006.

主要研究了面向数据库资源的网格安全技术,针对动态开放的数据库网络环境下资源共享和协作过程中确保信息安全的应用背景,提出了一套面向数据库资源的网格安全基础架构 DGSI 模型。介绍了授权、验证、信任等安全问题协议,并实现了协议的原型 Dart-DGSI。

[4] 叶志勇.基于语义的消息中间件 DART MQ[D].杭州:浙江大学,2006.

主要研究了异构网络环境下的分布式应用的消息中间件技术。提出并实现了一种基于 RDF 图的统一事件(消息)概念模型 Dart MQ,该模型支持包括关系数据结构、树型结构、图结构等各种格式的事件,以集成各种系统的异构消息。同时还设计了动态事件代理、动态的网络传输架构以适应各种不同的应用场景。

[5] Zheng X,Wu Z,Chen H,et al. A scalable probabilistic approach to trust evaluation [C]//4th International Conference on Trust Management (iTrust'2006),2006,LNCS 3986:423-438.

主要研究了语义网的可信任问题。提出了一种可扩展的概率信任评估方法,该方法综合了多种信息来源,在信任评估过程中考虑了四种成本(运营成本、机会成本、服务成本和咨询费用)和效用。该方法给予信任一个严格的概率解释,可帮助用户更好地根据自己的喜好选择合适的服务提供商。通过形式化的鲁棒性分析,检验了该方法的性能。

[6] Zheng X,Wu Z,Chen H,et al. Developing a composite trust model for multi-agent systems[C]//5th International Joint Conference on Autonomous Agents and Multiagent Systems (AAMAS'2006),2006:1257-1259.

主要研究了语义网的信任技术。提出了一种基于统计决策理论和贝叶斯序列分析的复合信任模型,以平衡信任评估过程中的成本和收益,并结合多种信息来源,帮助用户根据自己的选择做出正确的决策偏好。本文提出的模型从概率论的角度对信任进行了严格的数学解释。

[7] 张露.基于虚拟组织的大规模跨域协同平台及应用[D].杭州:浙江大学,2011.

主要研究了基于网格技术的跨域协同平台技术,设计了三层体系架构无缝、低耦合集成已有业务系统;提出了虚拟组织的新定义和跨域协同平台的安全模型;通过 OWL-S 给虚拟组织增加语义信息,设计实现基于角色授权证书的安全认证和基于角色的资源访问控制机制。实现了一个跨域协同原型平台。

[8] 张湘豫.基于云架构的高性能大规模网格监控系统的设计与实现[D].杭州:浙江大学,2012.

主要研究了基于云架构的高性能大规模网格监控系统技术。介绍了系统的详细设计与实现,重点介绍了基于 MongoDB 的海量监控数据存储技术。该技术支持高并发的读写请求,提供丰富的查询和检索接口,具有良好的可扩展性。还研究了基于一致性哈希的高效资源聚合技术。

(2)语义网格及中医药知识服务平台

研发了中医药语义网格服务平台 DartGrid，该平台包括 DartGrid 核心基础模块、DartQuery 语义查询系统、DartSearch 语义搜索系统、DartMapper 语义映射系统、DartSpora 数据挖掘系统，以及 Dart-Mashup 数据混搭系统等。平台能够动态集成大规模异质异构的数据库资源，实现虚拟组织的协同共建和数据共享。团队经历了早期的数据库网格技术，又融入到语义网技术的发展历程，开发了不同版本的 DartGrid，见文献[9-15]。研发成果总结在专著[16]中。基于中医药科学数据共享平台开发了知识服务平台原型系统，提供多层次的服务(包括中医药基础设施一体化服务、中医药信息共享服务、中医药知识服务、中医药知识社区服务以及中医药智能问答服务[17-21])。

[9] Chen H，Wu Z，Huang C，*et al*. TCM-Grid：Weaving a medical grid for traditional Chinese medicine[C]//International Conference on Computational Science（ICCS'2003），2003：1143-1152.

主要设计实现了中医药网格 TCM-Grid。目的是构建一个分布式系统，集成地理上分布的 TCM 信息和知识库，帮助实现健康专家、研究者、企业和个人共享中医药信息和知识。采用的方法是开发数据库网格以实现 TCM 数据库的集成、发现和细粒度共享；用知识库网格支持知识密集任务，同时由网格本体来实现网格智能。

[10] Xu J，Chen H，Wu Z. Knowledge Base Grid and its application in traditional Chinese Medicine[C]// 2003 IEEE International Conference on Systems，Man and Cybernetics（SMC'2003），IEEE，2003：2477-2482.

主要研究了一种通用的知识库网格技术并应用于中医药领域。该知识库网格由三大主要部分组成：虚拟开放知识库、知识库索引、支持 TCM 概念浏览和知识管理的语义浏览器。介绍了系统实现所用的知识表示方法和服务层次结构。

[11] 黄昶.Database Grid：面向网格的数据库资源管理平台[D]. 杭州：浙江大学，2004.

主要研究了动态开放的网络环境下的数据库网格关键技术。针对网格应用的数据管理需求，提出了一套解决数据库资源访问、语义发现、动态整合等一系列网格资源管理问题的解决方案。介绍了数据库网格原型系统以及在中医药领域的应用测试。

[12] 王恒.DartGrid V3 语义数据库网格的设计与核心模块实现[D]. 杭州：浙江大学，2006.

主要研究了通过重用和调整历史本体树来建设领域本体知识的技术。设计开发了 DartOnto 协同本体加工平台，包括语义集成，本体和数据的加工展示，以及对外查询接口。具体介绍了系统的本体层、本体引擎工具 OntoTool、服务器层和表现层（DartWiki、模型推理工具）等的设计实现。

[13] Chen H，Wang Y，Wang H，*et al*. Towards a Semantic Web of relational databases：a practical semantic toolkit and an in-use case from traditional Chinese medicine［C］// 5th International Semantic Web Conference(ISWC 2006)，2006：750-763.

主要介绍了一个应用程序开发框架 Dartgrid 和一组语义工具，以便于用语义 Web 技术集成异构关系数据库。其中 DartMapping 是一个可视化的映射工具，可以帮助 DBA 定义从异构关系模式到本体的语义映射。DartQuery 是一个基于本体的查询接口，帮助用户构造语义查询，能将 SPARQL 语义查询重写为一组 SQL 查询。DartSearch 是一个基于本体的搜索引擎，使用户能进行全文搜索，并在搜索结果之前进行语义导航。该工具包已被用于为中国中医科学院开发一个目前正在使用的应用程序,使得70多个遗留关系数据库通过一个包含70多个类和800个属性的本体进行语义连接,为中医社区提供集成的语义丰富的查询、搜索和导航服务。

[14]尹爱宁,陈华钧,何前锋,等.建立中医药虚拟研究院背景与方法[C]//第三届国际中医药工程学术会议论文集,2006:312-317.

主要提出了网上虚拟研究院的创新思路,即实现跨单位聚集科研实力和课题协作的新方法。探讨了虚拟研究院设立的背景和需求、基本特征与组织形式以及技术实现方法。

[15] Chen H,Mao Y,Zheng X,et al. Towards semantic e-Science for Traditional Chinese Medicine[J]. BMC Bioinformatics,2007,8(3):1-16.

主要研究了基于语义和知识构建动态可扩展的e-Science应用的综合方法。TCM是知识密集型学科领域,为中医药领域构建语义科学网,支持大规模的数据库集成和针对虚拟组织的服务协调。采用领域本体来集成TCM数据库资源,且在语义互联网上为用户提供浏览、搜索、查询和知识发现服务。开发了一组基于语义的工具集,为中医药科学家和研究人员提供信息共享和协同研究服务。

[16] 陈华钧,姜晓红,吴朝晖. DartGrid:支持中医药信息化的语义网格平台实现[M]. 杭州:浙江大学出版社,2011.

结合对中医药领域的应用需求分析,提出了基于语义网格构建面向中医药领域的e-Science环境,介绍了面向中医药领域的语义网格平台的具体实现(包括基于语义网格的数据集成与共享、海量中医药数据挖掘与分析等),详细阐述了其体系结构、技术特征和应用成果。

[17] 王超.基于知识集成引擎的中医药知识服务社区[D]. 杭州:浙江大学,2012.

主要研究了中医药知识服务虚拟社区平台架构及其关键技术。原型平台通过知识集成引擎集成了数据库查询、本体查询与搜索以及基于语义规则的推理引擎。为实现知识社区的开放性和灵活性,采用生动的Web用户接口为用户提供中医药信息的快速访问。

[18] 吴朝晖,姜晓红,陈华钧.知识服务:大数据时代下的中医药信息化发展趋势[J].中国中医药图书情报杂志,2013,37(2):2-5.

主要介绍了语义网、云计算、物联网、跨界服务等信息技术的发展趋势,分析了现有中医药信息化的现状,指出了中医药信息化工作将从以网格技术、搜索引擎为基础的信息共享转向基于云平台、大数据的跨界中医药知识服务的发展趋势。

[19] 于彤,于琦,李敬华,等.知识服务及其在中医药领域的应用[J].中国数字医学,2015,10(8):33-35.

主要阐述了知识服务的概念和性质,设计并实现了中医药知识服务平台,包括百科知识服务、知识搜索服务、知识发现服务、决策支持服务等中医药知识服务,为中医药科学研究、临床实践和新药研发提供了有力支持。

[20] 于彤,崔蒙,毛郁欣,等.基于移动互联网的中医养生知识服务研究[J].中国数字医学,2016,11(2):29-30,45.

主要调研了中医养生方面的移动应用程序,总结了中医养生移动应用程序的主要功能、知识内容、服务方式以及核心优势,分析存在的问题并提出研究思路。指出需要进一步建立综合性、科学性、大众性的中医养生知识库,为各种移动应用提供统一的支持。

[21]胡志强. 面向中医药领域的智能问答系统设计与实现[D]. 杭州:浙江大学,2020.

主要研究了面向中医药领域的智能问答系统的设计实现。提出了一种融合医药分词模型,提高了医药文本的分词性能;研究了不同任务下最佳性能的词向量训练方法;提出了 Bert-BiLSTM-CRF 实体识别模型,其对中医药命名实体识别具有高准确率;提出了一种新的文本语义匹配模型 Bert-Siamese,可达 0.925 的高 AUC 值。利用以上技术设计实现了一个面向中医药领域的智能问答系统,并以 Web 应用形式提供服务。

(3)云基础设施服务平台

研究了虚拟计算系统的核心关键技术,包括虚拟计算系统的性能分析和评价、基于在线迁移的性能优化、云资源调度和数据管理等[22-36]。开发实现了云基础设施服务平台 DartCloud,平台支持跨域的计算和存储资源的申请、部署、监管和调度,支持跨域的文件存储和共享,还研究了云平台的故障监测和维护技术[37-43]。主要研究和开发成果总结在专著[44]中。

[22] Ye K, Jiang X, Chen S, et al. Analyzing and modeling the performance in Xen-based virtual cluster environment[C]//12th IEEE International Conference on High Performance Computing and Communication (HPCC'2010),2010:281-288.

主要研究比较了 HPC 应用在 Xen 半虚拟化和全虚拟化的两种模式下的基本性能问题。创建了 16 个节点的虚拟集群系统,分析了 HPC 应用程序在虚拟化环境下的运行效率,评估了其在虚拟集群中的 MPI 扩展性,用 L2 Cache 失配、DTLB 失配、ITLB 失配等硬件特性辅助解释性能瓶颈。

[23] Ye K, Jiang X, Ye D, et al. Two optimization mechanisms to improve the isolation property of server consolidation in virtlized multi-core server[C]// 12th IEEE International Conference on High Performance Computing and Communication (HPCC'2010),2010:273-280.

主要研究了整合服务器负载在多核处理器上的隔离性问题。基于性能分析数据,提出了虚拟机级的优化机制来提升性能隔离性;研究了服务器整合场景下功能出错的服务器导致的故障隔离性,提出了一种核级的 Cache 敏感的优化方法提升故障隔离性。利用 Oprofile/Xenoprof 工具分析了硬件事件级的影响隔离性能的因素。

[24] 吴朝晖,叶可江,姜晓红,等. 一种缓存感知的多核处理器虚拟机故障隔离保证方法:201110008236.6[P].2012-12-05.

主要提出了一种缓存感知的多核处理器虚拟机故障隔离保证方法。当检测到异常虚拟机时,记录该故障虚拟机在处理器上的分配情况。当发现有其他虚拟机负载跟该故障虚拟机共享一块 L2 缓存时,就把故障虚拟机迁移到一块独立缓存所对应的核上。这就避免了其他正常虚拟机收到缓存的污染,降低了故障虚拟机对正常虚拟机运行的影响。

[25] Ye K, Jiang X, He Q, et al. Evaluate the performance and scalability of image deployment in virtual data center[C]// IFIP International Conference on Network and Parallel Computing(NPC'2010),2010,LNCS 6289:390-401.

主要研究了云数据中心的虚拟机部署问题。分析了数据中心典型应用服务器物理服务器上多虚拟机的映像可扩展性,进而分析了用不同的部署策略将 M 个虚拟机部署到 N 个物理服务器上的效率。得出以下结论:将单一虚拟机部署到一个物理机上时,存在资源瓶颈;对于某些特定应用,用更多物理机支持固定数量的虚拟机不一定效率更高;MPI 和网络通信开销会严重影响部署的效率。

［26］Ye K，Jiang X，Huang D，*et al*. Live migration of multiple virtual machines with resource reservation in cloud computing environments［C］// 4th International Conference on Cloud Computing（Cloud'2011），IEEE，2011：267-274.

主要研究了云计算环境中不同资源预留策略下在线迁移策略对源机器节点和目标机器性能的影响。用宕机时间、总迁移时间、负载性能等参数分析了并行迁移策略和负载敏感迁移策略的效率。基于实验结果,进一步提出了优化方法以提高在线迁移效率。

［27］Ye K，Jiang X，He Y，*et al*. vHadoop：A scalable hadoop virtual cluster platform for MapReduce-based parallel machine learning with performance consideration［C］// IEEE International Conference on Cluster Computing Workshops（Cluster'2012 Workshops），2012：152-160.

主要研究了 Hadoop 虚拟集群的性能,提出了面向大规模 MapReduce 并行数据处理应用的可扩展 Hadoop 虚拟集群平台 vHadoop。做了大量实验,以验证 vHadoop 平台的静态性能和动态性能。在平台上进一步针对两个典型数据集运行 6 个经典的并行集群算法,实验结果表明,平台满足预期的设计目标。

［28］Ye K，Jiang X，Ma R，*et al*. VC-Migration：Live migration of virtual cluster in the cloud［C］//13th ACM/IEEE International Conference on Grid Computing（Grid'2012），2012：209-218.

主要构建了一个系统框架 VC-Migration 以控制虚拟集群中虚拟机的迁移,研究了不同虚拟集群场景下的不同在线迁移策略的性能和开销,包括并发迁移策略、互相迁移策略、同构虚拟机迁移策略和异构虚拟机迁移策略等。在分析实验结果的基础上,还提出了几种优化策略以改进在线迁移性能。

［29］Jiang X，Yan F，Ye K. Performance influence of live migration on multi-tier workloads in virtualization environments［C］// 3rd International Conference on Cloud Computing，GRIDs，and Virtualization（Cloud Computing'2012），IEEE，2012：72-81.

主要研究了虚拟机在线迁移对虚拟机上工作负载的性能影响。做了大量实验,以工作负载在物理机上的性能为对照基础,研究了云环境中在线迁移对多层负载性能的影响。实验表明,频繁的在线迁移会严重影响负载性能,对于内存密集的工作负载,要避免在线迁移。实验还发现,虚拟机存在性能拐点,这为进一步研究迁移策略提供依据。

［30］吴朝晖,叶可江,姜晓红,等. 一种面向云数据中心的大规模虚拟机快速迁移决策方法：201310186581.8［P］. 2016-06-01.

主要提出了一种面向云数据中心的大规模虚拟机快速迁移决策方法。先对输入的初始方案和目标方案进行虚拟机到物理机映射关系的归类,消除两个方案中相同的映射关系,把初始方案快速转移至目标方案的问题转化为寻找从初始方案到目标方案的最佳匹配组合,执行递归,指导初始状态或目标状态为空。进行后处理,输出最终的迁移次数和具体迁移决策方案,最大程度减少迁移次数。

［31］叶可江. 虚拟计算系统的性能和能耗管理方法研究［D］. 杭州：浙江大学,2013.

主要研究了虚拟计算系统中的两个关键问题:低性能和高能耗。设计了一个基于典型应用场景的虚拟计算系统性能基准测试程序集 Virt-B;提出了一系列针对多机多核架构的性能调优策略和方法;提出了以虚拟机为粒度的云计算数据中心节能架构和方法;研究了虚拟机性能和能耗之间的权衡关系,提出了虚拟机负载性能约束下的最优节能整合模型及最优迁移决策算法。

[32] Ye K，Wu Z，Wang C，*et al*. Profiling-based workload consolidation and migration in virtualized data centres[J]. IEEE Transactions on Parallel and Distributed Systems(TPDS),2015, 26(3):878-890.

主要提出了一种基于轮廓分析的服务器整合框架。该框架既能减少数据中心的物理服务器数量,又能维持不同工作负载的满意性能。分析了不同工作负载在同一物理机上和在线迁移两种情况下的性能轮廓;设计了整合计划模型,该模型可以在给定一组工作负载时,计算最小化的物理机数量;设计了迁移计划模型,该模型可以在给定源/目标虚拟机的部署场景时,计算最小化虚拟机迁移数量。根据分析得到的负载性能轮廓数据,上述两个模型均能保证不同工作负荷的性能损失低于设定的阈值。

[33] 陈英芝. Spark Shuffle 的内存调度算法分析及优化[D]. 杭州:浙江大学,2016.

主要研究了分布式计算框架 Spark Shuffle 过程中不同任务间内存分配算法的优化方法。针对公平分配算法的不足,提出了基于溢出历史的自适应内存调度算法 SBSA,解决了任务对内存需求不均衡造成的低效率瓶颈问题。实验对比提出算法与先来先服务算法、公平分配调度算法的性能差异,验证了 SBSA 算法的有效性。

[34]何延彰. 弹性云平台的虚拟资源调度技术研究[D]. 杭州:浙江大学,2018.

主要研究了弹性云平台的资源调度管理技术。设计了一个基于虚拟机状态更细资源粒度的虚拟资源计费管理策略;提出了一个多目标虚拟机初始部署优化算法,同时考虑综合平均资源利用率 CARU 指标和综合资源利用均衡率 CRUB 指标;实现了一个大数据弹性计算平台 ScalaBD,可提供大数据存储、批量计算、流式计算、内存计算和工作流计算等多种服务形式。

[35] 马然. 高机密性高可用性的云存储系统研究[D]. 杭州:浙江大学,2013.

主要研究了兼顾机密性和可用性的云存储系统技术。提出了采用数据拆分和重建算法以及数据冗余策略提高数据的机密性和可用性;结合开源 HDFS 系统设计,实现了新的高机密性和可用性的 HCAFA 云存储原型系统,给出了对比 HDFS 和 HCAFA 的实验测试结果。

[36] He Y，Jiang X，Ye K，*et al*. HPACS:A high privacy and availability cloud storage platform with matrix encryption[C]// 10th International Symposium of Advanced Parallel Processing Technologies (APPT'2013),2013,LNCS 8299:132-145.

主要研究了云存储的数据隐私问题。设计并实现了一个兼顾高数据隐私和高可用性的云存储平台(HPACS)。平台建立在 Apache Hadoop 平台的基础上,在 HDFS 上集成了矩阵加密和解密模块,实现数据透明并加密传到不同服务器上,从服务器上取回后解密。实验在实现高隐私性和高可用性的同时,保证了合理的数据读写性能。

[37] 闫凤喜.跨域云平台的安装部署技术和在线迁移性能研究[D]. 杭州:浙江大学,2013.

主要研究了跨域云平台中的安装部署技术,解决了云平台中增减计算节点与镜像管理问题,设计实现了自动裸机部署工具以及自动的镜像管理系统,解决了虚拟机启动时复制镜像副本的低效问题,同时通过镜像的自动化补充,保证了系统对镜像的需求。

[38] 姜晓红,闫凤喜,陈忠忠,等. 一种云数据中心物理裸机快速部署操作系统的方法: 201310170073.0[P].2016-05-11.

主要提出了一种云数据中心中物理裸机快速部署操作系统的方法,包括从开启服务器 A,到裸机 B 从硬盘启动等七个步骤。该方法可以大大提高云数据中心物理裸机的装机速度。

[39] 黄鹏. 云平台虚拟计算资源的远程访问技术[D]. 杭州:浙江大学,2014.

主要研究并实现了 IP 地址资源严重受限条件下虚拟计算资源的远程访问技术。设计了 vr.cprocy 七层代理服务器,为 vnc4server 远程控制工具穿透内网,连接 DartCloud 云平台内部集群中的任意虚拟机。针对 vnc4server 传输桌面图像的弊端,基于 Web-based SSH,用多进程事件驱动技术设计实现了高并发量和吞吐率的 websshproxy 高性能代理服务器。

[40] 严海明. 云资源管理平台 DartCloud 的设计与实现[D]. 杭州:浙江大学,2014.

主要研究了云资源管理平台的设计实现技术,设计开发了基于 OpenNebula 系统的云资源管理平台 DartCloud,还提出基于遗传算法的虚拟机调度机制。解决了海量用户对弹性计算资源的租赁申请需求问题,实现了面向多租户异构应用的云计算 IaaS 服务。

[41] 杨红星. 云平台跨域分布式共享文件系统的设计与实现[D]. 杭州:浙江大学,2015.

主要研究了分布式文件系统的主流设计思想,设计实现了跨域分布式共享文件系统以支持跨地域集群的云平台数据管理需求。采用分级共享策略,使不同权限的本地用户与远程虚拟机实现文件交换。

[42] 姜晓红,杨红星,黄鹏,等. 跨域云平台的共享文件管理方法:201310139941.9[P]. 2015-11-18.

主要提出了一种用于跨域云平台的共享文件管理方法。在域中选出中心域,用于维护共享文件分布表。当某个域用户上传共享文件时,在中心域分布表上增加记录;当用户下载共享文件时,在中心域的分布表中查询该文件所在位置。用最小代价达到了跨域文件传输管理的目的。

[43] 陈忠忠. 云平台可维护性研究[D]. 杭州:浙江大学,2015.

主要研究了云平台的可维护性,在云平台的快速部署及监控系统的搭建、镜像管理策略的定制和对业务扩展性的支持这三方面做了深入的探讨。

[44] 代长波. 分布式系统自适应故障检测技术研究[D]. 杭州:浙江大学,2017.

主要研究了分布式系统的自适应故障检测技术。提出了一种新的自适应故障检测方法——DEMA-FD,它比传统心跳预测检测具有更好的准确性;设计了一种新的自适应检测协议——DLFDA,以动态调整检测结构以提高链路检测的覆盖率,同时使用 gossip 发布故障诊断结果,降低了检测负载;实现了一个通用可扩展的分布式自适应故障检测原型系统。

[45] 姜晓红,叶可江. DartCloud:云基础设施服务平台[M]. 北京:科学出版社,2015.

主要介绍了云基础设施服务平台的基本概念和背景,分析了各大开源云平台,深入研究了云资源调度技术、在线迁移技术、云数据管理技术、云能耗管理技术以及云系统性能评价研究等五大核心关键技术,最后介绍了一个跨域云基础设施服务平台 DartCloud 的功能和实现。

4.1 代表性学术论文全文

本节选取了中医药云平台与服务计算方向的 2 篇代表性学术论文"Towards a Semantic Web of Relational Databases: A Practical Semantic Toolkit and an In-Use Case from Traditional Chinese Medicine"和"Towards Semantic e-Science for Traditional Chinese Medicine"全文(分别于 2006 年和 2007 年发表于国际会议 *ISWC* 及国际期刊 *BMC Bioinformatics*)。

Towards a Semantic Web of Relational Databases: A Practical Semantic Toolkit and an In-Use Case from Traditional Chinese Medicine

Huajun Chen, Yimin Wang, Heng Wang, Yuxin Mao, Jinmin Tang, Cunyin Zhou, Ainin Yin, Zhaohui Wu
首发于 *ISWC 2006, LNCS* **4273**:750-763

Abstract

Integrating relational databases is recently acknowledged as an important vision of the Semantic Web research, however there are not many well-implemented tools and not many applications that are in large-scale real use either. This paper introduces the Dartgrid which is an application development framework together with a set of semantic tools to facilitate the integration of heterogenous relational databases using semantic web technologies. For examples, DartMapping is a visualized mapping tool to help DBA in defining semantic mappings from heterogeneous relational schemas to ontologies. DartQuery is an ontology-based query interface helping user to construct semantic queries, and capable of rewriting SPARQL semantic queries to a set of SQL queries. DartSearch is an ontology-based search engine enabling user to make full-text search over all databases and to navigate across the search results semantically. It is also enriched with a concept ranking mechanism to enable user to find more accurate and reliable results. This toolkit has been used to develop an currently in-use application for China Academy of Traditional Chinese Medicine (CATCM). In this application, over 70 legacy relational databases are semantically interconnected by an ontology with over 70 classes and 800 properties, providing integrated semantic-enriched query, search and navigation services to TCM communities.

1　Introduction

Up to date, many killer applications reported by the Semantic Web community often focus on processing the unstructured document data, using semantic annotation or various of learning, mining, and natural language processing techniques [1]. However, data in big organizations is normally stored in relational databases or other appropriately formatted documents. Over emphasizing on those applications, which handle unstructured document, may obscure the community from the fact that the essence of the Semantic Web comes from its similarity to a huge distributed database. To back up this idea, consider the following statements made by Tim Berners-Lee in 2005 about his vision of the future Semantic Web[①].

... The Semantic Web is not about the meaning of documents. It's not about marking up existing HTML documents to let a computer understand what they say. It's not about the artificial intelligence areas of machine learning or natural language understanding... **It is about the data which currently is in relational databases, XML documents, spreadsheets, and proprietary format data files, and all of which would be useful to have access to as one huge database...**

From this point of view, one of the way to realize the vision of Semantic Web is (i) to interconnect

---

①　http://www.consortiuminfo.org/bulletins/semanticweb.php.

distributed located legacy databases using richer semantics, (ii) to provide ontology-based query, search and navigation as one huge distributed database, and (iii) to add additional deductive capabilities on the top to increase the usability and reusability of data.

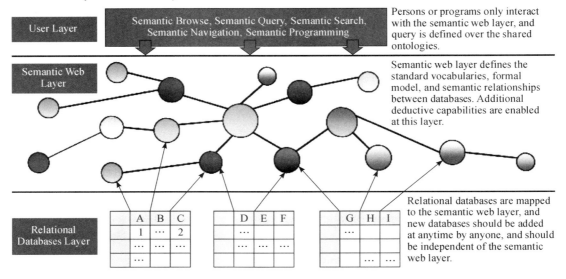

Figure 1　Towards a semantic web of relational databases.

Besides, since most of the data is currently stored in relational databases, for semantic web to be really useful and successful, great efforts are required to offer methods and tools to support integration of heterogeneous relational databases. Dartgrid is an application development framework together with a set of practical semantic tools to facilitate the integration of heterogenous relational databases using semantic web technologies. In specific, DartMapping is a visualized mapping tool to help DBA in defining semantic mappings from heterogeneous relational schemas to ontologies. DartQuery is an ontology-based query interface helping user to construct semantic queries, and capable of rewriting SPARQL semantic queries to a set of SQL queries. DartSearch is an ontology-based search engine enabling user to make full-text search over all databases and to navigate across the search results semantically. It is also enriched with a concept ranking mechanism to enable user to find more accurate and reliable results.

Building upon Dartgrid, we have developed and deployed a semantic web application for China Academy of Traditional Chinese Medicine (CATCM)②③. It semantically interconnects over 70 legacy TCM databases by a formal TCM ontology with over 70 classes and 800 properties. The TCM ontology acts as a separate semantic layer to fill up the gaps among legacy databases with heterogeneous structures, which might be semantically interconnected. Users and machines only need to interact with the semantic layer, and the semantic interconnections allow them to start in one database, and then move around an extendable set of databases. The semantic layer also enables the system to answer semantic queries across several databases such as "What diseases does this drug treat?" or "What kind of drugs can treat this disease?", not like the keyword-

---

②　http://ccnt.zju.edu.cn/projects/dartgrid/tcmgrid.html.
③　**Demo videos** http://ccnt.zju.edu.cn/projects/dartgrid/demo.

based searching mechanism provide by conventional search engines.

The paper is organized as follows. Section 2 talks about the system architecture and technical features. Section 3 elaborates on the implementation of the semantic mediator and the visualized semantic mapping tool. Section 4 introduces the TCM semantic portals which provide semantic query and search services. Section 5 reports the user evaluation and lessons learned from this developing life-cycle. Section 6 mentions some related works. Section 7 gives the summary and our future directions.

Please also note due to the special character of TCM research, in which the Chinese terminologies and definitions are not always interpretable, some figures in this paper contain Chinese search results and web interface. We have annotated all the necessary parts of the figures in English, and we expect it would be sufficient to understand the functionalities of this application.

2　System Architecture and Technical Features

2.1　System Architecture

As Figure 2 depicted, there are four key components in the core of DartGrid.

（1）**Ontology Service** is used to expose the shared ontologies that are defined using web ontology languages. Typically, the ontology is specified by a domain expert who is also in charge of the publishing, revision, extension of the ontology.

（2）**Semantic Registration Service** maintains the semantic mapping information. Typically, database providers define the mappings from relational schema to domain ontology, and submit the registration entry to this service.

（3）**Semantic Query Service** is used to process SPARQL semantic queries. Firstly, it gets mapping information from semantic registration service. Afterward, it translates the semantic queries into a set of SQL queries and dispatches them into specific databases. Finally, the results of SQL queries will be merged and transformed back to semantically-enriched format.

（4）**Search Service** supports full-text search in all databases. The search results will be statistically calculated to yield a *concepts ranking*, which helps user to get more appropriate and accurate results.

2.2　Technical Features

The following four features that distinguish this application from other similar semantic data integration tools, which will be introduced in detail in Section 6.

Semantic View and Visualized Semantic Mapping Tool. In our system, an ontology acts as the semantic mediator for heterogenous databases. Relational database schemas are mapped into corresponding classes or properties, and related by semantic relationship defined in this ontology. To be specific, the mappings are defined as *semantic views*, that is, each relational table is defined as a *view* over this shared ontology. Defining mappings is a labor-intensive and error-prone task. In our system, new database could be added into the system by using a visualized mapping tool. It provides many easy-of-use functionalities such as drag-and-drop mapping, mapping visualization, data source annotation and so on.

SPARQL Query Rewriting with Additional Inference Capabilities. A view-based query rewriting algorithm is implemented to rewrite the SPARQL queries into a set of SQL queries. This algorithm extends earlier

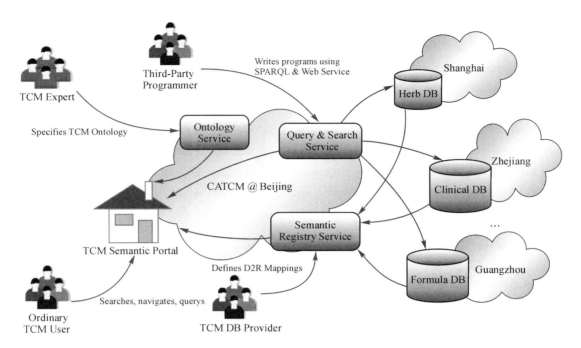

Figure 2　System Architecture and Usage Scenario.

relational and XML techniques for rewriting queries using views, with consideration of the features of web ontology languages. Otherwise, this algorithm is also enriched by additional inference capabilities on predicates such as *subClassOf* and *subPropertyOf*.

Ontology-based Semantic Query User Interface. A form-based query interface is offered to construct semantic queries over shared ontologies. It is automatically generated at runtime according to property definitions of classes, and will finally generate a SPARQL query.

Intuitive Search Interface with Concepts Ranking and Semantic Navigation. This Google-like search interface accepts one or more keywords and makes a complete full-text search in all databases. Users could semantically navigate in the search results, and move around an extendable set of databases based on the semantic relationships defined in the semantic layer. Meanwhile, the search system could generate a suggested list of concepts which are ranked based on their relevance to the keywords. Thereafter, users could explore into the semantic query interface of those concepts, and specify a semantic query on them to get more accurate and appropriate information.

3　Semantic Mediation

3.1　Semantic View and View-Based Mapping

In our system, databases are mediated and related by a shared ontology, and each relational table is mapped into one or more classes. For example, the mapping scenario in Figure 3 illustrates relational schemas from two sources(W3C and ZJU), and a shared ontology (a part of the foaf ontology).

Mappings are typically defined as views in conventional data integration systems in the form of GAV (global-as-view), LAV (local-as-view)[2]. Considering the case in this paper, GAV is to define each class or property as a view over relational tables, and LAV is to define each relational table as a view (or query) over the shared ontology. The experiences from conventional data integration systems tell us that LAV provides greater extensibility than GAV: the addition of new sources is less likely to require a change to the mediated schema [2]. In our TCM case, new databases are regularly added so total number of databases is increasing gradually. Therefore, the LAV approach is employed in our system, that is, each relational table is defined as a view over the ontologies. We call such kind of views as *Semantic View*.

The lower part of Figure 3 showcases how to represent the mappings as *semantic views* in a Datalog-like syntax. Like in conventional data integration, a typical *semantic view* consists of two parts. The left part is called the view head, and is a relational predicate. The right part is called the view body, and is a set of RDF triples. There are two kinds of variables in the view definitions. Those variables such as "?en, ?em, ?eh, ?pn, ?ph" are called distinguished variables, which will be assigned by an data or instance values from the database. Those variables such as "?y1, ?y2" are called existential variables.

In general, the body can be viewed as a query over the ontology, and it defines the semantics of the relational predicate from the perspective of the ontology. The meaning of semantic view would be clearer if we construct a *Target Instance* based on the semantic mapping specified by these views. For example, given a relational tuple as below, applying the View-4 in Figure 3 on this tuple will yield a set of RDF triples.

Relational Tuple:

w3c:emp("DanBrickley","danbri@w3.org",

"SWAD","http://swad.org","EU");

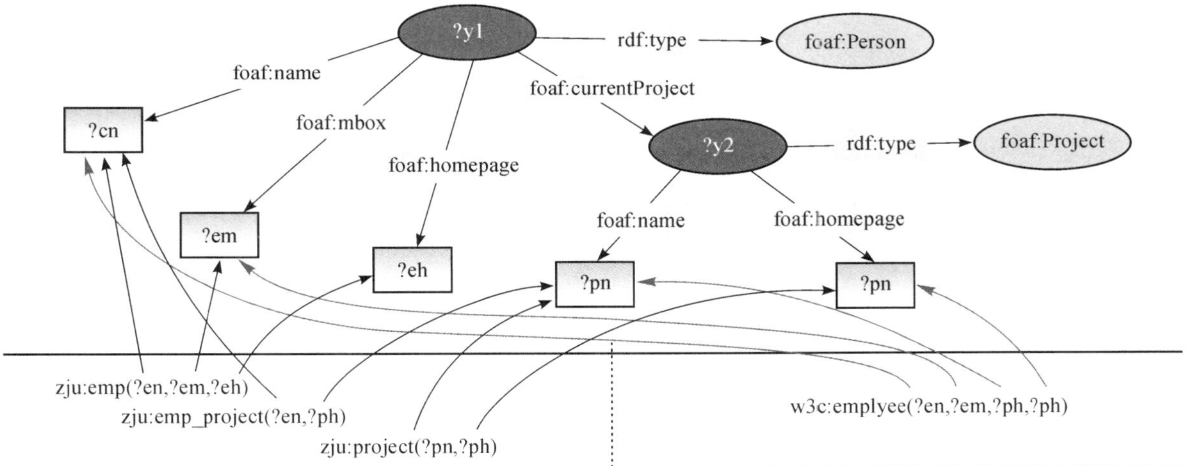

View-1:zju:emp(?en,?em,?eh):- (?y1,rdf:type, foaf:Person), (?y1, foaf:name,?en), (?y1, foaf:mbox,?em), (?y1, foaf:homepage,?eh).

View-2:zju:emp_project(?en,?ah):- (?y1,rdf:type, foaf:Person), (?y1, foaf:name,?en), (?y1, foaf:currentProject,?y2), (?y2, rdf:type, foaf:Project), (?y2, foaf:name,?pn).

View-3:zju:project(?an,?ah):- (?y2,rdf:type, foaf:Project), (?y2, foaf:name,?pn), (?y2, foaf:homepage,?ph).

View-4:w3:emp(?en,?em,?an,?ah):- (?y1,rdf:type, foaf:Person), (?y1, foaf:name,?en), (?y1, foaf:mbox,?em),(?y1, foaf:currentProject,?y2), (?y2, rdf:type, foaf:Project), (?y2, foaf:name,?pn), (?y2, foaf:homepage,?ph).

Figure 3　Mappings from two relational databases with different structures to an ontology. "?en, ?em, ?eh, ?pn, ?ph" are variables and represent "employee name", "employee email", "employee homepage", "project name", "project homepage", respectively.

Yielded RDF triples by Applying View-4:

```
_:bn1 rdf:type foaf:Person;
         foaf:name "Dan Brickley";
         foaf:mbox "danbri@w3.org";
         foaf:currentProject _:bn2.
_:bn2 rdf:type    foaf:Project;
         foaf:name "SWAD";
         foaf:homepage "http://swad.org".
```

One of the key notion is the newly generated blank node ID. As illustrated, corresponding to each existential variable ?y in the view, a new blank node ID is generated. For examples, $\_:bn1$, $\_:bn2$ are both newly generated blank node IDs corresponding to the variables ?y1, ?y2 in View-4 respectively. This treatment of existential variable is in accordance with the RDF semantics, since blank nodes can be viewed as existential variables. We give the formal definition of the semantic view as below. More detailed Fundamental aspects about *semantic view* could be found in another paper [3].

Definition 1. Semantic View. Let *Var* be a set of variable names. A typical semantic view is like the form: $R(\overline{X}):- G(\overline{X},\overline{Y})$, where:

(1) $R(\overline{X})$ is called the head of the view, and R is a relational predicate.

(2) $G(\overline{X},\overline{Y})$ is called the body of the view, and G is a RDF graph with some nodes replaced by variables in *Var*.

(3) The $\overline{X}$, $\overline{Y}$ contain either variables or constants. The variables in $\overline{X}$ are called distinguished variables, and the variables in $\overline{Y}$ are called existential variables.

3.2　Visualized Semantic Mapping Tool

The task of defining semantic mappings from relational schema to ontologies is burdensome and erroneous. Although we could develop tools to automate this process, it still can not be fully automated and require humans involvement, especially for integration of databases with different schema structures.

Figure 4 displays the visualized mapping tool we developed to facilitate the task of defining semantic views. It has five panels. The *DBRes* panel displays the relational schemas, and the *OntoSchem* panel displays the shared ontology. The *Mapping Panel* visually displays the mappings from relational schemas to ontologies. Typically, user drag tables or columns from DBRes panel, and drag classes or properties from OntoSchem panel, then drop them into the mapping panel to establish the mappings. By simple drag-and-drop operations, users could easily specify which classes should be mapped into a table and which property should be mapped into a table column. After these operations, the tool automatically generates a registration entry, which is submitted to the semantic registration service. Besides, user could use the *Outline* panel to browse and query previously defined mapping information, and use the *Properties* panel to specify some global information, such as namespace, or view the meta-information about the table.

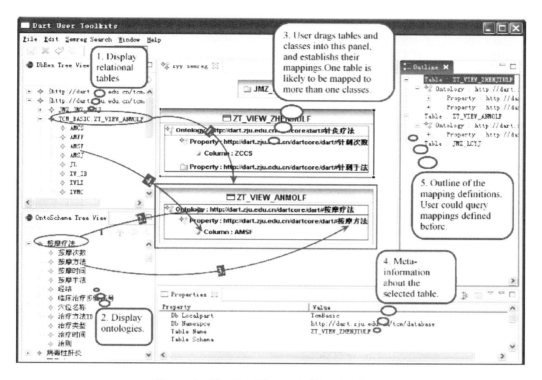

Figure 4　Visualized Semantic Mapping Tool.

4　TCM Semantic Portals

The semantic mediator is designed to separate data providers and data consumers so that they only need to interact with the semantic layer. For example, developers could write applications using the shared ontology without the need of any knowledge about databases. Besides that, our system also offer two different kinds of user interfaces to support query and search services.

4.1　Dynamic Semantic Query Interface

This form-like query interface is intended to facilitate users in constructing semantic queries. The query form is automatically generated according to class definitions. This design provides the extensibility of the whole system—when ontology is updated with the changes of database schema, the interface could dynamically adapt to the updated shared ontology.

Figure 5 shows the situation how a TCM user constructs a semantic query. Starting from the *ontology view panel* on the left, user can browse the ontology tree and select the classes of interest. A query form corresponding to the property definitions of the selected class will be automatically generated and displayed in the middle. Then user can check and select the properties of interests or input query constraints into the text boxes. Accordingly, a SPARQL query is constructed and could be submitted to the semantic query service, where the query will be rewritten into a set of SQL queries using mapping views contained in the semantic registration service. The query rewriting is a somewhat complicated process, and [3] gives the detailed introduction on the rewriting algorithm. In addition, user could define more complex queries. For example,

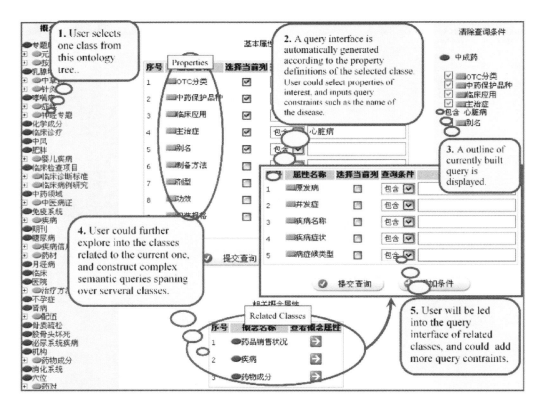

Figure 5 Dynamic Semantic Query Portal. Please note：because many Chinese medical terminologies are only available in Chinese language and they are not always interpretable，we have annotated all the necessary parts of the figures in English.

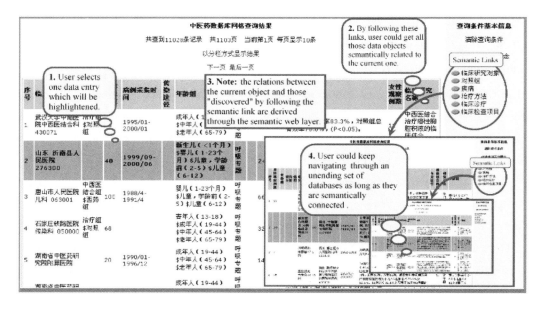

Figure 6 Semantic navigation through the query results.

depicted in the lower-middle part of Figure 5, user could follow the links leading to related classes of the current class, and select more properties or input new query constraints.

Figure 6 shows the situation in which a TCM user is navigating the query results. Starting from selecting one result highlighted, the user can find out all of the related data entries by following the semantic links. Please note that in this example, the relations between the search results and those "discovered" by following the semantic links, are derived from the semantic layer.

4. 2　Intuitive Search Interface with Concepts Ranking and Semantic Navigation

Unlike the semantic query interface, this Google-like search interface just accepts one or more keywords and makes a complete full-text search in all databases. Figure 7 shows the situation where a TCM user performs some search operations. Starting from inputting a keyword, the user can retrieve all of those data entries containing one or more hits of that keyword. Being similar to the case of the query interface, the user could also semantically navigate the search results by following the semantic links listed with each entries.

Meanwhile, the search system generates a list of suggested concepts which are displayed on the right part of the portal. They are ranked based on their relevance to the keywords. These concept links will lead the users to the dynamic query interface introduced in previous section. Thereafter, users could specify a semantic query on them to get more accurate and appropriate information. We call it as intuitive search because it could generate a list of concept suggestions to help user improve the search results.

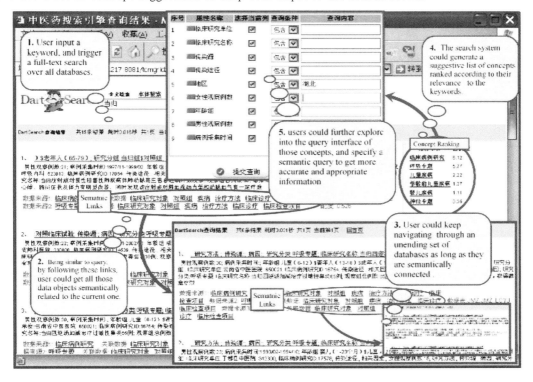

Figure 7　Intuitive Search Portal with Concept Ranking and Semantic Navigation.

5 User Evaluation and Lesson Learned

5.1 Feedbacks from CATCM

The first proof-of-concepts prototype was deployed during fall 2004. By using that prototype, we convinced CATCM partner to take the semantic web technologies to help them in managing their fast increasing TCM databases. After a thorough requirements analysis and with a careful redesign and re-engineering of the entire system, a more stable and user-friendly version was released in September 2005, and deployed at CATCM for open evaluation and real use.

Currently, the system deployed at CATCM provides access to over 70 databases including TCM herbal medicine databases, TCM compound formula databases, clinical symptom databases, traditional Chinese drug database, traditional Tibetan drug database, TCM product and enterprise databases, and so on. The TCM shared ontology includes over 70 classes, 800 data or object properties.

In general, users from CATCM reacted positively to the entire semantic web approach and our system. They indicated that the system provided an amazing solution for the semantic heterogeneity problem which had been troubling them for a long time. In particular, they gave high praise to the visualized semantic registration tool, and indicated that the features of semantic registration of new database considerably save them a lot of time when new database were developed and needed to be integrated.

They also gave positive comments to the semantic portals as well, especially the semantic navigation functionality. They indicated that semantic interconnections among different databases was indeed what they wanted. Nevertheless, we found most of the users prefer Google-like search to semantic query interface. Some of them complained that the learning cycle of using the semantic query interface was too long, although it could return more accurate results. They also said they would very like to use the concepts ranking functionality to get more accurate result by constructing further queries when the entries returned from search was overwhelming.

5.2 A Survey on the Usage of RDF/OWL Predicates

RDF/OWL has offered us a range of predicates, but not all of them are useful for relational data integration. We made a survey on the usage of RDF/OWL predicates for relational database integration, and the results are indicated in Table 1.

In this survey, we invited ten developers who are familiar with both semantic web technologies and our system. They are asked with the same questions: "From a practical view, what are those most important constructs do you think for relational data integration in semantic web?", and are requested to write down some explanation for the reason of their choice. We summarize their comments and the score result as follows.

Table 1　The results for the survey of predicates usage

Predicate	E1	E2	E3	E4	E5	E6	E7	E8	E9	E10	AVG
rdf:datatype	9	10	8	9	10	10	9	7	10	9	9.1
rdfs:subClassOf	8	8	7	9	9	8	8	9	10	7	8.3
rdfs:subPropertyOf	8	8	8	7	8	8	9	9	9	8	8.2
owl:inverseOf	8	8	7	8	7	9	8	9	7	9	8.0
owl:cardinality	7	8	7	7	6	7	9	7	7	9	7.4

Data type support was considered to be important, because most commercial RDBMS has well-defined and unique data type system. RDFS predicates *rdfs:subClassOf* and *rdfs:subPropertyOf* have higher scores because they could enhance the query processing with additional inference capabilities. OWL predicate *owl:inverseOf* is useful when defining relations in both directions which is a usual case in relation database integration. One of the developers indicated that predicate *owl:inverseOf* could help to find more efficient rewritings in some cases. Predicate *owl:cardinality* is useful in adding more constraints to ensure the data integrity.

Some other predicates are considered as useful include: *owl:TransitiveProperty*, *owl:Symmetric Property*, *owl:DatatypeProperty*, *owl:ObjectProperty*. Some of them thought both *owl:TransitiveProperty* and *owl:SymmetricProperty* could add additional deductive capabilities on top to yield more query results. *owl:DatatypeProperty* and *owl:Object Property* could be used to distinguish simple data value column and foreign key column.

6　Related Works

6.1　Semantic Web Context

In the Semantic Web community, semantic data integration has been always a noticeable research topic. In particular, there have been a number of works dealing with how to make contents of existing or legacy database available for semantic web applications. A typical one is D2RQ④. D2RQ is a declarative language to describe mappings between relational database schemata and OWL/RDFS ontologies, and is implemented as a Jena plugin that rewrites RDQL queries into SQL queries. The result sets of these SQL queries are transformed into RDF triples that are passed up to the higher layers of the Jena framework. RDF Gateway⑤ is a commercial software having similar functionalities. It connects legacy database resources to the Semantic Web via its *SQL Data Service Interface*. The *SQL Data Service* translates a RDF based query to a SQL query and returns the results as RDF data. Our system is different from D2RQ and RDF Gateway. We take the view-based mapping approach which has sound theoretical foundation, and we have visualized mapping tool and ontology-based query and search tool which are not offered by these two systems.

Some other works propose direct manipulation of relational data to RDF/OWL format, and then the data

---

④　http://www.wiwiss.fu-berlin.de/suh1/bizer/D2RQ.

⑤　http://www.intellidimension.com.

could be processed by OWL reasoners or be integrated by ontological mapping tool. D2RMap，KAON REVERSE⑥ and many other toolkits offer such kind of reverse engineering functionality. Cristian Perez de Laborda and colleagues [4] propose an ontology called "Relation OWL" to describe the relational schema as OWL，then use this OWL-representation to transform relational data items into RDF/OWL and provide query service by RDQL. The shortcoming of this kind of approaches is that they have to dump all the relational data into RDF/OWL format before querying，which would be impractical if the RDBMS contains huge volume of data. Moreover，they did not consider the issue of integrating heterogeneous databases using formal ontologies，which is one of the focuses of our solution.

Yuan An and colleagues [5] present an interesting paper concerning about defining semantic mappings between relational tables and ontologies within semantic web context. They introduce a tool which could automatically infer the LAV mapping formulas from simple predicate correspondences between relational schema and formal ontologies. Although completely automatic approach to define semantic mapping is difficult，it would be great enhancement to our visualized tool if some candidate mapping suggestions could be provided beforehand. That will be one of our future work.

The DOPE project (Drug Ontology Project for Elsevier) [6] explores ways to provide access to multiple life science information sources through a single semantic interface called DOPE browser. However，it is still a document management system，mainly concerning on thesaurus-based search，RDF-based querying，and concept-based visualization of large online document repositories. It can not answer semantic queries such as "What diseases does this drug treat?" or "What kind of drugs can treat this disease?". We've seen the authors of DOPE are considering it as one of their future work.

Piazza [7] is an interesting P2P-based data integration system with consideration of semantic web vision. But the current system has been implemented with the XML data model for its mapping language and query answering. However，we think P2P architecture would be a promising direction，and we are considering to extend our system to support P2P working mode and test its scalability and usability.

For other related works，Dejing Dou and colleagues [8] propose an ontology-based framework called OntoGrate. It can automatically transform relational schema into ontological representation，and users can define the mappings at the ontological level using bridge-axioms. Francois [9] considers theoretic aspect of answering query using views for semantic web and Peter Haase and Boris Motik introduce a mapping system for OWL-DL ontology integration [10].

6.2 Conventional Data Integration Context

Without considering the semantic web technologies，our solution can be categorized to the topic "answering query using view"，which has been extensively studied in database community [2] [11]. Most previous works has been focused on the relational case [2]，and XML case [12].

On the one hand，we believe it would be valuable for the semantic web community to take more consideration of the techniques that have been well studied in the data-base community such as answering query using view. On the other hand，we think that the semantic web research does raise a lot of new issues

---

⑥　http://kaon. semanticweb. org/alphaworld/reverse/view.

and challenges for database researchers. From our experiences, the challenges include: how to rank the data object just like the page rank of google? how to maintain highly evolvable and changeable schema mappings among an great number of and open-ended set of databases with no centralized control?

Moreover, a lot of work has been done in the area of ontology-based data integration [13]. Many of them took some ontological formalism such as DL to mediate heterogenous databases, and used the view-based mapping approach. In comparison with them, our implementation is the case of RDF/OWL-based relational data integration with a *semantic web vision in mind*.

7　Summary and Future Work

In this paper, we presented an in-use application of Traditional Chinese Medicine enhanced by a range of semantic web technologies, including RDF/OWL semantics and reasoning tools. The ultimate goal of this system is to realize the "web of structured data" vision by semantically interconnecting legacy databases, which allows a person, or a machine, to start in one database, and then move around an unending set of databases which are connected by rich semantics. To achieve this demanding goal, a set of convenient tools was developed, such as visualized semantic mapping tool, dynamic semantic query tool, and intuitive search tool with concepts ranking. Domain users from CATCM indicated that the system provided an amazing solution for the semantic heterogeneity problem troubling them for a long time.

Currently, although this project is complete, several updated functionalities are still in our consideration. To be specific, we are going to enhance the mapping tools with some heuristic rules to automate the mapping task as far as possible, just like the approach proposed by Yuan An and colleagues [5]. Otherwise, we will develop a more sophisticated mechanism to rank the data objects just like the page rank technology provided by popular search engines.

Acknowledgements

The authors' research is supported by China 973 subprogram "Semantic Grid for Traditional Chinese Medicine" (No. 2003CB316906), China NSF program (No. NSFC60503018) and the EU-IST-027595 NeOn project. We would thank the fruitful discussion and first hand evaluation from our colleagues and partners.

References

[1] Buitelaar, P., Olejnik, D., Sintek, M.: OntoLT: A protégé plug-in for ontology extraction from text. In: Proceedings of the International Semantic Web Conference (ISWC). (2003).

[2] Halevy, A. Y.: Answering queries using views: A survey. The VLDB Journal. 10 (2001) 270-294.

[3] Chen, H., Wu, Z., Wang, H., Mao, Y.: Rdf/rdfs-based relational database integration. In: ICDE. (2006) 94.

[4] de Laborda, C. P., Conrad, S.: Bringing relational data into the semantic web using sparql and relational owl. In: International Workshop on Semantic Web and Database at ICDE 2006. (2006) 55-60.

[5] An, Y., Borgida, A., Mylopoulos, J.: Inferring complex semantic mappings between relational tables and ontologies from simple correspondences. In: International Semantic Web Conference. (2005) 6-20.

[6] Stuckenschmidt, H., van Harmelen, F., de Waard et al, A.: Exploring large document repos- itories with rdf technology: The dope project. IEEE Intelligent Systems. 19 (2004) 34-40.

[7] Halevy, A. Y., Ives, Z. G., Madhavan, J., Mork, P., Suciu, D., Tatarinov, I.: The piazza peer data

management system. IEEE Trans. Knowl. Data Eng. 16-7（2004）787-798.

[8] Dou，D.，LePendu，P.，Kim，S.，Qi，P.：Integrating databases into the semantic web through an ontology-based framework. In：International Workshop on Semantic Web and Database at ICDE 2006.（2006）33-50.

[9] Goasdoue，F.：Answering queries using views：a krdb perspective for the semantic web. ACM Transaction on Internet Technology.（2003）1-22.

[10] Haase，P.，Motik，B.：A mapping system for the integration of owl-dl ontologies. In：IHIS'05：Proceedings of the first international workshop on Interoperability of heterogeneous information systems.（2005）9-16.

[11] Abiteboul，S.，Duschka，O.M.：Complexity of answering queries using materialized views，. In：The Seventeenth ACM SIGACT-SIGMOD-SIGART symposium on Principles of database systems.（1998）254-263.

[12] Yu，C.，Popa，L.：Constraint-based xml query rewriting for data integration. In：2004 ACM SIGMOD international conference on Management of data.（2004）371-382.

[13] Wache，H.，Vögele，T.，Visser，U.，Stuckenschmidt，H.，Schuster，G.，Neumann，H.，Hubner，S.：Ontology-based integration of information—a survey of existing approaches. In Stuckenschmidt，H.，ed.：IJCAI01 Workshop：Ontologies and Information Sharing.（2001）108-117.

Towards Semantic e-Science for Traditional Chinese Medicine

Huajun Chen, Yuxin Mao, Xiaoqing Zheng, Meng Cui, Yi Feng, Shuiguang Deng, Aining Yin, Chunying Zhou, Jinming Tang, Xiaohong Jiang, Zhaohui Wu

首发于 *BMC Bioinformatics*,2007,8(3):1-16

Abstract

Background: Recent advances in Web and information technologies with the increasing decentralization of organizational structures have resulted in massive amounts of information resources and domain-specific services in Traditional Chinese Medicine. The massive volume and diversity of information and services available have made it difficult to achieve seamless and interoperable e-Science for knowledge-intensive disciplines like TCM. Therefore, information integration and service coordination are two major challenges in e-Science for TCM. We still lack sophisticated approaches to integrate scientific data and services for TCM e-Science.

Results: We present a comprehensive approach to build dynamic and extendable e-Science applications for knowledge-intensive disciplines like TCM based on semantic and knowledge-based techniques. The semantic e-Science infrastructure for TCM supports large-scale database integration and service coordination in a virtual organization. We use domain ontologies to integrate TCM database resources and services in a semantic cyberspace and deliver a semantically superior experience including browsing, searching, querying and knowledge discovering to users. We have developed a collection of semantic-based toolkits to facilitate TCM scientists and researchers in information sharing and collaborative research.

Conclusion: Semantic and knowledge-based techniques are suitable to knowledge-intensive disciplines like TCM. It's possible to build on-demand e-Science system for TCM based on existing semantic and knowledge-based techniques. The presented approach in the paper integrates heterogeneous distributed TCM databases and services, and provides scientists with semantically superior experience to support collaborative research in TCM discipline.

1　Background

Traditional Chinese Medicine (TCM) is a medical science that reflects traditional Chinese culture and philosophical principles. As a kind of complex medical science, TCM embodies rich dialectical thought, puts the human body into a large system for observation and adjusts the relations among formations, factors and variables to remain in a healthy status. Recent advances in Web and information technologies with the increasing decentralization of organizational structures have resulted in massive amount of TCM information resources (literature, clinical records, experimental data, etc.). The vast amount of TCM information resources today is distributed among many specialized databases like medical formula database, electronic medical record database, clinical medicine database, and so on [1]. For example, the Consortium for Globalisation of Chinese Medicine (CG-CM) is a global non-profit organization, with a mission of advancing the field of Chinese herbal medicine to benefit human kind of through joint efforts of the academic institutions, industries and regulatory agencies around the world. Members of CG-CM have TCM information resources of their own. Many TCM scientists and biologists begin to use bioinformatics methods to analyze

TCM contents from different points like biochemistry, genetics and molecular biology, so more and more biology databases have been introduced into TCM research. The information in those databases is potentially related to each other within a TCM knowledge-based system, and it is necessary for TCM scientists to reuse them in a global scope. There is an increased emphasis on integration of heterogeneous information resources in present of such a new setting. TCM scientists need to perform dynamic data integration over hundreds of or even thousands upon thousands of geographically distributed, semantically heterogeneous data sources that are subject to different organizations.

Besides the emerging information resources like databases, many scientific methods and processes in TCM have been enclosed as services (e-learning services, information analysis services, data mining services, etc.) by different organizations. There are many bioinformatics services available on-line, which TCM scientists can use to improve their research from the point of biology. Service oriented science [2] has the potential to increase individual and collective scientific productivity by making powerful information tools available to all and thus enabling the widespread automation of data analysis and computation. Scientists and applications are able to access Web services to finish specific tasks or gain information. As scale increases, creating, operating, and even accessing services become challenging. Services are designed to be composed under some contexts, that is, combined in service workflows to provide functionality that none of the component services could provide alone. There is an increased requirement on coordination of various TCM services to support collaborative and on-demand scientific activities.

E-Science is the term applied to the use of advanced computing technologies to support global collaboration for scientists [3]. However, complete and seamless TCM e-Science is impeded by the heterogeneity and distribution of the independently designed and maintained information and service resources. The use of domain knowledge provides a basis for full interoperability in a distributed environment like the Web. As the foundation of the Semantic Web [4], ontologies [5] are the specification of conceptualisations, used to help programs and humans share knowledge. Encoding domain knowledge in terms of ontologies provides a possible approach to overcome the problem of semantic heterogeneity of both information and service resources. As before-mentioned, there are many information resources in the TCM discipline and most of them exist in terms of databases. Formal semantics in ontologies has provided a feasible way to integrate scientific information resources in a conceptual information space. Besides, some semantic mark-up languages like OWL-S [6] are used to describe services with more precise semantics. Richer semantics helps to provide automation or semi-automation of such activities as verification, simulation, configuration, composition, and negotiation of services. From this point of view, the research in knowledge-based approaches especially the semantic techniques has pointed out a new direction to realize the vision of e-Science for TCM.

A number of approaches for e-Science in biology or medicine have been proposed or developed. Stevens *et al.* in [7] aim to exploit Grid techniques especially the Information Grid to achieve e-Science for bioinformatics. They present the myGrid platform that provides middleware layers to satisfy the needs of bioinformatics. The myGrid platform is building high level services for data and application integration such as resource discovery, workflow enactment and distributed query. Tao *et al.* in [8] illustrate through a Semantic Web based knowledge management approach the potential of applying Semantic Web techniques in an e-Science pilot project called GEODISE for the domain of Engineering Design Search and Optimization. They design advice mechanisms based on semantic matching, to consume the semantic information and facilitate service discovery, assembly and configuration in a problem solving environment. They have shown the potential of using semantic technologies to manage and reuse knowledge in e-Science. Roure *et al.* in [9] analyze the state of the art and the research challenges involved in developing the computing infrastructure for e-Science. They propose the future e-Science research infrastructure, which is termed the Semantic Grid and a conceptual architecture for the Semantic Grid is presented, which adopts a service-oriented perspective. They consider the requirements of e-Science in the data/computation, information and knowledge layers. Clearly, e-Science is a widely open research area and there is still much room for improvement on all existing approaches, especially for achieving on-demand e-Science in knowledge-intensive domain like TCM.

In this paper, we address the before-mentioned issues by applying semantic techniques and standards such as RDF[10] and OWL [11] to enable database integration and service coordination towards the full richness of e-Science vision of TCM science over the Internet. To achieve this vision, we propose an approach (1) to model on domain knowledge and develop large-scale domain ontology (2) to interconnect distributed databases using richer semantics as one huge virtual database, and (3) to coordinate scientific services by semantic-driven workflow. We present a dynamic and extendable approach to build on-demand e-Science applications for knowledge-intensive disciplines like TCM based on the semantic techniques. We recognize TCM research as information gathering and process workflows. We have designed and developed the approach as a layered structure to satisfy the TCM research requirements in e-Science. The proposed methods aiming at facilitating the integration and reuse of distributed TCM database and service resources in cyberspace, and deliver a semantically superior experience to TCM scientists. We have developed a collection of semantic-based toolkits to facilitate TCM scientists and researchers in information sharing and collaborative research.

2 Results

System architecture

Briefly, we illustrate the abstract architecture of our approach in Figure 1. In our approach, a TCM e-Science system is composed of client side and server side. We have designed and developed the server side as a layered structure including resource layer, semantic layer and function layer.

- The resource layer mainly supports the typical remote operations on the contents of resources on the Web and querying the meta-information of databases and services. The services in this layer extend some core Grid [12,13] services from the Globus [14] platform. We build the whole e-Science system on these Grid services that provide the basic communication and interaction mechanism for TCM e-Science. There are two services in this layer. *Resource Access Service* supports the typical remote operations on the contents of databases and execution of services. To relational databases, the operations contain query, insertion, deletion, and modification. Resource Information Service supports inquiring about the meta-information of database or service resources including: relational schema definition, DBMS descriptions, service descriptions, privilege information, and statistics information.
- The semantic layer is mainly designed for semantic-based information manipulation and integration.

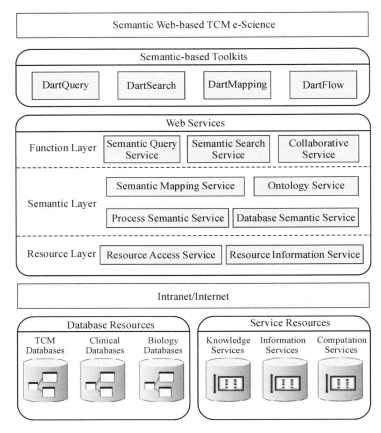

Figure 1   Architecture. The abstract architecture of Semantic Web e‑Science for TCM.

This layer is composed of two sub‑layers. The lower layer contains two services. *Process Semantic Service* is used to export services as OWL‑S descriptions. *Database Semantic Service* is used to export the relational schema of databases as RDF/OWL semantic description. The upper layer contains two services. *Ontology Service* is used to expose the shared TCM ontology and provide basic operations on the ontology. Ontology is used to mediate and integrate heterogeneous databases and services on the Web. Semantic Mapping Service establishes the mappings from local resources to the mediated ontology. *Semantic Mapping Service* maintains the mapping information and provides the mechanism of registering and inquiring about the information.

• The function layer delivers a semantically superior experience to users to support scientific collaborative research and information sharing. *Semantic Query Service* accepts semantic query，inquires Semantic Mapping Service to determine which databases are capable of providing the answer，and then rewrites the semantic queries in terms of database schema. A semantic query is ultimately converted into a set of SQL queries. The service wraps the results of SQL queries by semantics and returns them as triples. *Semantic Search Service* indexes all databases that have been mapped to mediated ontology and accepts semantic‑based full‑text search. The service uses the standard classes and instances from the TCM ontology as the lexicon in establishing indexes. *Collaborative Service* discovers and coordinates various services in a process work‑flow to supports research activities in a virtual community for TCM scientists.

Note that we differentiate two kinds of services. The services in this architecture are fundamental services to support the whole e-Science system, whereas there are many common services treated as Web resources for e-Science process. At the client side, the e-Science system provides a set of semantic-based toolkits to assist scientists to perform complex tasks during research. We call this architecture *Dart* (Dynamic, Adaptive, RDF-mediated and Transparent) [15], which is an abstract model for TCM e-Science. A detailed description of the service-oriented architecture is provided in the Methods section.

2.2 TCM domain ontology

Recent advent of the Semantic Web and bioinformatics has facilitated the incorporation of various large-scale online ontologies in biology and medicine, such as UMLS [16] for integrating biomedical terminology, Gene Ontology [17] for gene product and MGED Ontology [18] for microarray experiment. As the backbone of the Semantic Web for TCM, a unified and comprehensive TCM domain ontology is also required to support interoperability in TCM e-Science.

To overcome the problem of semantic heterogeneity and encode domain knowledge in reusable format, we need an integrated approach to develop and apply a large-scale domain ontology for the TCM discipline. In collaboration with the China Academy of Traditional Chinese Medicine (CATCM), we have taken more than five years in building the world's largest TCM domain ontology [19].

We divide the whole TCM domain into several sub-domains. The TCM ontology is developed collaboratively by several branches of the CATCM as categories. A category is a relatively independent ontology corresponding to a relatively closed sub-domain, compared with the ontology corresponding to the whole domain. There are 12 categories in the current knowledge base of the TCM ontology. Each category is corresponding to a sub-domain (Basic Theory of TCM, Formula of Herbal Medicine, Acupuncture, etc) of TCM. We list the characterization of content of each category in Table 1. Considering medical concepts and their relationships from the perspective of TCM discipline, we define the knowledge system of the TCM ontology by two components: concept system and semantic system (see Figure 2). The concept system contains content classes that represent the domain knowledge of the TCM discipline and four kinds of basic implemental classes (name class, definition class, explanation class, and relation class) to define each content class. The semantic system concerns the basic semantic type and semantic relationship of class. A class has literal property and object property. The range of a literal property is a literal or string, whereas the range of an object property is a class. A content class has five object properties (see Table 2) with each related with a class. Relation class has two properties: the range of the former is semantic relationship and the range of the latter is content class. Content classes are related with each other through semantic relationship. In this way, all content classes in the TCM ontology have the unified knowledge structure whereas different instances of content class have various contents and relationships.

There are more than 20,000 classes and 100,000 instances defined in the TCM ontology and the ontology has become a distributed large-scale knowledge base for TCM domain knowledge. The ontology has become large enough to cover different aspects of the TCM discipline and is used to support semantic e-science for TCM. As a large-scale domain ontology, the TCM ontology is used to integrate various database resources in a semantic view and provide formal semantics to support service coordination in TCM e-Science.

Table 1 TCM ontology categories. The initial categories defined in the TCM ontology corresponding to the sub-domains of TCM.

Categories
The Basic Theory of Traditional Chinese Medicine
The Doctrines of Traditional Chinese Medicine and Relevant Science
Chinese Materia Medica (Herbal Medicine)
Formula of Herbal Medicine
Humanities
Medicinal Propagation and Other Resources
Cause and Mechanism of Disease and Diagnosis
Therapeutic Principles and Treatments
Informatics and Philology
Acupuncture
Prevention
Diseases

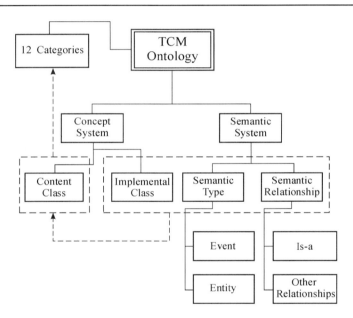

Figure 2 Semantic system framework. The semantic system framework of the TCM ontology.

Table 2 Content class structure. The structure of content class in the TCM ontology

Class Property		Property Value
hasNames	Name Class	
hasDefinitions	Definition Class	
hasExplanations	Explanation Class	
hasRelatedClasses	Relation Class	Semantic Relationship
		Content Class
hasSemanticTypes	Semantic Type	

2.3 TCM database integration

We use ontology semantics to integrate distributed TCM databases as a global virtual database. We have developed a set of semantic-based toolkits for scientists to integrate and use information in distributed TCM databases.

2.4 DartMapping

In our approach，before-mentioned domain ontology acts as a semantic mediator for integrating distributed heterogeneous databases. Relational schemata of distributed TCM databases are mapped to the TCM ontology according to their intrinsic relations. To facilitate the process of semantic mapping between the schemata of local databases and the semantics of the mediated ontology，we have developed a visual semantic mapping tool called *DartMapping* for integrating relational databases in a Semantic Web way（see Figure 3）. The tool provides two major functions：establishing semantic mapping from heterogeneous relational database to a mediated ontology semi-automatically，especially mapping for composite schema with complex join between tables，and converting relational databases schema to ontology statements based on the semantic mapping information.

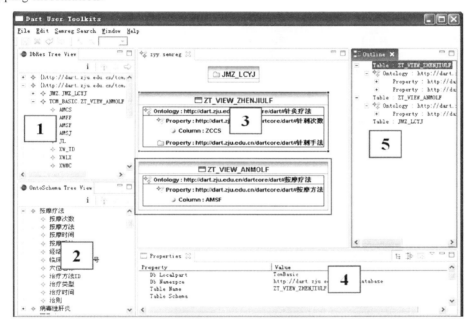

Figure 3 DartMapping. The default user interface for DartMapping.

Figure 3 depicts how we use DartMapping to establish mapping between ontology and database schema. Relational database schema is displayed in hierarchy including the names of databases，tables and the corresponding fields（1）. The class hierarchy and class properties of the mediated ontology are displayed below（2）. Classes and properties are displayed as labels in the panel. User drags tables and classes into the main panel（3），and establishes their mappings directly. One table is likely to be mapped to more than one class. The meta-information about the selected table is shown under the main panel（4）. The right panel shows the outline of the mapping definitions（5）. A mapping definition can be exported as XML files and reused by applications. Besides，users are able to query mapping information defined previously in DartMapping. TCM scientists are able to map local databases to the mediated TCM ontology with

DartMapping. Distributed and heterogeneous databases including TCM databases (e. g. herbal medicine formula database), clinical databases (e. g. EHR database) and biology databases (e. g. neuron database) are integrated as knowledge sources for TCM scientists to carry out research. TCM scientists are able to perform searching and querying over the integrated databases to gain useful information in research.

2.5 DartSearch

We developed a database search engine called *DartSearch* to enable full-text search over distributed databases. Scientists are able to perform searching through the integrated databases to get required information as we do in search engines like Google [20]. However, search here is different with Google-like search. The search process is performed based on the semantic relations of the ontology. We call it *semantic search*, which is searching for data objects rather than Web pages. Semantics is presented in two aspects in DartSearch:

- We construct a domain-specific lexicon for segmentation based on the TCM ontology. Each term in the lexicon is a class or instance in the ontology plus its part of speech. When we segment a piece of information from database, only the words that appear in the TCM ontology are segmented whereas other words are discarded as irrelevant information to TCM semantic search.

- Unlike keyword-based index in traditional search engine, we construct index for classes or instances in databases. The semantic relations between those classes or instances are encoded as part of the index.

In this way, scientists are able to search with more accurate constraints and get more relevant information from search results. For example, if a TCM scientist wants to find some TCM formulas that cure *influenza*, then he can use influenza as a keyword to perform a semantic search. The search returns TCM-specific information and the information that doesn't contain the keyword influenza but contains terms related to influenza is also returned. We connect directly-matched information and relevant information by using semantic relations in the ontology.

We provide users with a Google-like search interface to perform semantic search (see the bottom left panel in Figure 4) in DartSearch. The result of a semantic search request is shown in Figure 4 with *gene* used as the keyword. The statistics information about the search result (e. g. the number of items) is displayed (1). DartSearch lists the items in a descending order according to their matching degrees to the keywords of the search (2). Each item in the list is a piece of information from databases that have been mapped to TCM ontology classes (3). At the bottom of each item, there are the classes the item is mapped to (4), the classes relevant to the mapping classes (5) and the matching degree to the keyword. The classes and relevant classes are connected by semantic relations in the ontology. The schemata of a database are allowed to be mapped to several categories of the TCM ontology. Categories that relevant to the search result are listed in a descending order according to their matching degrees to the search (6).

2.6 DartQuery

Generally, semantic search only gives us a coarse set of result. If scientists want to get more exact information, they are able to perform querying instead of searching in the semantic layer. A Web-based query tool called *DartQuery* is provided for scientists to query over distributed TCM databases dynamically (see Figure 5). Relevant categories generated during semantic search imply the possible scopes from within scientists perform semantic query. They are able to select the category with the largest matching degree to

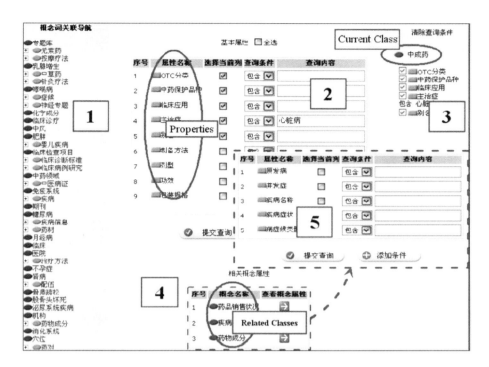

Figure 4　DartSearch. The default user interface for DartSearch.

construct a semantic query statement. To enable querying in the semantic layer，we use the SPARQL [21] query language. Every query in SPARQL is viewed as an ontology class definition，and processing a query request is reduced as computing out ontology instances satisfying the class definition [22]. The statement of a semantic query about the properties（name，usage，composition，etc.）of a TCM formula that cures influenza is as follows：

```
SELECT ?fn ?fu ?fc ?dn ?dp ?ds
WHERE {
?y1 rdf: type tcm: Formula_of_Herbal_Medicine
?y1 tcm: name ?fn
?y1 tcm: usage_and_dosage ?fu
?y1 tcm: composition ?fc
?y1 tcm: cure ?y2
?y2 tcm: name "influenza"
?y2 tcm: pathogenesis ?dp
?y2 tcm: symptom_complex ?ds
}
```

Such a query in SPARQL is constructed dynamically. A form-like query interface is used to facilitate users in constructing semantic query statements in Web browser. The user interface incorporates an open-source AJAX framework [23]，which enables immediate data update without refresh Web pages in web browsers. DartQuery generates querying forms automatically according to the class definitions in a category. Scientists who want to query something are able to construct a query statement by selecting classes and properties from the forms in the query interface. Figure 5 depicts the process how a user constructs a semantic

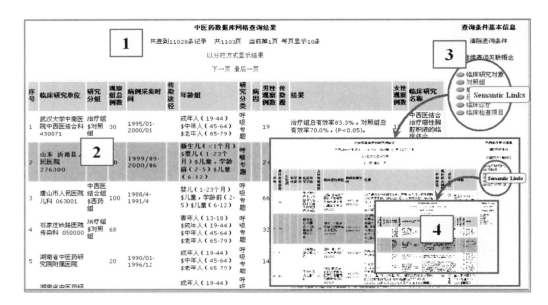

Figure 5 DartQuery. The default user interface for DartQuery.

query about **traditional patent medicine**. Starting from the ontology view panel on the left, the user is able to browse the hierarchy tree and select the relevant classes (1). A query form corresponding to the property definitions of the selected class is automatically generated and displayed in the middle. Users could select properties of interest, and inputs query constraints such as the **efficiency** of the medicine (2). An outline of the currently-built query including the current class is displayed (3). Users could further explore into the classes related (e.g. **disease**) to the current one, and construct more complex semantic queries spanning over several classes (4). Users are led into the query interface of related classes, and could add more query constraints (5).

The SPARQL query statement is submitted to the system and converted into a SQL query plan according to the mapping information between database schemata and the mediated ontology. The SQL query plan is then dispatched to specific databases for information retrieval. The query returns all satisfactory records from databases that have been mapped to the ontology. Since the query result from databases is just a record set without any semantics, the system converts the record set into a data stream in RDF/XML format and the semantics of the result is fully presented. Figure 6 depicts the situation in which a user is navigating the query result. The statistics information about the query result is displayed (1). User selects one data object, which is highlighted (2). By following semantic links, user could get all those data objects semantically related to the current one (3). Note that the relations between the selected object and those discovered by following semantic links are derived from the ontology in the semantic layer. User could keep on navigating through a collection of databases as long as they are semantically connected (4).

2.7 TCM service coordination

Ontology semantics are used to support dynamic and ondemand service coordination in a VO. Scientists are able to discover, retrieve and compose various services to achieve complex research tasks in a visual environment.

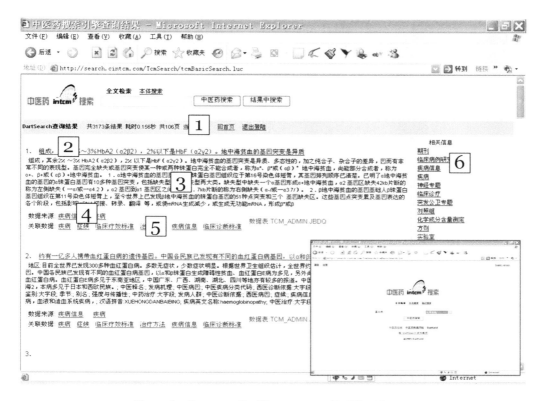

Figure 6　Query result. The query result of DartQuery.

2.8　Knowledge discovery service

There are various services in a TCM VO and we mainly recognize three kinds of services: computation services, information services, and knowledge services. Computation services are services that execute computational jobs or analyze scientific data. Information services are services that manipulate and provide specific information. Semantic query service and semantic search service mentioned-before are two typical information services. Knowledge services are services that apply information to solve domain-specific problems or discover facts. Different services are used to support different kinds of tasks for TCM research.

One of the most important knowledge services for TCM research is the knowledge discovery service. The distributed databases integrated under the ontology contain much implicit domain knowledge that is hard to be discovered manually by human-being and thus require some intelligent methods to assist scientists to discover the implicit knowledge. For example, a formula of herbal medicine is composed of several individual drugs. In database of herbal medicine formula, we get the components of a formula directly; however, the same individual drug may appear in Several formulas, and then the correlation between two individual drugs in various formulas can't be acquired directly by querying or searching. Notice that, according to TCM theory, a relatively fixed combination of several individual drugs is called a paired-drug when such a combination is able to strengthen their medical effects, or lessen the toxicity and side effects of some drugs. Implicit knowledge such as "paired-drug" is more likely to be discovered by data mining, instead of directly querying or searching information resources. Our method integrates several semantic-based data mining algorithms like the associated and correlated pattern mining [24] to achieve knowledge discovery on distributed databases.

Scientists are able to select knowledge discovery service according to the requirements of the research task and perform knowledge discovery over a selective set of information from distributed databases.

2.9 DartFlow

Besides database integration, a sophisticated e-Science system should also support service coordination for scientists, which is a significant part of TCM e-Science. Similarly with bioinformatics, TCM scientific research often requires coordination and composition of service resources. We have applied semantic techniques to achieve dynamic and on-demand service coordination in a VO and developed a Web-based service coordination tool (see Figure 7) called *DartFlow* [25]. DartFlow provides a convenient and efficient way for scientists to collaborate with each other in research activities. It offers interfaces to allow researchers to register, query, compose and execute services in the semantic layer.

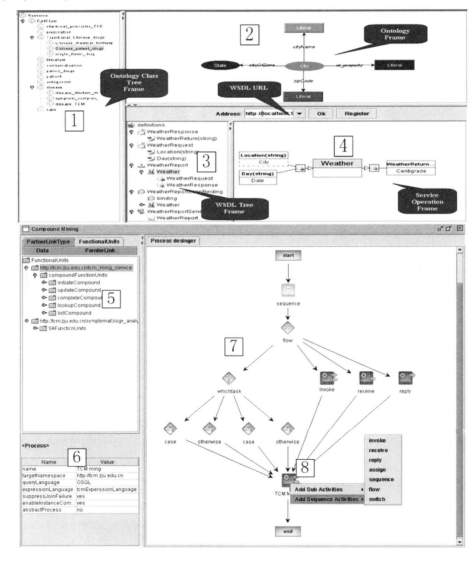

Figure 7   DartFlow. The user interface of DartFlow.

Service providers register component Web service into the VO before service composition. DartFlow integrates a service registration portal for scientists to register new services. The class hierarchy (1) and class properties (2) of the mediated ontology are displayed graphically. Service description (e. g. the input and output parameters) is displayed in hierarchy (3). Similarly with semantic mapping in database integration, service providers create mappings between ontology classes and service descriptions (4). The mapping information is stored in the repository of the portal. Automatic service discovery and service match-making are achieved based on semantics. So far DartFlow has been full of a collection of scientific services, which are all provided by different TCM research institutes.

When a VO has been filled with various applied service, scientists are able to build serviceflow to achieve complex research tasks in DartFlow. We should retrieve enough services in order to compose a serviceflow. If scientists want to query services, they submit a service profile (e. g. a service to analyze TCM clinical data) to the portal specifying their requirements. The portal invokes suitable match-making agent to retrieve target services for users (5). The agent has been implemented according to some semantic-based service matchmaking algorithm. Scientists are able to compose retrieved services (6) into a serviceflow in the workspace (7) to achieve a research task. In order to enhance the flexibility and usability of serviceflow, DartFlow supports both static activity node and dynamic activity node in serviceflow (8): the former refers to those nodes combined with specific applied services at build-time; and the latter refers to those nodes combined with semantic information. After a serviceflow is designed graphically, the corresponding OWL-S file is generated according to the service mapping information. Scientists are able to validate the serviceflow from both logic aspect and syntax aspect with a validator in DartFlow and the validated serviceflow will be executed ultimately.

2. 10　TCM collaborative research scenario

The proposed semantic-based approach is able to support TCM scientists to perform research collaboratively in a VO. TCM scientists are able to use the semantic-based toolkits before-mentioned in Web browsers anywhere to solve problems and finish tasks. We illustrate the application of our approach through the following collaborative research scenario as several steps (see Figure 8):

2. 11　Task-driven information allocation

Information resources are often related to perform a research task. Grouping task-related information resources is a precondition for achieving collaborative research. Given a research task, TCM scientists are able to perform semantic search or construct semantic query to allocate information according to the task context. A TCM scientist, said, Wang is performing a research task about *the impact of herbal medicine formula on gene expression*. As a TCM scientist, Wang is not familiar about biology especially gene, so he needs to find some initial information about gene before starting to conduct experiments. He is able to perform semantic search over distributed databases in DartSearch about gene as well as its relations with TCM. DartSearch will return a general result about gene and its relation with TCM. If Wang wants more exact results about current research progress about herbal medicine formula and gene, he can perform semantic query in DartQuery. The semantic search in DartSearch has implied that the required information is mainly located in categories Formula of Herbal Medicine and Diseases. Then Wang is able to perform

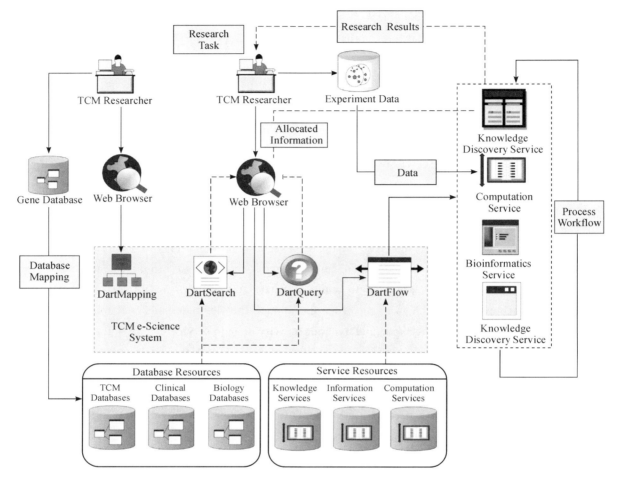

Figure 8 **Scenario. A scenario about TCM collaborative research based on the TCM e-Science system.**

semantic query within the databases that have been integrated under these two categories. Wang constructs semantic query statements dynamically in DartQuery and the query returns a collection of literature about herbal medicine formula and gene.

2.12 Collaborative information sharing

After reading a batch of relevant papers，Wang decides to perform further research about the relations between herbal medicine formula and gene expression. However，he finds the information he allocated is insufficient for his task，and it means the TCM VO lacks the required information. Scientists are able to allocate only a very small sub-set of information or services in the field of TCM. It's impossible for a single scientist to deal with all the domain information. Scientists can share information collaboratively in a VO based on the semantic e-Science system. Wang can communicate with other scientists in the VO to ask for required information. Fortunately，an institute in the VO has developed a new database that contains information about gene expression. The institute registers the database into the VO by creating semantic mappings with DartMapping. Then Wang is able to get further information about gene expression by querying the database.

2. 13　Scientific service coordination

Wang selects suitable services according to his research requirements and designs a serviceflow in DartFlow to achieve his research goal (see Figure 8). The first knowledge discovery service in the serviceflow is used to discover some underlying rules from the allocated information. The result of knowledge discovery has shown that there exists underlying relation between Sini decoction (a kind of herbal medicine formula) and glutathione S-transferase (GST) gene expression from many research papers. Wang starts to conduct experiments on the impacts of Sini decoction on GST gene expression. The experiment data is submitted to the computation service in the serviceflow. He also uses bioinformatics services such as BLAST in the serviceflow to deal with the works related with GST gene. The final result of the serviceflow has shown that *Sini decoction has strong impacts on GST gene expression*. The serviceflow here may involve a recursive process in order to refine the result.

3　Discussion

Due to the bottleneck of information extraction and NLP, the proposed approach is inclined to structured information resources rather than unstructured or semi-structured resources. However, much information is involved in those resources, which we can't integrate into the TCM e-Science system well with the current method. Although we could extract schemata from unstructured or semistructured resource and map those to the mediated ontology in a similar way as database integration, there leaves much work to be done for the purpose. We have provided a set of semantic-based toolkits to assist TCM scientists to reuse information and carry out research. Although the tools are implemented and used based on web browser, the process of interaction may be still a little bit complex to TCM scientists who have no knowledge of semantics. As TCM is a traditional science and there are also many TCM scientists who are even not familiar with computer and Internet. To those scientists, we should improve the usage and convenience of the system to satisfy their requirements well.

4　Conclusion

We have presented a comprehensive and extendable approach that is able to support on-demand and collaborative e-Science for knowledge-intensive disciplines like TCM based on semantic and knowledge-based techniques. The semantic-based e-Science infrastructure for TCM supports large-scale database integration and service coordination in a virtual organization. We have developed a collection of semantic-based toolkits to facilitate TCM scientists and researchers to achieve information sharing and collaborative research. We illustrate the application of the proposed approach through a TCM collaborative research scenario. Based on the proposed approach, we have built a fundamental e-Science platform for TCM in CATCM and the system currently provides access to over 50 databases and 800 services in practice. The result has shown that integrating databases and coordinating services with a large-scale domain ontology is an efficient approach to achieve on-demand e-Science for TCM and other similar application domains, such as life science and biology.

5   Methods

5.1   TCM ontology engineering

The TCM ontology is a basic element to achieve semantic e-Science for TCM, therefore the quality of the ontology directly affects the e-Science. We should develop the TCM ontology according to some criteria based on the agreement among the participant institutes. The development of ontologies is a modelling process that needs the cooperation of ontology engineers (also called ontologists) who should have sufficient understanding of the domain knowledge. To our experience, ontology construction is a complex and labor-intensive activity.

First, we employ a layered privilege model in ontology development. Users that play different roles in the process of ontology development hold different privileges. There are mainly four kinds of privileges: reader, editor, checker and administrator.

- Ontology readers are able to browse all the contents of the ontology.
- Ontology editors are able to input, modify and delete instances within a category but have no privilege to manipulate the classes of the category.
- Ontology checkers own the privilege to manipulate both classes and instances in a category.
- Ontology administrators have the global privilege to all categories of the whole ontology.

Then, we could develop the ontology according to the following procedure:

- Analyze and determine knowledge sources. The scientific control of the conceptual glossary of a discipline is the most important issue in NLP. It's necessary to analyze specialized lexicons as the knowledge sources of ontology contents.
- Construct an upper-level conceptual framework. Comprehensive analysis and research of the disciplines is needed before the ontology design. A domain oriented conceptual framework is constructed to address all the knowledge engineering problems and instruct editing ontology content.
- Determine and assign developing tasks. Developing a large-scale ontology is a laborious work that requires collaborative efforts. We divide a large-scale ontology into categories and assign developing tasks to participants by category according to the complexity of each category.
- Extend conceptual hierarchy. Checkers create low-level class hierarchy.
- Materialize ontology contents. Editors extract and acquire domain knowledge from various sources, and formalize knowledge into instances.
- Check and revise contents. Checkers check each instance in the category they take charge of to make sure that there is no error or contradiction in newly input contents.
- Publish ontology by using user interface. The ontology is published as Web service and users are able to browse and query the ontology through Web browsers.

Step 4 to step 6 is a recursive process. Follow this general procedure and we are able to develop a large-scale domain ontology for e-Science system.

5.2   View-based semantic mapping

The semantic-based e-Science system allocates database information and integrates heterogeneous databases together under the TCM ontology by creating semantic views. A relational table is mapped into one or more classes of the ontology and a table field is mapped to a class property. Implicit relationships between database resources are interpreted as semantic relations in the ontology.

According to the conventional data integration literature [26], view-based approach has a well-understood foundation and been proved to be flexible for heterogeneous data integration. There are two kinds of view in conventional data integration systems, GAV (global-as-view) or LAV (local-as-view). Considering the Semantic Web situation, GAV is to define each class or property as a view over relational tables, and LAV is to define each relational table as a view (or query) over the mediated ontology. The experiences from conventional data integration systems tell us that LAV provides greater extensibility than GAV: the addition of new sources is less likely to require a change to the mediated schema [26]. In the field of TCM, new databases are regularly added so total number of databases is increasing gradually.

Therefore, the LAV approach is employed in our method, that is, each relational table is defined as a view over the ontologies. We call such kind of views as *semantic view*, and such kind of mappings from relational database to ontology as *semantic mapping*. Like that in conventional data integration, a typical semantic view consists of two parts: the view head, which is a relational predicate, and the view body, which is a set of RDF triples. In general, the view body is viewed as a query over the ontology, and it defines the semantics of the relational predicate from the perspective of the ontology. The meaning of semantic view would be clearer if we construct a *target instance* based on the semantic mapping specified by these views. In this way, different TCM databases can be integrated under the shared TCM ontology. Scientists needn't care about the actual structure of database resources and they just operate on the semantic layer. More detailed aspects about semantic view and semantic mapping could be found in [27].

5.3 Semantic-based service matchmaking

A service is abstracted as service description including input and out parameters. If the service descriptions are mapped to ontology classes, service matchmaking and composition can be achieved automatically and dynamically based on semantics. Ideally, given a user's objective and a set of services, an agent would find a collection of services requests that achieves the objective. We use a semantic-based method to achieve dynamic service matchmaking and composition in DartFlow. Assume X and Y are two ontology classes. We represent the matching degree of class X to class Y as Similarity(X, Y). If X can provide all the properties that Y embodies, they are totally matched. If X embodies Y, they are partially matched. They only partially provide the properties that value of Similarity(X, Y) ranges from 0 to 1. The value 0 means X is not semantically similar to Y at all, and the value 1 means X is the same as Y. Note that Similarity(X, Y) and Similarity(Y, X) represent different matching degrees. Different relations between X and Y result in different formulas of similarity evaluation.

Service matchmaking is to match a service request against a collection of services. As services are mapped to ontology classes by service providers, service matchmaking is reduced into calculating the semantic similarity of ontology classes. Given a service $S = (I, O)$ and a service request $R = (I_r, O_r)$, we can calculate the matching degree between S and R, which is denoted as $\Omega(S, R)$. $\Omega(S, R)$ is mainly determined by the similarity between I and I_r, and the similarity between O and O_r. Our algorithm ensures the value of a matching degree ranging from 0 to 1. Service composition is also performed based on semantic similarity.

Given a service A = (I_a , O_a) in the serviceflow and a collection of candidate services, the service B = (I_b , O_b) will be selected as the subsequent service of A in the serviceflow as long as $\Omega(A, B)$ is the largest among the candidate services. More detailed aspects about the algorithm could be found in [25]. Given a representation of services as actions, we can exploit AI planning techniques for automatic service composition by treating service composition as a planning problem [28].

Competing interests

The authors declare that they have no competing interests.

Authors' contributions

The semantic-based approach was developed jointly by all authors and implemented by YM, HC, CZ, JT and SD. HC, YM, XZ, YF and SD have designed the system architecture, developed general concepts, participated in the manuscript writing and coordinated the study. The TCM ontology was mainly designed by HC, MC, AY and YM. The database integration method was mainly designed and developed by HC, YM, JT and CZ. The service coordination method was mainly developed by SD, HC and YM. The knowledge discovery method was mainly designed and developed by YF. All authors read and approved the final version of the manuscript.

Acknowledgements

HC's work is funded by NSFC under Grant No. NSFC60503018 and Zhejiang Provincial Natural Science Foundation of China (No. Y105463), YM, XZ, YF, SD, CZ's work are supported by subprogram of China 973 project (No. 2003CB317006), ZH's work is funded under National Science Fund for Distinguished Young Scholars of China NSF program (No. NSFC60525202), and the Program for New Century Excellent Talents in University of Ministry of Education of China (No. NCET-04-0545).

This article has been published as part of *BMC Bioinformatics* Volume 8 Supplement 3, 2007: Semantic e-Science in Biomedicine. The full contents of the supplement are available online at http://www. biomedcentral. com/1471-2105/8?issue = S3.

References

[1] Feng Y, Wu Z, Zhou X, Zhou Z, Fan W: Knowledge Discovery in Traditional Chinese Medicine: State of the Art and Perspectives. Artif Intell Med 2006,38(3):219-236.

[2] Foster I: Service-Oriented Science. Science 2005,308(5723):814-817.

[3] De Roure D, Hendler JA: E-Science: The Grid and the Semantic Web. IEEE Intell Syst 2004,19(1):65-71.

[4] Berners-Lee T, Hendler J, Lassila O: The Semantic Web. Sci Am. 2001, 284(5): 34-43.

[5] Gruber T: A Translation Approach to Portable Ontology Specifications. Knowl Acquis 1993,5(2):199-220.

[6] OWL-S [http://www. w3. org/Submission/OWL-S/].

[7] Stevens R, Robinson A, Goble CA: myGrid: Personalised Bioinformatics on the Information Grid. Bioinformatics 2003,19(Suppl 1):i302-i304.

[8] Tao F, Shadbolt N, Chen L, Xu F, Cox S: Semantic Web based Content Enrichment and Knowledge Reuse in e-Science. Proceedings of 3rd International Conference on Ontologies, DataBases, and Applications of Semantics for Large Scale Information Systems: 25-29, October 14, 2004: Agia Napa, Cyprus 2004:654-669.

[9] Research Agenda for the Semantic Grid: A Future e-Science Infrastructure [http://www. semanticgrid. org/v1. 9/

semgrid. pdf].

[10] Resource Description Framework（RDF）[http://www.w3.org/ TR/rdf-concepts/].

[11] Web Ontology Language（OWL）[http://www.w3.org/TR/owl- features/].

[12] Foster I，Kesselman C.（Eds）：The Grid：Blueprint for a New Computing Infrastructure Morgan Kaufmann，San Francisco，CA；1999.

[13] Foster I，Kesselman C，Tuecke S：The Anatomy of the Grid：Enabling Scalable Virtual Organizations. Lecture Notes in Computer Science 2001，2150：1-26.

[14] Foster I，Kesselman C：Globus：A Metacomputing Infrastructure Toolkit. Int J Supercomp Appl 1997，11(2)：115-128.

[15] Chen H，Wu Z，Mao Y，Zheng G：DartGrid：a semantic infrastructure for building database Grid applications. Concurr Comp-Pract E 2006,18(14)：1811-1828.

[16] Bodenreider O：Unified medical language system（umls）：integrating biomedical terminology. Nucleic Acids Res 2004,32(D)：D267-D270.

[17] Ashburner M，Ball CA，Blake JA，Botstein D，Butler H，Cherry JM，Davis AP，Dolinski K，Dwight SS，Eppig JT，Harris MA，Hill DP，Issel-Tarver L，Kasarskis A，Lewis S，Matese JC，Richardson JE，Ringwald M，Rubin GM，Sherlock G：Gene Ontology：tool for the unification of biology. Nat Genet 2000,25：25-29.

[18] Whetzel P，Parkinson H，Causton H，Fan L，Fostel J，Fragoso G，Game L，Heiskanen M，Morrison N，Rocca-Serra P，Sansone SA，Taylor C，White J，Stoeckert C：The MGED Ontology：a resource for semantics-based description of microarray experiments. Bioinformatics 2006,22(7)：866-873.

[19] Zhou X，Wu Z，Yin A，Wu L，Fan W，Zhang R：Ontology Development for Unified Traditional Chinese Medical Language System. Artif Intell Med 2004,32(1)：15-27.

[20] Google [http://www.google.com]

[21] SPARQL Query Language for RDF [http://www.w3.org/TR/rdf- sparql-query/].

[22] Chen H，Wang Y，Wang H，Mao Y，Tang J，Zhou C，Yin A，Wu Z：Towards a Semantic Web of Relational Databases：a Practical Semantic Toolkit and an In-Use Case from Traditional Chinese Medicine. Proceedings of the 5th International Semantic Web Conference：5-9，Nov.，2006；Athens，GA，USA 2006：750-763.

[23] Qooxdoo Open Source AJAX Framework [http://qooxdoo.org].

[24] Zhou Z，Wu Z，Wang C，Feng Y：Efficiently Mining Both Association and Correlation Rules. Proceedings of the 3rd International Conference on Fuzzy Systems and Knowledge Discovery：24-28，Sep.，2006；Xi'an，China 2006：369-372.

[25] Deng S，Wu J，Li Y，Wu Z：Service Matchmaking Based on Semantics and Interface Dependencies. Proceeding of the 7th International Conference on Web-Age Information Management：17-19，June，2006；Hong Kong，China 2006：240-251.

[26] Halevy AY：Answering queries using views：A survey. VLDB J 2001,10：270-294.

[27] Chen H，Wu Z，Wang H，Mao Y：Rdf/rdfs-based relational data- base integration. Proceedings of the 22nd International Conference on Data Engineering：20-23，Oct.，2006；Atlanta，Georgia，USA 2006：94.

[28] Wu D，Parsia B，Sirin E，Hendler J，Nau D：Automating DAML-S Web Services Composition Using SHOP2. Proceedings of the 2nd International Semantic Web Conference：20-23，Oct.，2003；Sanibel Island，FL，USA 2003：195-210.

4.2 学位论文摘要

本节摘录了中医药云平台与服务计算方向 2004—2020 年共 19 份学位论文资料信息(其中博士学位论文 1 份,硕士学位论文 18 份)。

4.2.1 Database Grid:面向网格的数据库资源管理平台

黄昶(指导教师:吴朝晖)

2004 年硕士学位论文

网格是下一代 Internet 上的计算平台。它的核心任务是管理分布在 Internet 广域环境中的各种类型的软硬件资源,为基于 Internet 的分布式应用提供一个统一的、虚拟的共享资源的计算平台。作为网格计算模型的一个重要组成部分,网格上的数据管理一直以来是网格研究的一个热点。目前网格数据管理的研究对象主要集中在基于文件的信息资源,很少涉及数据库资源。然而,来自科学和商业领域的大量网格应用迫切需要数据库系统的支持。因此,如何将数据库资源并入现有的网格架构,满足更加广泛的网格应用的数据管理需求,已经成为一项亟待解决的难题。

本文从动态开放的网格环境下数据的资源共享与协同管理的应用需求背景出发,综合了现有 Internet 下的数据资源的信息共享与语义整合解决方案,提出了数据库网格的概念。数据库网格是一个基于现有网格体系标准(OGSA)的,面向动态、开放分布式计算环境的数据库资源管理平台。数据库网格以数据库资源的语义融合为主线,提出了一套解决数据库资源访问、语义发现、动态整合等一系列网格资源管理问题的方案。本文阐述了数据库网格的基本思想、服务分层模型框架,并以协议的方式定义了网格环境下数据库资源的共享行为规则。本文介绍的数据库网格协议是课题研究的核心内容,旨在为数据库资源管理问题提供一套可参考的规范。本文还介绍了依照数据库网格协议,设计并实现的数据库网格原型系统 DartGrid,并介绍了 DartGrid 在传统中医药研究领域的一个应用测试床。最后,本文进行了总结,提出了进一步的工作,并且对 Database Grid 的发展进行了展望。

4.2.2 知识库网格模型的研究

徐杰锋(指导教师:吴朝晖)

2004 年硕士学位论文

语义互联网的出现将产生大量网上知识库资源。如何发现、组织、管理这些知识库资源,并提供高可靠性的可扩展服务是一个亟待解决的问题。网格技术以其成熟的互联网分布式计算服务体系,承诺对网络资源的广泛共享和协同使用,为上述问题的解决提供了良好的基础技术支撑。

知识库网格 DartGrid/KG 是一个针对语义互联网中知识库资源的共享、管理和协同使用的网格体系,它结合了语义互联网和网格的观点,以服务的方式对外提供了知识库管理、操作、查询等一系列接口。本文主要围绕知识库网格这个创新性概念,对其模型进行深入研究,着重描述了知识库网格的拓扑结构以及模型实现的若干关键技术。文章的主要工作如下。

本文探讨了知识库网格 DartGrid/KG 的系统组成。在知识库网格中,知识服务器是最基本的单元,它包括本体知识服务器、规则服务器、案例服务器等类型,是知识库网格的信息和知识来源。本体论服务器用于指导知识的分类、管理和维护。知识库目录服务器则提供了知识服务器的注册、发现、管理等功能。语义浏览器,作为知识库网格的客户端,提供了知识浏览、查询、简单推理、节点管理等功能。

本文定义了知识库网格的服务模型和核心协议族。DartGrid/KG 的服务模型扩展于开放网格服务体系 OGSA,并增加了知识库网格特有的本体论服务、规则推理服务和案例推理服务。本体论服务、语义注册和发现是 DartGrid/KG 的核心,与之对应的语义注册协议、本体论查询协议、本体论验证协议和本体论融合协议也是本文的一个重点。

本文描述了知识库网格的实现及其在中医药研究中的应用。DartGrid/KG 作为信息网格 DartGrid 的语义支撑,提供了资源的动态语义注册、分布式语义查询和知识级语义浏览。目前系统已经基本实现,并在中医药研究中得到了充分的应用。

今后的工作重点将放在对多种本体论语言的兼容,分布式推理的完善与实现,以及知识级通信协议的设计上。

4.2.3 DartGrid V3 语义数据库网格的设计与核心模块实现

王恒(指导教师:吴朝晖、陈华钧)
2006 年硕士学位论文

在互联网飞速发展的背景下,数据库应用体现出了不同于以往的新特点,新的需求应运而生。海量数据及数据孤岛的产生,严重阻碍了科学数据的有效共享。

本文从这一背景出发,在传统的数据集成解决方案的基础上引入了语义技术和网格技术,提出了基于语义的数据库网格的概念,作为异质异构数据库集成的一种解决方案。

在基于语义的数据库网格理论中,传统数据资源网格服务化和语义化对异质异构数据库集成有着重要的意义。实现传统数据资源网格服务化的关键问题,是数据资源网格虚拟组织的组成、角色及各自职责的定义问题;而实现传统数据资源语义化的关键问题,是基于语义视图的语义映射和查询重写的思想。

DartGrid 平台是基于语义的数据库网格的一个实现。本文通过对 DartGrid V3 平台的系统核心构架、核心模块、核心算法、外围辅助工具及遇到的问题等多个方面进行分析,对基于语义的数据库网格系统的功能性、实用性、易用性进行了探讨。

通过将 DartGrid V3 平台与当前语义和网格研究领域一些相似或相关的研究工作进行对比,说明了基于语义的数据库网格及其实现 DartGrid V3 的特色,并对一些技术上的选择做出了分析。

最后,本文还简单介绍了基于语义的数据库网格的一个实际应用——中医药数据共享平台。

4.2.4 基于 GSI 的数据库网格安全基础架构

王闯(指导教师:吴朝晖、陈华钧)
2006 年硕士学位论文

网格是下一代 Internet 上的计算平台,其核心任务是管理分布在 Internet 广域环境中的各种类型的数据与服务资源,并为基于 Internet 的分布式应用提供一个统一的、虚拟的共享资源的计算平台。作为数据存储与管理的常用媒介,数据库在网格计算中扮演着重要的角色,由广域分布的、众多的、自治的数据库组成的网格环境称为数据库网格。在这样的环境中,数据库资源被广泛共享,而且动态组合成虚拟组织,用以解决某一个领域的问题或者提供专门的数据服务。

本文首先介绍了数据库网格环境的概念与特点,然后从动态开放的数据库网格环境下资源共享与协作过程中确保信息安全的应用需求背景出发,综合现有 Internet 下的数据资源的信息共享与整合管理的安全解决方案,提出了一套面向数据库资源的网格安全基础架构:Database Grid Security Infrastructrue(DGSI)模型。DGSI 是一个基于 GSI 验证机制,符合网格体系标准,针对数据库资源,面向网格环境的信息保护与共享安全的基础架构,旨在为解决网格环境下的数据库资源授权、验证、信任等问题提供一套可参考的设计与实现。

本文阐述了数据库网格安全管理的基本思想,描述了数据库网格环境安全架构 DGSI 的重要组成及一系列关于授权、验证、信任等安全问题的协议,并实现了原型系统 Dart-DGSI。本文还介绍了 Dart-DGSI 在中医药研究中的一个应用场景。最后,本文进行了总结并提出了进一步的工作展望。

4.2.5 基于语义的消息中间件 DART MQ

叶志勇(指导教师:吴朝晖、陈华钧)

2006 年硕士学位论文

在分布式计算环境中,为了集成分布式应用,开发者需要为异构网络环境下的分布式应用提供有效的通信手段。在这样的需求下,越来越多的分布式应用采用消息中间件来构建,通过消息中间件来进行消息的交互。消息中间件技术发展到现在,我们迫切希望消息中间件能够提供统一的消息交换格式,实现消息的按需、高效、可靠传输。

在本文中,我们采用语义网技术,将消息中间件交换的事件(消息)所涉及的各种概念整合到一起,建立了统一的事件概念模型,集成各种系统的异构消息。在系统内部,每个事件被表示为一个 RDF 图。因此,本系统可以同时支持各种格式的事件,包括关系数据结构、树型数据结构以及图状数据结构等,其表达能力非常强。当事件被发布时,系统首先将其转换成 RDF 格式,然后再对其进行进一步的处理。而对于事件接收者而言,所有的事件都是 RDF 格式的。

本文还定义了一个动态的事件代理调度策略,在客户端进入系统后,首先通过代理调度服务选择合适的事件代理负责对客户端的消息传输。

另外,我们设计了动态的网络传输架构,支持多种网络传输协议以适应各种不同的应用场景。在 DART MQ 中,底层的网络传输协议实现是对用户透明的。客户端加入系统后,DART MQ 会根据客户端对消息传输的具体要求自动选择最佳的网络传输协议。另外,考虑到网络的不稳定性,当消息传输性能不符合要求时,系统还支持在消息传输过程中对网络传输协议进行迁移。

4.2.6 基于虚拟组织的大规模跨域协同平台及应用

张露(指导教师:陈华钧、姜晓红)

2011 年硕士学位论文

随着科技与社会的进步,工作流技术在现代企业的管理中发挥了越来越大的作用,企业之间的合作日趋频繁,规模越来越大。这些企业在地理上广域分布且拥有各自独立的业务系统,相互之间缺乏有效的信息交换,没有统一的、自动化的、协同化的机制来协调彼此之间的各种软硬件资源。

本文将网格技术、OWL-S 语义技术相结合并应用到工作流技术中,设计并实现了基于虚拟组织的大规模跨域协同平台。

首先,本文简要介绍了工作流技术、网格技术、OWL-S 语义技术、富互联网应用技术的发展现状。分析跨域协同平台的需求,结合当前最新的计算机应用技术,提出跨域协同平台的架构设计。本文设计的三层体系架构将已有业务系统无缝地、低耦合地集成在一起,解决跨域系统的协同问题。

本文的重点是提出了虚拟组织的新的定义和跨域协同平台的安全模型,对所采用的技术、框架、实现等多方面做了分析介绍。通过 OWL-S 给虚拟组织增加语义信息,针对 GSI 访问控制模型的缺陷,设计并实现基于角色授权证书的安全认证以及基于角色和资源的访问控制机制。

最后是对跨域协同平台的实现的简要介绍。

4.2.7　基于知识集成引擎的中医药知识服务社区

王超(指导教师:陈华钧)
2012 年硕士学位论文

中医药信息是几千年中华文明的一块瑰宝,但其知识体系极其庞大并且表达非常复杂。考虑如何由古籍分散、非系统化的知识和积累了数千年的经验案例抽象成为系统化的可分析的科学知识,一直是中医药信息化发展的重中之重。虚拟社区是当今信息化网络中一种全新的用户交互的社交网络形态,既具有便于用户访问的开放性,又有集成知识、寓教于乐的灵活性。

本文首先介绍了中医药知识服务社区平台的架构。该架构通过知识集成引擎集成了关系数据库的 SQL 查询、RDF/OWL 本体库中的本体查询及搜索,借助于语义规则推理引擎,采用生动的 Web 用户接口,为用户提供中医药信息的快速访问。知识社区的表现形式主要包括中医基础五行理论的 flex2D/3D 模型推理展示、中医药 3D 虚拟社区和 2D 中医药多媒体游戏。

接下来分别以知识服务社区的各个展示形式进行介绍。中医基础五行理论的 flex2D/3D 动态模型推演及病机推理展示,采用前台 flex 交互的 j2ee 开发框架,基于中医药专家创建的用于抽象化语义表达的五行理论本体模型及由中医药基础理论中抽取出来的一阶逻辑规则,通过推理机对语义本体知识库进行语义推理,并应用 flex 2D/3D 开发库开发出相应的展示模型;中医药 3D 虚拟社区采用了虚拟现实的技术,利用三维建模工具 3DMax 和三维模型整合工具 virtools 进行社区搭建,模拟社区场景和人物角色,创建了一个全新的以用户为第一人称,用户和电脑、用户和用户之间可以进行交互的虚拟世界,是第一个以中医药知识为背景的 3D 虚拟社区,主要用于促进中医药事业的大众推广;2D 中医药多媒体游戏是采用 flash 前端技术开发的一套具有中医药知识特性的中药农场游戏,通过高人气、低门槛的 SNS 游戏方式增加知识教育类产品的亲和力。

4.2.8　基于云架构的高性能大规模网格监控系统的设计与实现

张湘豫(指导教师:陈华钧、姜晓红)
2012 年硕士学位论文

网格系统通过一体化架构、规范化接口、标准化服务等手段,实现了计算资源、存储资源、服务资源、数据资源等各种资源的集成共享和跨域协同,充分利用了互联网上大量的闲置资源。网格环境下各类资源具有大规模、异构以及地域分布广泛等特点,资源可以动态地加入或者离开网格虚拟组织,构建一个高性能大规模的全局监控系统具有非常重要的意义。

为了满足网格监控系统对高可用性、高可扩展性、高实时性和高效性等需求,我们提出了一个基于云架构的高性能大规模网格监控系统。本文介绍了该系统的详细设计与实现,并着重介绍了海量监控数据存储和资源聚合两个关键技术。

本文采用了基于 MongoDB 的海量存储技术来存储资源状态监控数据,解决了以往监控系统只能保持最近一段时间的监控数据、监控数据孤立且不能产生更多价值的问题。该存储架构提供了丰富灵活的数据模型,能够支持高并发的读写请求,提供高效的存储和访问以及丰富的查询和检索接口,有良好的可扩展性,能适应集群规模的不断增长。本文还通过采用基于一致性哈希的高效易扩展资源聚合技术,解决了以往资源聚合技术采用树形结构带来的实时性低、易出现单点故障等问题。该聚合技术能够自动分配资源与索引服务器的对应关系,易于实现负载均衡,增加或者减少索引服务器对已有结构改变小,同时能够自动检测和处理故障机器。

4.2.9　高机密性高可用性的云存储系统研究

马然(指导教师:姜晓红)
2013 年硕士学位论文

随着云计算技术的不断发展,云存储目前也成为计算机领域的研究热点,其相关技术是解决海量数据存储问题的有效方案。研究如何提高云存储系统的机密性和可用性,对于保障云存储过程中的数据安全、进一步促进云存储技术发展具有重大意义。然而现存的主流云存储系统在安全保障机制方面,尤其是在保证数据的机密性和可用性方面手段单一。

本文针对上述不足,对高机密性、高可用性的云存储系统展开了研究,主要贡献包括:

(1)提出了采用数据拆分和重建算法以及数据冗余策略提高数据的机密性与可用性;

(2)结合数据拆分和重建算法以及开源 HDFS(Hadoop 分布式文件系统)设计了新的数据块控制流程,实现了 HCAFS(高机密性和可用性文件系统)云存储原型系统;

(3)对 HDFS 和 HCAFS 进行了大量的性能对比测试,给出了测试结果及分析;

(4)为了更好地监控文件系统的表现,设计和实现了云服务监控与管理平台。

4.2.10　跨域云平台的安装部署技术和在线迁移性能研究

闫凤喜(指导教师:姜晓红)
2013 年硕士学位论文

近年来,云计算快速发展,已经成为互联网行业一个全新的产业。云计算的三种服务模式即 IaaS、PaaS 和 SaaS 共同构成了云计算产业的生态环境。其中,IaaS 作为云计算生态环境的基础,为企业用户享受云服务提供了多重选择:租用云提供商的虚拟机,或者利用虚拟化与开源云平台搭建自己的私有云。本课题作为一个 863 项目,主要工作就是基于各合作单位的物理资源,利用虚拟化技术与开源云管理平台,搭建一个跨域的实验云平台,完成一个基于 Web 的面向个人及企业用户的跨域云管理接口。整个项目被称为"跨域云平台"。本文从课题的背景、意义、架构、IaaS 的关键技术等方面对"跨域云平台"进行了详细的介绍。总体来说,本文的主要贡献如下。

(1)深入分析了 XEN 与 OpenNebula 的实现原理,并以此为切入点,讲述了"跨域云平台"的实现原理。

(2)基于 OpenNebula 在添加计算节点与镜像管理方面的诸多不足,对 Open Nebula 进行了优化,提高了平台的可用性。

(3)为了验证"跨域云平台"在迁移方面的性能,在"跨域云平台"之上进行了一系列在线迁移实验,探索在线迁移对多层工作负载(multi-tier workload)的影响,并最终为在线迁移策略提供了重要依据。

4.2.11　虚拟计算系统的性能和能耗管理方法研究

叶可江(指导教师:吴朝晖、姜晓红)

2013 年博士学位论文

虚拟计算系统是基于虚拟化技术构建起来的新一代计算系统,是对传统计算理论和模式的一次重要创新。它通过引入虚拟机管理器层,消除了底层硬件体系结构和上层系统软件之间的紧密耦合关系,实现了多种资源的动态组合和透明共享,提高了物理资源的使用效率,并为用户提供了个性化和普适化的使用环境。虚拟化技术最典型的应用场景就是云计算。但当把虚拟化技术大规模推广到实际的云计算数据中心的时候,还需要解决两个关键的挑战问题。①低性能问题。性能的损耗是虚拟化技术带来的一个最突出的问题。随着云计算的不断普及,大量的传统应用程序将逐步迁移到云中运行。如何对不同类型的典型应用程序在虚拟化环境下的运行性能进行量化分析和建模优化是一个重要挑战。②高能耗问题。云计算的一个典型特征就是计算资源和存储资源高度集中,这对云数据中心的能耗管理提出了很高的要求。区别于传统的数据中心节能方法,如何利用虚拟机的特性对云数据中心的能耗进行分布式管理是另一个重要的挑战。

针对这两个挑战,学术界已经开始了不少前期研究,但尚存一些不足。基于此,本文提出了一系列新的方法,旨在解决虚拟计算系统的"性能"和"能耗"这两个核心挑战问题,即从虚拟计算系统的性能评估与分析、虚拟计算系统的性能调优策略与方法、虚拟计算系统的能耗管理方法以及虚拟计算系统的性能和能耗权衡关系等四个方面开展系统性研究工作。本文工作的创新点总结如下。

(1)提出了一个基于典型应用场景的虚拟计算系统性能基准测试程序集 Virt-B。基准测试程序集(Benchmark)的缺失是造成虚拟计算系统性能量化评估困难的一个最关键的原因。本文通过对虚拟化技术的典型应用案例进行梳理和总结,归纳出虚拟化技术的六大典型应用场景,分别是单机虚拟化、服务器整合、虚拟机部署、虚拟机在线迁移、计算密集型(MPI)虚拟集群和数据密集型(MapReduce)虚拟集群。本文针对这六大典型应用场景,详细定义了其评测指标和负载,并且开展了大量的性能量化分析工作,为本领域的研究人员提供第一手详实的性能测试数据。此外,本文设计并开发了一个测试环境自动构建和测试负载自动生成的工具来辅助测试。

(2)提出了一系列针对多机多核架构的虚拟计算系统性能调优策略和方法。在详细全面的性能测试数据基础上,本文继续提出了相应的针对多机多核虚拟计算系统的性能调优策略和方法。特别地,针对多虚拟机环境,提出了一种基于资源预留的多虚拟机在线迁移优化方法以及虚拟集群迁移控制框架和策略;针对多核处理器环境,提出了一种负载感知的虚拟机性能隔离性优化方法和一种缓存感知的虚拟机故障隔离性优化方法。在真实的虚拟化环境下的真实负载测试结果表明,所提出的几种优化方法,都能有效提升虚拟机在多机多核环境下的运行性能。

(3)提出了两种以虚拟机为粒度的云计算数据中心节能架构和方法。数据中心虚拟化之后,传统的节能方法将不能直接应用于虚拟化云计算数据中心。这是因为虚拟机的能耗不能通过电表直接测量。本文对虚拟化云计算数据中心的节能挑战和方法进行全面的分析与探讨,并基于此进一步提出了两个以虚拟机为粒度的云数据中心节能架构,即基于资源监控的虚拟计算系统节能架构和基于负载轮廓分析的虚拟计算系统节能架构。前者易于实现,但无法保证虚拟机负载的性能。后者则通过对虚拟机负载进行事先的轮廓分析,在虚拟机动态调整时能保证虚拟机负载的性能。两种方法都能有效降低虚拟化云数据中心的能耗。

(4)研究了虚拟计算系统中虚拟机性能和能耗之间的权衡关系,提出了虚拟机负载性能约束下的最优节能整合模型及最优迁移决策算法。由于不同类型的虚拟机负载整合在一起时的性能表现不同,因此如何选择最优的整合匹配,使各种应用程序的性能达到最佳,同时使得所占用的物理机个数最少是一个挑战。同时,不同的应用程序在虚拟机迁移时导致的性能开销是不同的。因此,在制定大规模虚拟机迁移决策的时候,需要考虑这些特征。基于这些考虑,本文提出了一个最优化模型,用于解决应用程序性能约束下的最优节能整合,同时提出了一个多项式时间算法,用于解决大规模虚拟机的最优化迁移,最大程度地降低整体迁移的开销。

4.2.12 云平台虚拟计算资源的远程访问技术研究与实现

黄鹏(指导教师:姜晓红、陈华钧)

2014 年硕士学位论文

云计算是近年来 IT 领域的一个热门话题,普遍被业内人士认为是下一代互联网技术的基础,将会影响到整个互联网产业的格局。当前,国内外都涌现出一批成熟的云计算产品,这极大地推动了整个 IT 产业的进步。

浙江大学 CCNT 实验室也开展了云计算的相关研究工作,并设计和开发了 DartCloud 云平台。与其他成熟平台不同,DartCloud 受限于互联网 IP 地址的不足,提供的虚拟机只有局域网 IP。为了穿透内网,本文设计了七层代理服务器,使得互联网用户能够使用浏览器突破内网的限制,远程连接云平台中的任意虚拟机。

本文的主要工作和贡献如下。

(1)针对 IP 地址资源匮乏的问题,设计并实现了 vncproxy 代理服务器。它属于七层代理服务器,主要是为 vnc4server 远程控制工具穿透内网,连接 DartCloud 云平台内部集群中的任意虚拟机。本文主要介绍 vncproxy 代理服务器的设计思路以及采用的技术,确保 vncproxy 代理服务器能满足用户的需求。

(2)针对 vnc4server 传输桌面图像的弊端,我们选择 Web-based SSH 作为另一种选择,并设计和实现了 websshproxy 高性能代理服务器。本文主要介绍 websshproxy 代理服务器的设计思路以及采用当前流行的多进程事件驱动技术,使得 websshproxy 具有很高的并发量和吞吐率。

(3)设计和开发了 DartCloud 云平台管理员端软件,集成云资源管理、监控等功能,通过浏览器完成大部分工作,这极大地方便了我们的管理员监控和管理整个云平台资源。

4.2.13　云资源管理平台 DartCloud 的设计与实现

严海明(指导教师:姜晓红、李石坚)
2014 年硕士学位论文

随着云计算的不断发展和普及,IaaS(Infrastructure as a Service,基础设施即服务)的相关技术成为当下研究的热点。本文的 DartCloud 云资源管理平台是在 OpenNebula 开源云资源管理平台上的二次开发和改进,主要解决了 OpenNebula 缺少基础设施资源的租赁管理(以下称为业务管理)功能,以及它对云数据中心资源综合利用率低等问题。本文的工作得到了国家高技术研究发展计划(863 计划)课题"基于海量语言资源的语言翻译分布并行处理技术"的资助和支持,主要贡献如下。

(1)设计与实现了 DartCloud 业务管理子平台。具体包括前端视图层、业务消息的接收与处理以及底层基础设施资源的管理、调度和分配等功能模块。通过消息队列缓冲机制来实现高并发下的消息缓冲,设计了资源预留机制和资源时隙表数据结构来实现云数据中心资源的管理,并在此基础上实现了业务的调度算法以及虚拟机到服务器的映射模型。因此,DartCloud 在 OpenNebula 的基础上解决了海量用户对弹性计算资源的租赁申请需求,并实现了面向多租户异构应用的云计算 IaaS服务。

(2)针对多租户环境下应用的异构性,提出了一个基于遗传算法的虚拟机调度机制。具体包括设计与实现了染色体的分组编码机制,基于轮盘赌算法的个体选择机制,以及基于双亲、双子单点的染色体交叉框架。最后,与 OpenNebula 平台使用的经典算法进行对比实验,结果显示 DartCloud在提高服务器资源的综合利用率、搭建绿色节能数据中心等方面具有明显优势和潜在价值,从而进一步解决了数据中心多租户异构应用背景下所带来的效率和能耗问题。

4.2.14　云平台可维护性研究

陈忠忠(指导教师:姜晓红)
2015 年硕士学位论文

因云计算的兴盛与普及,越来越多的企业选择引入云计算技术以改造原有的企业数据中心,一些企业则开始租赁大厂商的云服务。学术界和业界研究人员投入了相当多的精力,专注于提高云平台的安全性和资源利用率,但对于云平台的可维护性,却很少有人涉及。本文通过对 DartCloud 云平台搭建的实践和思考,研究了云平台的可维护性,主要包括云平台的快速部署及监控系统的搭建、镜像管理策略的定制和对业务扩展性的支持。

本文工作得到了 863 项目"互联网语言翻译系统研制"的资助和支持。本文的工作和贡献如下。

(1)对云平台的可维护性做了全面阐述,并在云平台的快速部署及监控系统的搭建、镜像管理策略的定制和对业务扩展性的支持这三方面做了深入的探讨。

(2)分析了 OpenNebula 和 Xen 的实现原理,给出了从物理裸机到一个云平台的搭建指南,针对现有部署效率低下的问题,提出并实现了批量部署和自动化部署策略,加速云平台的搭建和部署,提高了云平台扩展性和部署效率。相关专利已受理公开。

(3)实现了基于 Ganglia 的云资源监控管理系统,提供各虚拟机、各物理服务器的 CPU 利用率等指标,为性能调优提供基本依据。

(4)提出并实现了一个完整的镜像管理解决方案,其中主要包括分级镜像权限控制、镜像版本管理和基于增量复制策略的镜像自动化管理这三个部分。相关专利已受理公开。

(5)通过实现的 DartCloud 资源监控系统采集实验数据,深入分析了云平台中 scale-up 和 scale-out 两种资源扩展方法在大数据并行计算应用上的性能差异,为综合提高资源利用率和减少成本的性能调优管理提供了依据。研究成果已写成论文并发表在会议论文集上。

4.2.15 云平台跨域分布式共享文件系统的设计与实现

杨红星(指导教师:姜晓红)
2014 年硕士学位论文

随着云计算和大数据技术的兴起,互联网产业正颠覆着传统的商业模式和生活方式,跨领域、跨行业的大数据共享云平台开始广泛应用于各个领域。而支持共享文件需求的跨域云管理系统目前还没有开源系统实现。本文的研究工作是国家 863 计划课题"基于互联网海量资源的语言翻译分布并行处理技术"的一部分,目的是在跨域的云环境中提供方便灵活的共享文件系统,满足跨地域多协同单位在云环境下的分级文件共享需求。本文在跨域的云平台 DartCloud 环境中设计实现了一个跨域分布式共享文件系统。主要贡献如下。

(1)分析和研究了分布式文件系统的两种主流设计思想,分析比较了两种设计思想的优缺点;分析了在 DartCloud 云平台环境下跨域分布式共享文件系统的应用需求,指出现有文件系统的不足。

(2)设计和实现了跨域分布式共享文件系统。该系统能够很好地满足跨地域集群的云平台数据管理需求。同时系统采用分级共享策略,根据用户权限设置分享级别。此外,该文件共享系统也打通了与云平台虚拟机的连接,从而方便了用户本地主机和远程虚拟机的文件交换。

(3)对 DartCloud 云平台相关子系统进行了设计与开发工作,包括 Topology 网络拓扑系统和 DartCloudDemo 翻译并行系统。通过这两个子系统,可以方便地查询到云平台的网络拓扑结构,以及自动化地协同运行各家单位的翻译系统。

4.2.16 Spark Shuffle 的内存调度算法分析及优化

陈英芝(指导教师:姜晓红)
2016 年硕士学位论文

随着分布式计算框架的不断发展和普及,Spark 以其先进的设计理念,迅速成为开源社区的热门研究项目。对于大数据计算框架而言,Shuffle 过程的设计优劣和性能高低直接影响着整个系统的性能和吞吐量。本文研究的主要内容为 Spark Shuffle 过程中不同任务间内存分配算法的分析与优化。在分析已有 Shuffle 优化算法的基础上,发现各任务对内存需求不均衡而造成 Shuffle 运行效率低的瓶颈。针对公平分配内存调度算法的不足,本文提出了一种基于溢出历史的自适应内存调度算法,并通过典型实验证明本文算法能有效提高内存利用率和程序运行效率,提高 Spark 系统的整体运行性能。本文的主要贡献如下。

(1)阐述了分布式计算的主流框架 MapReduce,包括 MapReduce 的编程模型、现状和不足。通过介绍 Spark 的设计理念分析了 Spark 对 MapReduce 模型的改进,比较了两者的优缺点。

(2)研究了 Spark Shuffle 的概念、发展及优化过程,通过阅读分析 Spark Shuffle 的源码,研究了 Shuffle 内存调度的思想,指出了公平分配算法存在的不足。

(3)提出了基于溢出历史的自适应内存调度算法 SBSA,解决了 Spark Shuffle 公平分配内存调度算法影响 Shuffle 运行效率的问题。本算法详细设计了空闲内存的计算方式、关键 Task 可从空闲内存借用的内存比例以及任务可用内存的最大阈值。

(4)通过典型实验比较了 SBSA 算法与先来先服务算法、公平分配调度算法的性能差异。实验结果证明,本算法可以大大提高数据分布不均匀的应用程序的执行效率。从综合表现来看,本算法能充分利用空闲内存资源,提高资源利用效率,在一定程度上缓解目前内存资源不足的问题。

4.2.17　分布式系统自适应故障检测技术研究

代长波(指导教师:姜晓红)
2017 年硕士学位论文

可靠稳定的分布式系统被广泛用于军事、医疗以及金融等众多领域,然而随着系统规模和复杂度的不断增加,故障的发生概率也逐渐增加,故障检测作为保证分布式系统可靠运行的基础组件之一,具有重要的研究意义。本文主要针对故障检测的自适应性和可扩展性,研究能自适应于系统和网络状态的故障检测器以及基于链路故障的自适应检测协议。

心跳检测是分布式系统故障检测中最常用的技术,本文基于 EMA(指数移动平均)和方差比进行心跳预测,提出一种新的自适应故障检测器——DEMA-FD。该检测器比传统心跳预测检测器具有更好的准确性,而且能根据故障检测器的服务质量(Quality of Service,QoS)基本评价指标进行调整,满足不同分布式应用的故障检测需求。经理论证明,在部分同步系统中 DEMA-FD 可以实现一个 $\diamond P$ 类故障检测器。本文随后对 DEMA-FD 进行了实验验证。

传统故障检测器存在将链路故障等同于节点故障的问题,极大地影响了故障定位和快速修复。本文提出一种新的自适应检测协议——DLFDA。该协议中每个节点同时拥有 k 个检测者进行故障类型诊断,能够准确区分链路故障和节点故障。DLFDA 协议将一种新的权责累积故障检测器 DA-FD 作为直接检测。该检测器利用 DEMA-FD 中心跳预测算法的自适应性,基于指数函数输出一个随时间累积的决策值,用户通过设定阈值灵活调整检测强度。另外,DLFDA 协议能够动态调整检测结构以增加链路检测的覆盖率,同时使用 gossip 发布故障诊断结果,降低了检测负载。最后对 DLFDA 协议进行了实验验证,结果表明其符合理论设计要求。

本文最后设计了一个通用可扩展的分布式自适应故障检测系统原型。该原型具有三层架构,三层分别是成员管理、信息同步以及自适应故障检测。系统功能上层次分明,模块之间耦合性较低,通过统一接口可以快速扩展。

4.2.18　弹性云平台的虚拟资源调度技术研究

何延彰(指导教师:姜晓红)

2018 年硕士学位论文

传统互联网数据中心存在物理机资源利用率低下、难以适应业务发展需求、管理复杂和运维成本居高不下等难题,以服务的形式通过互联网交付给用户虚拟资源的云计算数据中心应运而生。云计算采用计算机集群硬件和软件的形式构成云数据中心,它拥有资源池化、弹性服务、按需计费和泛在接入四大特征。虚拟化技术和云资源管理技术是云计算的两大关键技术,相应地带来了虚拟资源的高效整合和虚拟资源的弹性伸缩两大挑战。针对以上两点挑战,我们设计实现了一个跨域的云资源租赁平台 DartCloud,以优化云数据中心的虚拟机放置问题,并在虚拟机上层搭建弹性大数据计算平台 ScalaBD。本文的贡献主要可以归纳为以下几方面。

(1)实现 DartCloud 平台为用户提供虚拟机集群的租赁服务。在管理层,实现了基于时间状态的虚拟机镜像自动补充守护进程和一个外网穿透内网的 Web-based SSH 代理服务器。在业务层,提出了一个基于虚拟机状态更细资源粒度的虚拟资源计费策略,分为预付费模式和按需计费模式。

(2)提出了一个多目标虚拟机初始部署优化算法,同时考虑云数据中心的综合平均资源利用率 CARU 和综合资源利用均衡率 CRUB 两个评价指标,解决了多租户应用场景下虚拟机在各个维度资源的异构性所带来的虚拟机性能、物理机资源利用率和数据中心能耗等多方面的问题。实验中对比了 CPUPack、MemPack 和 Stripping 三个常用部署方法,结果表明我们的算法能提高 5% 左右的综合平均资源利用率,并获得最好的综合资源利用均衡率 8%。

(3)大数据弹性计算平台 ScalaBD 能提供大数据存储、批量计算、流式计算、内存计算和工作流计算等多种服务形式。在存储方面,我们实现了基于矩阵加密的高私密性和高可用性的存储平台。在批量计算方面,我们分析了 Hadoop 集群的资源扩展性问题,包括资源横向扩展和纵向扩展两个方面。实验中,运行 WordCount、RegexMatch、TeraSort 基准测试程序和 Mahout 并行机器学习应用来进行分析。结果表明,在 CPU 密集型应用中,纵向资源扩展获得更好的性能,而在 I/O 密集型应用中,横向资源扩展性能更好。最后,结合虚拟机集群配置参数和大数据计算框架参数,提出双层参数调节器的概念来进一步提高集群的资源利用率并降低集群的租赁费用。

4.2.19　面向中医药领域的智能问答系统设计与实现

胡志强(指导教师:姜晓红)

2020 年硕士学位论文

随着自然语言处理技术和深度学习技术的飞速发展,医疗人工智能进入了高速发展阶段,中医药的智能化迎来了新的发展机遇。中医药智能问答系统是中医药智能化的一个重要应用。本文基于中医药知识库和中医药知识图谱三元组,设计并实现了一个面向中医药领域的智能问答系统。

本文主要贡献如下。

(1)为克服现有单分词模型的不足,提出了一种融合医药分词模型,通过融合三种单分词模型,提高了医药文本上的分词性能。

（2）研究了不同任务下的最佳性能词向量训练方法，并通过内部评估任务和外部评估任务对医药领域词向量的性能进行了评估，为针对不同任务选择合适的医药领域词向量提供了参考依据。

（3）根据真实场景下用户问题的特点，提出三种中医药命名实体识别方法。将 Bert-BiLSTM-CRF 模型用于中医药命名实体识别任务，达到 0.956 的高 F1 值。

（4）提出一种使用 Siamese 网络对 Bert 进行微调的 Bert-Siamese 文本语义匹配模型，用于医药问题语义匹配任务，达到 0.925 的高 AUC 值，比 Bert 基线模型高 14.5%。将 HNSW 算法用于本系统的问题匹配，极大地提高了海量问题中语义最相近问题的检索效率。

（5）结合以上研究，设计并实现了一个面向中医药领域的智能问答系统，并以 Web 应用的形式提供服务。

4.3　学术论文摘要

本节摘录了中医药云平台与服务计算方向 2003—2016 年共 18 篇主要学术论文（分别发表在《中国中医药信息杂志》、《中国中医药图书情报杂志》、*TPDS*、*HPCC*、*CLOUD* 等国内外期刊和会议论文集上）。

4.3.1　Knowledge Base Grid: A Generic Grid Architecture for Semantic Web

Zhaohui Wu, Huajun Chen, Jiefeng Xu

首发于 *Journal of Computer Science & Technology*, 2003, 18(4): 462-473

The emergence of semantic web will result in an enormous amount of knowledge base resources on the web. In this paper, a generic Knowledge Base Grid Architecture (KB-Grid) for building large-scale knowledge systems on the semantic web is presented. KB-Grid suggests a paradigm that emphasizes how to organize, discover, utilize, and manage web knowledge base resources. Four principal components are under development: a semantic browser for retrieving and browsing semantically enriched information, a knowledge server acting as the web container for knowledge, an ontology server for managing web ontologies, and a knowledge base directory server acting as the registry and catalog of KBs. Also a referential model of knowledge service and the mechanisms required for semantic communication within KB-Grid are defined. To verify the design rationale underlying the KB-Grid, an implementation of Traditional Chinese Medicine (TCM) is described.

4.3.2　TCM-Grid: Weaving a Medical Grid for Traditional Chinese Medicine

Huajun Chen, Zhaohui Wu, Chang Huang, Jiefeng Xu

首发于 *ICCS*, 2003, *LNCS* 2659: 1143-1152

We present a TCM-Grid for Traditional Chinese Medicine (TCM). The purpose of the TCM-Grid is to aid the development of distributed systems that help health professionals, researchers, enterprizes and personal users to retrieve, integrate and share TCM information and knowledge from geographically decentralized TCM database resources and knowledge base resources in China. Our approach involves developing a Database Grid for discovering and accessing TCM database resources coordinately and a Knowledge Base Grid supporting TCM knowledge sharing globally. With our application experience, we argue that nowadays' Grid architecture is not enough: we need Database Grid to support finely granular data sharing and integration, and we also need a Knowledge Base Grid to support knowledge-intensive task. We also recommend a Grid Ontology effort to enable Grid intelligence.

4.3.3　Knowledge Base Grid and Its Application in Traditional Chinese Medicine
Jiefeng Xu, Huajun Chen, Zhaohui Wu
首发于 *SMC*,2003,3:2477-2482

Knowledge Base Grid enables worldwide sharing and coordinated using of knowledge base resources which are distributed around the Internet. By constructing large-scale web knowledge bases, Knowledge Base Grid supports on-demand and intelligent services satisfying personal needs and expectations such as personal health consultation. In this paper, we introduce a generic knowledge base grid for Traditional Chinese Medicine (TCM). Its framework consists of three main parts: Virtual Open Knowledge Base in which TCM knowledge has been well organized, Knowledge Base Index that indexes the TCM knowledge services, and a Semantic Browser that supports TCM concepts browsing and TCM knowledge management. The implementation of TCM Knowledge Base Grid includes TCM knowledge representation and services hierarchy.

4.3.4　建立中医药虚拟研究院背景与方法
尹爱宁,陈华钧,何前锋,范为宇,刘静,郑国轴,王恒,范宽,景鲲
首发于《第三届国际中医药工程学术会议论文集》,2006:312-318

本文系统地讨论了中医药虚拟研究院设立的背景与需求、基本特征与组织形式、技术实现方法、机制创新以及对完成国家基础性工作平台项目的促进作用;提出了中医药科研课题实力的聚集与课题协作的新方法。希望能够推广应用。

4.3.5　A Scalable Probabilistic Approach to Trust Evaluation
Xiaoqing Zheng, Zhaohui Wu, Huajun Chen, Yuxin Mao
首发于 *iTrust*,2006,*LNCS* 3986:423-438

The Semantic Web will only achieve its full potential when users have trust in its operations and in the quality of services and information provided, so trust is inevitably a high-level and crucial issue. Modeling trust properly and exploring techniques for establishing computational trust is at the heart of the Semantic Web to realize its vision. We propose a scalable probabilistic approach to trust evaluation which combines a variety of sources of information and takes four types of costs (operational, opportunity, service charge and consultant fee) and utility into consider during the process of trust evaluation. Our approach gives trust a strict probabilistic interpretation which can assist users with making better decisions in choosing the appropriate service providers according to their preferences. A formal robust analysis has been made to examine the performance of our method.

4.3.6　Developing a Composite Trust Model for Multi-Agent Systems
Xiaoqing Zheng, Zhaohui Wu, Huajun Chen, Yuxin Mao
首发于 *AAMAS*,2006:1257-1259

The Semantic Web, conceived as a collection of agents, brings new opportunities and challenges to trust research. Enabling trust to ensure more effective and efficient interaction is at the heart of the Semantic Web vision. We propose a composite trust model based on statistical decision theory and Bayesian sequential analysis to balance the costs and benefits during the process of trust evaluating, and combine a variety of sources of information to assist users with making the correct decisions in selecting the appropriate service providers according to their preferences. The model proposed by this paper gives trust a strict mathematical interpretation in terms of probability theory.

4.3.7 Analyzing & Modeling the Performance in Xen-Based Virtual Cluster Environment

Kejiang Ye, Xiaohong Jiang, Siding Chen, Dawei Huang, Bei Wang
首发于 *HPCC*,2010:273-280

Virtualization technology is currently widely used due to its benefits on high resource utilization, flexible manageability and powerful system security. However, its use for high performance computing (HPC) is still not popular due to the unclearness of the virtualization overheads. It's worthy to evaluate the virtualization cost and to find the performance bottleneck when running HPC applications in virtual cluster. We first evaluate the basic performance overheads due to virtualization. Then we create a 16-node virtual cluster and perform a performance evaluation for both para-virtualization and full virtualization. After that, we evaluate the MPI (Message Passing Interface) scalability to investigate the impact of MPI and network communication between virtual machines. In addition to the macro assessment, we use the Oprofile/Xenoprof to investigate the architecture characterization like CPU cycle, L2 cache misses, DTLB misses and ITLB misses, which is an auxiliary explanation to the performance bottleneck. Experimental results indicate that performance overheads of virtualization are acceptable for HPC, para-virtualization is very suitable for HPC due to the high virtualization efficiency and efficient inter-domain communication. Finally, we use the non-linear regression modeling technology to present a performance model for network latency and bandwidth to predict the performance in virtual cluster environment.

4.3.8 Evaluate the Performance and Scalability of Image Deployment in Virtual Data Center

Kejiang Ye, Xiaohong Jiang, Qinming He, Xing Li, Jianhai Chen
首发于 *NPC*,2010,*LNCS* 6289:390-401

Virtualization technology plays an important role in modern data center, as it creates an opportunity to improve resource utilization, reduce energy costs, and ease server management. However, virtual machine deployment issues arise when allocating virtual machines into single or multiple physical servers. In this paper, we explore the performance and scalability issues for virtual machine deployment in a virtualized data center. We first evaluate the image scalability when allocating multiple VMs per physical server using four typical servers in data center. Then we investigate how the overall efficiency will be affected when deploying M virtual machines into N physical machines with different deployment strategies. Experimental results show that (i) there is a resource bottleneck when deploying single type virtual machine server into single physical server, except for composite workloads; (ii) more physical machines do not always benefit for some specific applications to support a fixed number of virtual machines; (iii) MPI and network communication overheads affect the deployment efficiency seriously.

4.3.9 Two Optimization Mechanisms to Improve the Isolation Property of Server Consolidation in Virtualized Multi-Core Server

Kejiang Ye, Xiaohong Jiang, Deshi Ye, Dawei Huang

首发于 *HPCC*,2010:281-288

Virtualization brings many benefits such as improving system utilization and reducing cost through server consolidation. However, it also introduces isolation problem when running multiple virtual machine workloads in one physical platform. Additionally, with the advent of multi-core technology, more and more cores are built into one die in today's data center that will share and compete for the resource like cache. It's worthy to study the isolation of server consolidation in modern multi-core platform. However, to our knowledge there is little work done on the isolation property especially the fault isolation property when one of the virtual machine workloads is attacked in server consolidation. In this paper, we study the isolation property from the performance perspective and provide two optimization methods to improve the isolation property. We first define the isolation property and quantify the performance isolation in consolidation and propose a VM-level optimization method. Then we study the fault isolation by introducing a misbehavior virtual machine in server consolidation scenario and propose a core-level cache aware optimization method to improve the fault isolation. Experimental results show that our two optimization methods can effectively improve the performance isolation and fault isolation with 29.39% and 19.52% respectively. What's more, Oprofile/Xenoprof toolkits are used to find out the factors affecting isolation property from the hardware events level.

4.3.10 Live Migration of Multiple Virtual Machines with Resource Reservation in Cloud Computing Environments

Kejiang Ye, Xiaohong Jiang, Dawei Huang, Jianhai Chen, Bei Wang

首发于 *CLOUD*,2011:267-274

Virtualization technology is currently becoming increasingly popular and valuable in cloud computing environments due to the benefits of server consolidation, live migration, and resource isolation. Live migration of virtual machines can be used to implement energy saving and load balancing in cloud data center. However, to our knowledge, most of the previous work concentrated on the implementation of migration technology itself while didn't consider the impact of resource reservation strategy on migration efficiency. This paper focuses on the live migration strategy of multiple virtual machines with different resource reservation methods. We first describe the live migration framework of multiple virtual machines with resource reservation technology. Then we perform a series of experiments to investigate the impacts of different resource reservation methods on the performance of live migration in both source machine and target machine. Additionally, we analyze the efficiency of parallel migration strategy and workload-aware migration strategy. The metrics such as downtime, total migration time, and workload performance overheads are measured. Experiments reveal some new discovery of live migration of multiple virtual machines. Based on the observed results, we present corresponding optimization methods to improve the migration efficiency.

4. 3. 11　Performance Influence of Live Migration on Multi-Tier Workloads in Virtualization Environments

Xiaohong Jiang, Fengxi Yan, Kejiang Ye

首发于 *Cloud Computing*, 2012: 72-81

Live migration is a widely used technology for load balancing, fault tolerance, and power saving in cloud data centers. Previous research includes significant research work in the performance improvement of live migration. However, little work has been done to investigate the influence of live migration on virtual machine workloads that users care about most. We notice that these workloads can be classified into two categories: single-tier workloads and multi-tier workloads which is a typical type for internet applications. We conduct a series of deliberate experiments to investigate the influence of live migration on multi-tier workloads in a cloud environment and also on traditional physical machines for comparison. Our experimental results show that multi-tier workloads on virtual machines can work as well as those on traditional physical machines. However, in an unstable environment, if virtual machines migrate constantly, live migration will cause a profound performance decrease on multi-tier workloads. Also, it is best to avoid migrating virtual machines that are hosting memory intensive workloads in a virtualization environment due to bad downtime performance. Further, we perform experiments trying to find the turning point of the performance of a virtual machine, which might provide support evidence for future research on live migration policy.

4. 3. 12　vHadoop: A Scalable Hadoop Virtual Cluster Platform for MapReduce-Based Parallel Machine Learning with Performance Consideration

Kejiang Ye, Xiaohong Jiang, Yanzhang He, Xiang Li, Haiming Yan, Peng Huang

首发于 *ICCCW*, 2012: 152-160

Big data processing is currently becoming increasingly important in modern era due to the continuous growth of the amount of data generated by various fields such as particle physics, human genomics, earth observation, etc. However, the efficiency of processing large-scale data on modern virtual infrastructure, especially on the virtualized cloud computing infrastructure, is not clear. This paper focuses on the performance of hadoop virtual cluster and proposes a scalable hadoop virtual cluster platform vHadoop for the large-scale MapReduce-based parallel data processing. We first describe the design and implementation of *vHadoop* platform. Then we perform a series of experiments to investigate both the static and dynamic performance of *vHadoop* platform, such as the performance characterization of cross-domain hadoop virtual cluster and live migraiton of hadoop virtual cluster. After that, we use the *vHadoop* platform to process 6 typical parallel clustering algorithms, such as *Canopy*, *Dirichlet*, *Fuzzy k-Means*, *k-Means*, *MeanShift*, *MinHash*, etc., on two typical datasets. Experimental results verify the efficiency of *vHadoop* platform to process the MapReduce-based parallel machine learning applications.

4.3.13 VC-Migration: Live Migration of Virtual Clusters in the Cloud

Kejiang Ye, Xiaohong Jiang, Ran Ma, Fengxi Yan
首发于 *ICGC*,2012:209-218

Live migration of virtual machines (VM) has recently become a key ingredient behind the management activities of cloud computing system to achieve the goals of load balancing, energy saving, failure recovery, and system maintenance. However, to our knowledge, most of the previous live VM migration techniques concentrated on the migration of a single VM which means these techniques are insufficient when the whole virtual cluster or multiple virtual clusters need to be migrated. This paper investigates various live migration strategies for virtual clusters (VC). We first describe a framework VC-Migration to control the migration of virtual clusters. Then we perform a series of experiments to study the performance and overheads of different migration strategies for virtual clusters, including concurrent migration, mutual migration, homogeneous VC migration, and heterogeneous VC migration. After that, we present several optimization principles to improve the migration performance of virtual clusters. The HPCC benchmark is selected to represent the virtual cluster workloads, and the metrics such as downtime, total migration time, and workload performance are measured. Experimental results reveal some new discoveries which are useful to the future development of new migration mechanisms and algorithms to optimize the migration of virtual clusters.

4.3.14 HPACS: A High Privacy and Availability Cloud Storage Platform with Matrix Encryption

Yanzhang He, Xiaohong Jiang, Kejiang Ye, Ran Ma, Xiang Li
首发于 *APPT*,2013,*LNCS 8299*:132-145

As the continuous development of cloud computing and big data, data storage as a service in the cloud is becoming increasingly popular. More and more individuals and organizations begin to store their data in cloud rather than building their own data centers. Cloud storage holds the advantages of high reliability, simple management and cost-effective. However, the privacy and availability of the data stored in cloud is still a challenge. In this paper, we design and implement a High Privacy and Availability Cloud Storage (HPACS) platform built on Apache Hadoop to improve the data privacy and availability. A matrix encryption and decryption module is integrated in HDFS, through which the data can be encoded and reconstructed to/from different storage servers transparently. Experimental results show that HPACS can achieve high privacy and availability but with reasonable write/read performance and storage capacity overhead as compared with the original HDFS.

4.3.15 知识服务:大数据时代下的中医药信息化发展趋势

吴朝晖,姜晓红,陈华钧
首发于《中国中医药图书情报杂志》,2013,37(2):90-93

论文介绍了语义网、云计算、物联网、跨界服务等信息技术的发展趋势,分析了现有中医药信息化的现状,指出了中医药信息化工作将从以网格技术、搜索引擎为基础的信息共享转向基于云平台、大数据的跨界中医药知识服务的发展趋势,并列举了中医药知识服务的实践。

4.3.16　Profiling-Based Workload Consolidation and Migration in Virtualized Data Centers

Kejiang Ye, Zhaohui Wu, Chen Wang, Bingbing Zhou, Weisheng Si, Xiaohong Jiang, Albert Y. Zomaya

首发于 *IEEE Transactions on Parallel and Distributed Systems*,2015,26(3):878-890

Improving energy efficiency of data centers has become increasingly important nowadays due to the significant amounts of power needed to operate these centers. An important method for achieving energy efficiency is server consolidation supported by virtualization. However, server consolidation may incur significant degradation to workload performance due to virtual machine (VM) *co-location* and *migration*. How to reduce such performance degradation becomes a critical issue to address. In this paper, we propose a profiling-based server consolidation framework which minimizes the number of physical machines (PMs) used in data centers while maintaining satisfactory performance of various workloads. Inside this framework, we first profile the performance losses of various workloads under two situations: running in *co-location* and experiencing *migrations*. We then design two modules: (i) consolidation planning module which, given a set of workloads, minimizes the number of PMs by an integer programming model, and (ii) migration planning module which, given a source VM placement scenario and a target VM placement scenario, minimizes the number of VM migrations by a polynomial time algorithm. Also, based on the workload performance profiles, both modules can guarantee the performance losses of various workloads below configurable thresholds. Our experiments for workload profiling are conducted with real data center workloads and our experiments on our two modules validate the integer programming model and the polynomial time algorithm.

4.3.17　知识服务及其在中医药领域的应用

于彤,于琦,李敬华,杨硕,张竹绿

首发于《中国数字医学》,2015,10(8):33-35

目的:通过发展中医药知识服务,促进中医药知识与经验的保护与传承。方法:根据服务计算理论,阐述知识服务的概念和性质,设计并实现中医药知识服务平台。结果:中医药知识服务平台整合中医药知识资源,实现了百科知识服务、知识搜索服务、知识发现服务、决策支持服务等中医药知识服务模式。结论:中医药知识服务平台面向中医专家和社会大众提供知识服务,为中医药科学研究、临床实践和新药研发提供了有力支持。

4.3.18　基于移动互联网的中医养生知识服务研究

于彤,崔蒙,毛郁欣,高宏杰,于琦,李敬华,朱玲,张竹绿

首发于《中国数字医学》,2016,11(2):29-30,45

目的:采用移动互联网技术,促进中医养生知识的共享与传播。方法:通过文献检索和互联网搜索等手段,对中医养生方面的移动应用程序进行了调研。结果:对中医养生移动应用程序的主要功

能、知识内容、服务方式以及核心优势进行总结,分析其中存在的问题并提出研究思路。结论:中医养生领域已出现了很多移动应用程序,它们普遍具有安装和使用方便等特点,但知识内容尚缺乏专业性和权威性。需要进一步建立综合性、科学性、大众性的中医养生知识库,为各种移动应用程序提供统一的支持。

4.4 学术著作和标准

本节主要介绍了中医药云平台与服务计算方向于 2011 年由浙江大学出版社出版的一部著作《DartGrid:支持中医药信息化的语义网格平台实现》,摘录了著作前言和一级目录信息;同时介绍了团队参与制定的《中药制药过程工艺语义框架》国际标准。

4.4.1 DartGrid:支持中医药信息化的语义网格平台实现

陈华钧,姜晓红,吴朝晖
首发于浙江大学出版社,2011

前言

近年来,以 Web 2.0 为代表的网络新应用层出不穷,并推动着计算机各方面技术的进一步发展。这些应用的一个典型特征是数据驱动。例如博客、播客以及各种社会计算网站,如 Facebook、YouTube、Flickr、Twitter、Google Social Graph、Microsoft Connection 等,由用户产生的各种类型的 Web 数据已经远远超过了传统的 Web 网站。各种应用所产生的数据都已经达到或将要达到 Petabytes 甚至更大的规模。这些网络数据还具有跨域和异构的特征。数据驱动型网络应用的核心需求是有效整合、聚合,乃至融合由多个管理域产生的多种异质异构数据,并支持大规模的并发访问。

语义网格,将以语义 Web 为代表的语义技术和以网格计算为代表的体系架构技术结合起来,通过规范化描述明确表达包括计算、存储、数据库、服务等各种信息资源的内涵语义,提供开放、安全、有序、可扩展的管理体系架构来解决和实现复杂网络环境下跨多个机构的大规模分布式协同计算和数据共享问题。语义网格为应对上述互联网新的挑战提供了新的思路和技术方法。

DartGrid 是由浙江大学计算机学院自主研发的语义网格平台软件系统。DartGrid 主要面向中医药信息化等数据驱动型网络应用领域的一些新需求,并结合语义 Web 技术和网格技术等新兴互联网技术研制。其主要技术包括数据的语义集成技术、语义搜索技术、流程服务的语义组合技术、语义网格中的分布式数据挖掘与知识发现等,旨在为语义网格提供一套综合信息管理平台。

DartGrid 平台的主要开发背景是中医药信息化。DartGrid 可以有效地支持数据与知识密集型领域中的知识表示、管理与问题求解,而中医药领域是一个典型的数据与知识密集型领域。本书结合对中医药领域的应用需求分析,提出基于语义网格构建的、面向中医药领域的 e-Science 环境,并就基于语义网格的数据集成与共享、海量中医药数据挖掘与分析等,详细阐述了其体系结构、技术特征以及应用成果。

本书的组织结构如下:第 1 章介绍了语义网格的基本概念以及 DartGrid 的功能与技术;第 2 章对 DartGrid 所涉及的关键技术进行了系统性的介绍;第 3 章结合中医药应用实例介绍了 DartQuery 语义查询系统;第 4 章针对中医药信息搜索的需求,介绍了 DartSearch 语义搜索系统;第

5 章介绍了 DartMapping 语义映射系统；第 6 章针对中医药海量数据的特征介绍了 DartSpora 海量数据挖掘系统；第 7 章介绍了一个基于语义的数据 Mashup 系统；第 8 章结合中医药的信息服务化需求，介绍了一个服务管理系统。本书既可以作为互联网技术领域的研究者和实践者的参考读物，也可以为从事中医药信息化工作的科研人员提供参考。

本书是浙江大学 CCNT 实验室的教师和学生多年的努力成果，以下老师和同学为本书的撰写或与本书相关的项目研发做出过贡献，在此一并表示感谢，他们是：邓水光、于彤、周春英、毛郁欣、封毅、张宇、王俊健、张小刚、付志红、秘中凯、密金华、刘森、盛浩、陶金火、杨克特、卢宾、郑耀文、梁欣颖、刘明魁、顾佩钦、张露、张湘豫等。本书还是浙江大学与中国中医科学院信息研究所多年合作的成果之一，在此向中国中医科学院的崔蒙研究员、尹爱宁、刘静、李园白、雷蕾等同仁给予我们的长期支持表示感谢！

本书相关研究内容受到如下项目资助：科技部"973"语义网格专项（No. 2003 CB317006）、国家杰出青年基金（No. NSFC60533040）、科技部现代服务业支撑计划（2006BAH02401）、科技部"863"计划（2006AA01A122，2009AA011903，2008AA01Z141），国家自然科学基金项目（No. NSFC 61070156，NSFC60873224）、浙江省科技重大项目（2008C03007）。在此一并表示感谢！

目录

4.4.2　《中药制药过程工艺语义框架》ISO 标准

中医药作为中国的国粹，近年来在欧美国家产生的影响力越来越大，尽早尽快建立中药生产相关国际标准就尤为迫切。基于这样的认识，我们联合浙江大学药学院现代中药研究所和中医药科学院中医药信息研究所，经近一年的讨论酝酿，早在 2017 年 8 月就向国际标准化组织（ISO）提交了《中药制药过程工艺语义框架》标准提案，2017 年在英国召开的 ISO 国际会议上做了报告，2018 年 2 月即通过了 NP 投票，正式立项。随后两年里，经过众多国际专家讨论修改，ISO 于 2020 年 1 月正式发布了该标准（ISO/TS 23303：2020 Health informatics—Categorial Structure for Chinese materia medica products manufacturing process），即《中药制药过程工艺语义框架》ISO 标准。

该标准主要围绕现代中药制药过程及控制体系，针对相关数学模型及理论进行了标准化研究，提炼和梳理了现代中药制药过程中的关键步骤及其涉及的对象之间的语义关联关系，定义了中药制药过程工艺的语义分类框架。率先构建覆盖中药智能制造全流程的概念语义框架，为中药智能制造的系列标准构建起到引导作用，为实现中药智能制造提供参考。

作为中药生产领域的第一个国际标准,《中药制药过程工艺语义框架》ISO 标准成为我国中药生产领域的标志性成果。该国际标准的正式发布将为中药智能制造控制和持续改进提供科学依据,对推进中医药的国际化具有重大意义。

4.5 发明专利

本节摘录了中医药云平台与服务计算方向 4 项相关发明专利(于 2012—2016 年得到授权)。

4.5.1 一种缓存感知的多核处理器虚拟机故障隔离保证方法

吴朝晖,叶可江,姜晓红,何钦铭

专利号:ZL201110008236.6;授权公告号:CN102053873B;授权公告日:2012-12-05

本发明涉及计算机系统结构领域的系统级虚拟化技术及多核处理器上的虚拟机调度技术,公开了一种缓存感知的多核处理器虚拟机故障隔离保证方法,包括故障检测器对所有运行中的虚拟机进行状态异常监控和心跳信息检测。当检测到异常虚拟机时,隔离调度器首先记录该故障虚拟机在处理器核上的分配情况。当发现有其他虚拟机负载跟该故障虚拟机共享一块 L2 缓存时,隔离调度器把故障虚拟机迁移到一块独立缓存所对应的核上,其他正常虚拟机根据缓存敏感性特征进行 VM-core 调度。本发明提出了故障虚拟机在多处理器上的动态隔离调度的方法,避免了其他正常虚拟机受到缓存的污染,降低了故障虚拟机对正常虚拟机的运行影响,提升了系统的整体隔离性。

4.5.2 跨域云平台的共享文件管理方法

姜晓红,杨红星,黄鹏,吴朝晖,严海明

专利号:ZL201310139941.9;授权公告号:CN103248674B;授权公告日:2015-11-18

本发明公开了一种用于跨域云平台的共享文件管理方法,在域中选出中心域,用于维护共享文件分布表。当某个域用户上传共享文件时,可在中心域分布表上增加记录;当用户下载共享文件时,可在中心域的分布表中查询该文件所在位置。从而实现了使用最小代价达到跨域文件传输管理的目的。同时通过在每个虚拟机内设置 public 文件夹,对应共享文件中心,显示其中"是否是文件副本"字段为"no"的部分共享文件分布表。用户上传、下载文件时,只需要把文件复制到该文件夹中,就能实现虚拟机和本机对文件操作的无缝对接。

4.5.3 一种云数据中心中物理裸机快速部署操作系统的方法

姜晓红,闫凤喜,陈忠忠,吴朝晖

专利号:ZL201310170073.0;授权公告号:CN103297504B;授权公告日:2016-05-11

本发明公开了一种云数据中心中物理裸机快速部署操作系统的方法,包括:①开启一个服务器 A,在服务器 A 上安装 dnsmasq 服务和"裸机部署 Daemon";②裸机 B 加电开机并以 PXE 方式启动,服务器 A 为裸机 B 分配 IP 地址;③服务器 A 传送一个 Ramdisk 至裸机 B;④裸机 B 运行所述 Ramdisk;⑤服务器 A 上的"裸机部署 Daemon"服务挂载来自裸机 B 的 iSCSI target,将所述 iSCSI target 划分为操作系统主分区和操作系统 swap 分区;⑥服务器 A 上的"裸机部署 Daemon"服务将一个预先定义好的操作系统镜像文件复制到步骤⑤划分的操作系统主分区中,修改所述操作系统主分区中的 grub 启动文件;⑦裸机 B 上的 Ramdisk 执行服务器 A 操作完成的通知后,执行重启命令,裸机 B 从硬盘启动。采用本发明的方法可大大提高装机效率。

4.5.4　一种面向云数据中心的大规模虚拟机快速迁移决策方法

吴朝晖,叶可江,姜晓红,李翔
专利号:ZL201310186581.8;授权公告号:CN103246564B;授权公告日:2016-06-01

　　本发明涉及计算机系统结构领域的系统级虚拟化技术及虚拟机迁移技术,公开了一种面向云数据中心的大规模虚拟机快速迁移决策方法。先对输入的初始方案和目标方案进行虚拟机到物理机映射关系的归类,然后进行预处理操作,消除初始方案和目标方案中相同的映射关系,接着把从初始方案快速转移至目标方案的问题转化为寻找从初始方案到目标方案的最佳匹配组合,执行递归,直到初始状态或目标状态为空,则执行结束,最后进行后处理,减去重复计算的迁移次数,并输出最终的迁移次数和具体迁移决策方案。本发明提出的大规模虚拟机快速迁移的决策方法,能最大程度减少虚拟机的迁移次数,降低虚拟机迁移开销,加快虚拟机迁移执行。

附录　代表性演讲报告

互联网技术新进展
及中医药科学数据建设中的应用思考

吴朝晖
浙江大学计算机学院
2011年10月27日 上海

提纲

- ☐ 中医药科学数据系统建设回顾
- ☐ 互联网技术及应用进展
  - 语义互联网与知识技术
  - 服务计算与云计算
  - SNS与社会计算
- ☐ 未来发展的若干思考与初步实践
  - 中医药复杂知识建模
  - 中医药知识服务平台
  - 中医药虚拟知识社区（Social 3D）

中医药信息系统建设回顾

中医药研发回顾概述

十余年研发坚持

八十多个应用程序开发

五十余名研究生培养（其中近10名博士生）

一百余篇相关论文发表

技术发展脉络

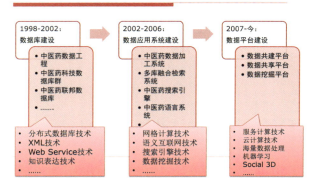

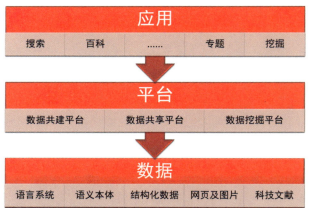

中医药搜索引擎

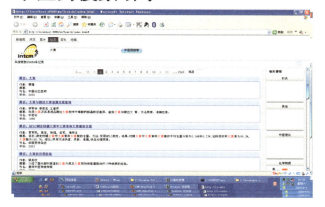

中医药知识百科

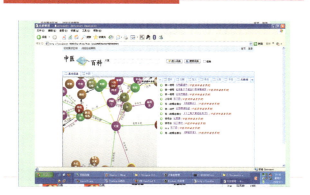

中医药知识挖掘与分析

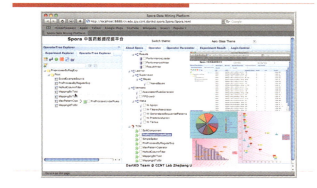

临床疾病库查询系统

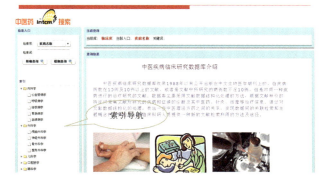

药理实验库查询系统

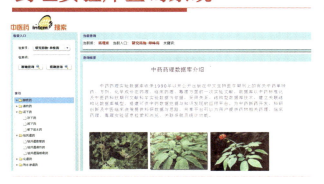

中医药知识专题

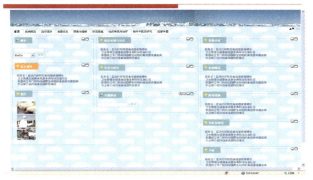

数据挖掘的相关研究工作

- ☐ 中医方剂配伍规律的知识发现
- ☐ 中医药效的知识发现
- ☐ 中医证候基因关系的知识发现
- ☐ 中医药数据预处理的探索
- ☐ 基于网格及云技术平台的数据挖掘

中医方剂配伍规律的知识发现

- ☐ 采用有效的高频集数据挖掘方法，进行中药复方的配伍规律研究
- ☐ 得到了常用药物组方配伍与药物间相互作用的知识
- ☐ 为进一步探讨分析中药复方的组成配伍规律及药物间的相互作用奠定了技术方法基础

各库中用药频次排在前20的单味药比较

排序	中国方剂	新药品种	成方制剂标准	排序	中国方剂	新药品种	成方制剂标准
1	甘草	甘草	甘草	11	陈皮	黄芪	冰片
2	当归	当归	黄芪	12	半夏	木香	连翘
3	人参	茯苓	当归	13	干姜	桔梗	柴胡
4	白术	陈皮	川芎	14	黄芪	党参	白术
5	防风	冰片	黄芩	15	附子	大黄	红花
6	黄芩	川芎	茯苓	16	大黄	地黄	麦冬
7	木香	白术	丹皮	17	枳壳	防风	地黄
8	川芎	白芍	金银花	18	麝香	红花	陈皮
9	茯苓	黄芩	白芍	19	桔梗	山药	党参
10	黄连	熟地黄	大黄	20	柴胡	香附	三七

中医方剂药对知识发现图示

高频药对指利用高频集算法挖掘出的药对

匹配药对指中药药对数据库里已经收录的药对

找到的高频药对等于匹配药对，说明验证了已有药对

找到的高频药对在药对数据库中没有出现，说明是可能的新药对

高频药对频次	匹配药对名称	高频药对名称	高频药对频次	匹配药对名称	高频药对名称	高频药对频次	匹配药对名称	高频药对名称
		白术	2596	当归、黄芪	当归、黄芪	2004		当归、木香
		人参	2522		人参、白茯苓	1941		当归、人参、白术
		川芎	2321	白术、陈皮	白术、陈皮	1909		当归、茯苓
3523		当归、白术	2210	当归、白芍	当归、白芍	1906		当归、桂心
3049	人参、黄芪	人参、黄芪	2142		人参、防风	1897		连黄芩、黄连
2853		参、茯苓	2127		防风、川芎			
		风	2079	人参、半夏	人参、半夏			
			2076	乳香、没药	乳香、没药			
			2025		当归、黄芩	1836		人参、陈皮

中医药效的知识发现

- ☐ 采用了基于分层聚类的**KDD**方法
- ☐ 探究了中药药物的功效机理问题
- ☐ 得到了单味药间按照功效相似性分类的结果

中药药效知识发现的部分结果

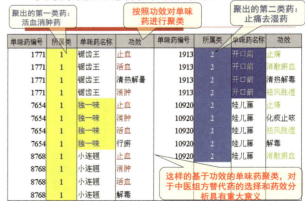

聚出的第一类药：活血消肿药

按照功效对单味药进行聚类

聚出的第二类药：止痛去湿药

单味药编号	所属类	单味药名称	功效	单味药编号	所属类	单味药名称	功效
1771	1	锯齿王	止血	1913	2	开口箭	止痛
1771	1	锯齿王	活血	1913	2	开口箭	消散瘀血
1771	1	锯齿王	清热解暑	1913	2	开口箭	清热解毒
1771	1	锯齿王	消肿	1913	2	开口箭	祛风胜湿
7654	1	独一味	止血	10920	2	娃儿藤	止痛
7654	1	独一味	消肿	10920	2	娃儿藤	化痰止咳
7654	1	独一味	活血	10920	2	娃儿藤	祛风胜湿
7654	1	独一味	行瘀	10920	2	娃儿藤	解毒
8768	1	小连翘	止血	10920	2	娃儿藤	消散瘀血
8768	1	小连翘	消肿				
8768	1	小连翘	活血				
8768	1	小连翘	解毒				

这样的基于功效的单味药聚类，对于中医组方替代药的选择和药效分析具有重大意义

中医证候基因关系的知识发现

- ☐ 提出了一种基于分布式字聚类和信息抽取的文本挖掘方法
- ☐ 首创了中医证候与基因相关关系的研究
- ☐ 为生命科学的发展提供了新知识和新方法

中医证候基因关系知识挖掘的图示

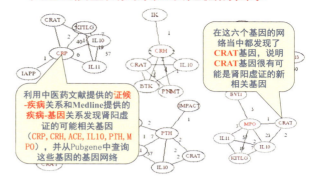

肾阳虚证的相关基因的基因网络

中医药数据预处理的探索

- ☐ 药物组成等字段的自动结构化
- ☐ 功效等字段缺失值的填补

利用KDD算法填补的功效与原有功效的比较（部分结果）

方剂中已知功效（假设缺失）	利用KDD算法计算出的功效
补肾益肺、清热化痰、止咳平喘	清热化痰、健脾益气、止咳平喘
温肾壮阳、补益精血	温肾壮阳、补气养血
补气养血、调经散寒	补气养血、通经散寒
补肾壮腰、固精止遗、调经	补肾壮腰、固精止遗
滋补强壮、助力固精	滋补强壮、助气固精
益气补血、滋补肝肾	补气健脾、滋补肝肾
滋阴补气、益肾填精	滋阴补气、填精益髓
清热生津、益气养阴	补中益气、养阴生津
补肾健脾、养心安神	敛肺补肾、养心安神

开发的部分挖掘应用程序

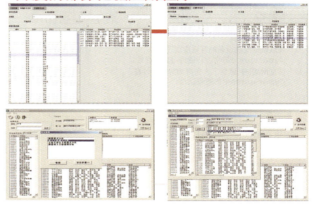

中医药数据挖掘平台 Spora

- ☐ **平台定位：在前人工作基础上，为中医药知识发现提供方便、灵活、可定制的新一代操作平台**
- ☐ **核心思想：面向组件的架构**
  - ■ 基于流程组合的思想，以操作符组合为核心
  - ■ 集成各类操作符
    - ☐ 各类open source的数据挖掘算法
    - ☐ 新开发的数据预处理操作符：规则替换、字段拆分
- ☐ **其他技术特点：**
  - ■ 基于C/S快速原型工具
  - ■ 基于Ajax的界面交互技术

数据挖掘平台Spora截图

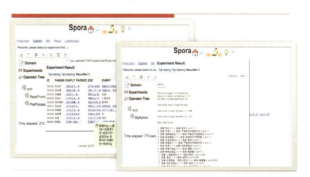

互联网技术及应用新进展

未来的互联网

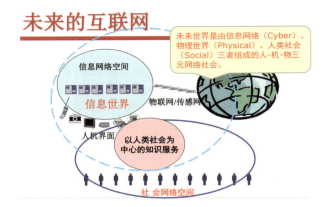

未来世界是由信息网络（Cyber）、物理世界（Physical）、人类社会（Social）三者组成的人-机-物三元网络社会。

互联网深广度发展带来新问题与新挑战

- 互联网→数据共享变得容易，用户可用数据激增。
- 移动互联网→ 实现了Cyberspace与人连接的可持续性。
- 物联网→泛在设备的互联实现了Cyberspace与物理环境连接的可通性。
- 社交网络 → 建立了人类群体的社会性在Cyberspace中的可表达性。

智能系统的复杂性急剧增强
个性化、智能化、自适应性需求迫切
海量数据的智能分析与挖掘问题突出
呼唤新理论、新方法、新技术

主要相关技术

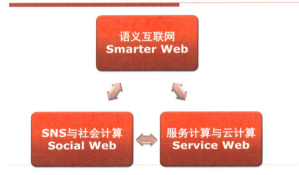

语义互联网的提出

2001年，Tim Berners-Lee, James Hendler和Ora Lassila在Scientific American上正式提出并阐述了语义互联网的概念。

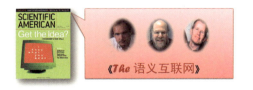

Tim Berners-Lee, James Hendler and Ora Lassila, The 语义互联网, Scientific American, May 2001。

语义互联网的提出

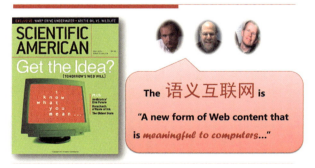

The 语义互联网 is "A new form of Web content that is *meaningful to computers...*"

语义互联网的关键技术

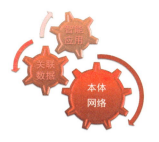
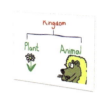

语义互联网的关键技术

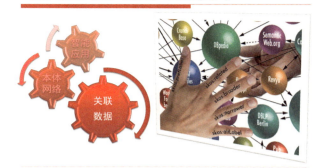

语义互联网的关键技术

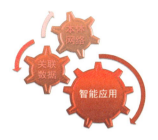
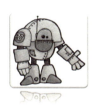

本体网络

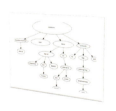

领域本体用于精确地
表达领域的概念结构
· SNOMED CT
· Gene Ontology

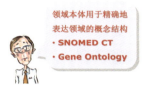

本体网络

面向领域的本体联网

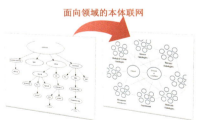

实现某个领域
中全部本体资
源的互联

本体网络

面向领域的本体联网　　　全球范围的本体联网

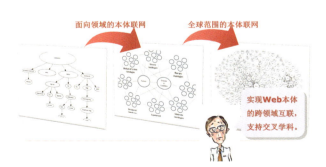

实现Web本体
的跨领域互联,
支持交叉学科。

互联数据

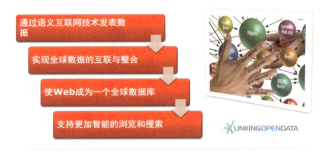

- 通过语义互联网技术发表数据
- 实现全球数据的互联与整合
- 使Web成为一个全球数据库
- 支持更加智能的浏览和搜索

互联数据

☐ **2007，W3C组织Linking Open Data（LOD）工程：**

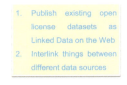

1. Publish existing open license datasets as Linked Data on the Web
2. Interlink things between different data sources

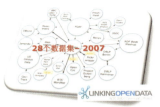

28个数据集-2007

互联数据

☐ **2011，LOD的知识体系日趋成熟，出现专著和大量科技文献**

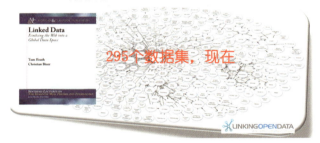

295个数据集，现在

信息语义：
语义互联网：Smart Web

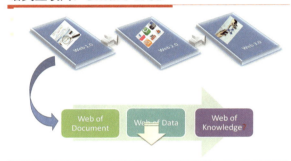

信息语义：
语义互联网：Smart Web

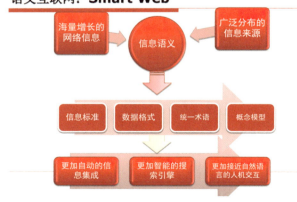

- 海量增长的网络信息 → 信息语义 ← 广泛分布的信息来源
- 信息标准 / 数据格式 / 统一术语 / 概念模型
- 更加自动的信息集成 / 更加智能的搜索引擎 / 更加接近自然语言的人机交互

语义互联网与 生命医学

☐ 在国际上，语义互联网技术在生命科学领域引起极大的重视。原因：
  - 生命科学领域是知识密集型领域，大量信息需要复杂的知识表达方法才能描述；
  - 生命科学领域已经产生了巨大的、多样化的数据资源，迫切需要进行集成和共享，以支持深层次的知识发现研究；
  - 生命科学领域的信息资源大部分是基于Web的。

☐ 从2006年起，由MIT, Harvard, Yale, Lily Pharmaceutics等组织牵头，全球多个高等研究机构和医药企业参与的一个大项目，主要目的是研究如何利用语义互联网技术到脑科学和 neuroscience area.
  - Details can be found: http://esw.w3c.org/topics/HCLS

支持对脑疾病机理的研究

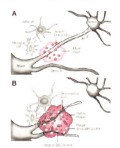

Alzheimer's disease is characterized by neural degeneration. Among other things, there is damage to dendrites and axons, parts of nerve cells.

What resources do we have available to learn more about biological processes in dendrites?

主要方法：

☐ 用语义和本体集成来自多个领域和多个机构的资源

· Integration and analysis of heterogeneous data sets
· Hypothesis, Genome Pathways, Molecular Properties, Disease, etc.

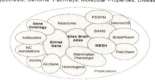

From molecular level to behavior level

The Knowledge Semantics Continuum

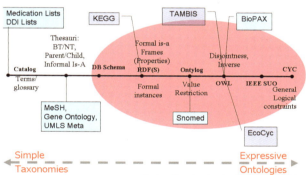

Ontology Dimensions based on McGuinness and Finin

语义互联网对于生命与医学信息的好处

☐ **Fusion of data across many scientific disciplines**
  ■ 融合多学科的数据
☐ **Easier recombination of data**
  ■ 更简单的数据重组
☐ **Querying of data at different levels of granularity**
  ■ 在不同粒度层次查询数据
☐ **Capture provenance of data through annotation**
  ■ 跟踪数据来源
☐ **Data can be assessed for inconsistencies**
  ■ 通过跨数据集的推理寻找数据之间的不一致性
☐ **Knowledge discovery from semantic network formed by integrating cross-institutional, cross-dispinaries data sources.**
  ■ 跨多个数据集的知识发现。

云计算的概念——**Google**

（1）数据在云端
· 不怕丢失
· 不必备份
· 海量存储

（2）软件和服务在云端
· 不必下载
· 自动升级

（3）无所不在的云计算
· 浏览器即客户端
· 任何设备登录
· 随时随处从云中获取数据

（4）无限强大的云计算
· 无限空间
· 无限速度

云概念——《福布斯》

　　云计算的理想在计算机发展的早期就已经出现，其概念其实非常简单，即通过互联网提供软件与服务，并由网络浏览器界面来实现。用户不需要安装服务器或任何客户端软件，可在任何时间、任何地点、任何设备(前提是接入互联网)上随时随意访问云中的数据和软件。

新概念层出不穷

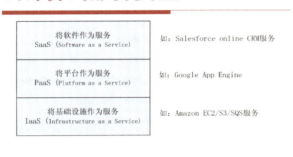

云计算的技术背景

云计算是并行计算(Parallel Computing)、分布式计算(Distributed Computing)和网格计算（Grid Computing）的发展，或者说是这些计算机科学概念的商业实现。

云计算是虚拟化(Virtualization)、效用计算(Utility Computing)、IaaS(基础设施即服务)、PaaS(平台即服务)、SaaS(软件即服务)等概念混合演进并跃升的结果。

云计算的服务类型

将软件作为服务 SaaS (Software as a Service)	如：Salesforce online CRM服务
将平台作为服务 PaaS (Platform as a Service)	如：Google App Engine
将基础设施作为服务 IaaS (Infrastructure as a Service)	如：Amazon EC2/S3/SQS服务

云计算的特点

超大规模　　　　高可扩展性

虚拟化

高可靠性　　　　按需服务

极其廉价

通用性

互联网的未来发展趋势：
The Social Trends：Web of People

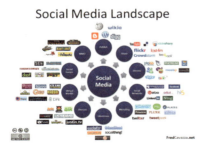

什么是社会计算

☐ 传统的社会计算泛指采用计算机仿真的方法对社会群体进行建模和模拟，以便对一些社会现象进行分析、预测和辅助决策的方法。例如：

- 人工社会系统
- 群集智能系统
- ......

☐ **典型应用，如：**

- 智能交通系统
- 公共卫生
- ......

什么是社会计算

□ 新一代的社会计算研究主要得益于互联网的发展，特别是**Web 2.0**的发展，使得互联网的社交功能发展得到充分发挥，由此出现一系列新的社会计算研究课题和应用：

- Social Web→ Social Bookmarking, Social Recommendation, Social Searching, Social Tagging, WiKi, Micro Blogging……
- SNS → Mobile SNS
- Social Software → Enterprise Social Computing
  □ IBM Lotus Greenhouse, Google Wave……
- Social 3D → Second Life, HiPiHi

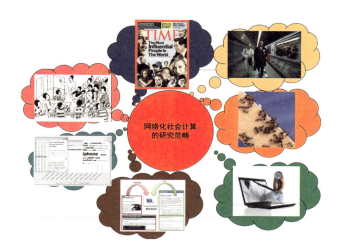

未来发展的若干思考与初步实践

三个方面的思考

中医药复杂知识建模

中医药知识服务平台

中医药虚拟知识社区

中医药领域复杂知识建模

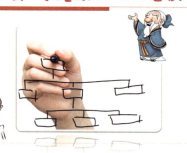

中医药领域总体模型

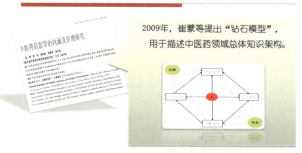

2009年，崔蒙等提出"钻石模型"，用于描述中医药领域总体知识架构。

中医药领域总体模型

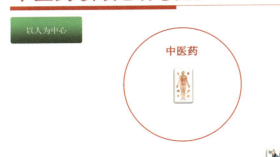

中医药领域总体模型

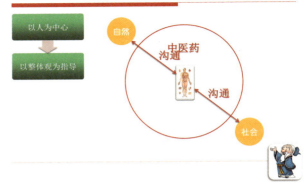

中医药领域总体模型

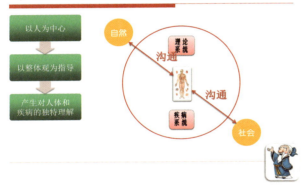

中医药领域总体模型

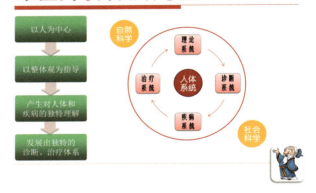

中医药领域知识建模问题

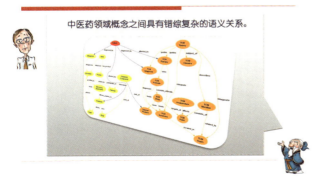

中医药领域知识建模问题

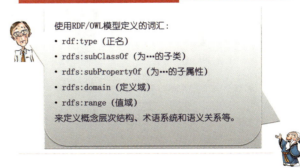

中医药领域知识建模问题

中医药领域具有复杂的概念层次结构和术语系统。

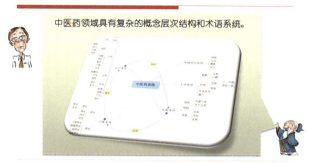

中医药领域知识建模问题

使用SKOS本体中定义的词汇：

· skos:prefLabel （正名）

· skos:altLabel （异名）

· skos:defination （定义）

· skos:broader （上位词）

· skos:narrower （下位词）

· skos:relatedTo （关联词），

来定义概念层次结构、术语系统和语义关系等。

中医药领域知识建模问题

中医药领域广泛采用中华传统文化特有的思维方式。

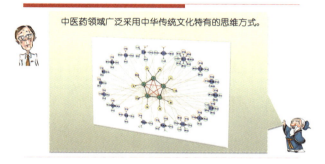

中医药领域知识建模问题

提出一系列面向本体设计的语义模式：

· 结构模式 （Structural Patterns）

· 逻辑模式 （Logical Patterns）

· 文字模式 （Literal Patterns）

· 内容模式 （Content Patterns）

对中医药中广泛使用的传统思维模式进行建模：

· 取象比类

· 方剂配伍…

中医药领域知识建模问题

中医药领域涉及到意义复杂的概念和复杂的领域逻辑。

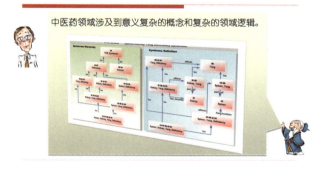

中医药领域知识建模问题

使用OWL中的知识表达构件：

· owl:intersectionOf，owl:unionOf

· owl:complementOf

· owl:oneOf

· owl:allValueFrom，owl:someValueFrom

· owl:inverseOf,

· owl:sameAs, owl:differentFrom

对中医药领域的复杂知识进行建模。

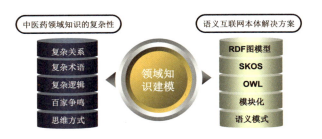

中医药领域复杂知识建模

TCMOnto

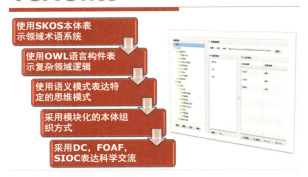

中医药知识服务平台

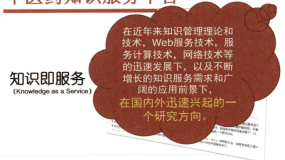

知识即服务
(Knowledge as a Service)

基于语义互联网实现知识服务

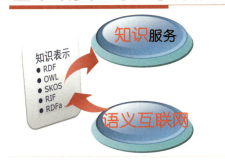

基于语义互联网实现知识服务

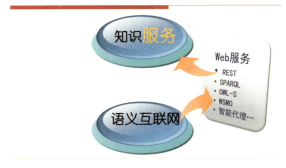

基于语义互联网实现知识服务

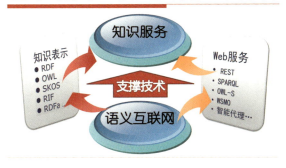

基于语义互联网实现知识服务平台的基本思路

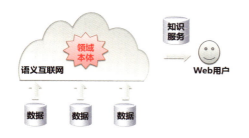

基于语义互联网实现知识服务

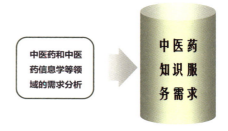

基于语义互联网实现知识服务

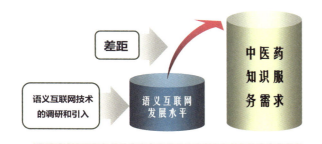

基于语义互联网实现知识服务

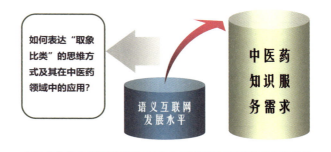

基于语义互联网实现知识服务

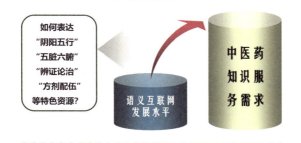

基于语义互联网实现知识服务

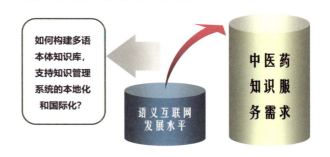

基于语义互联网实现知识服务

如何将中医药领域的各类数据库映射为合适的语义互联网知识库?

语义互联网发展水平

中医药知识服务需求

基于语义互联网实现知识服务

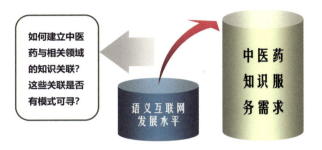

如何建立中医药与相关领域的知识关联?这些关联是否有模式可寻?

语义互联网发展水平

中医药知识服务需求

基于语义互联网实现知识服务

· 本体设计模式
· 知识管理模式
· 知识关联模式
· 智能行为模式
· 智能应用模式

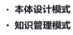
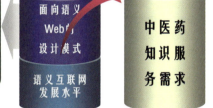

面向语义Web的设计模式

语义互联网发展水平

中医药知识服务需求

知识服务平台的解决方案

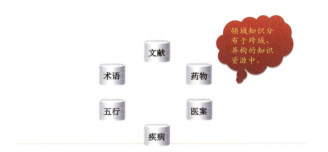

文献

术语

药物

五行

医案

疾病

领域知识分布于跨域、异构的知识资源中。

知识服务平台的解决方案

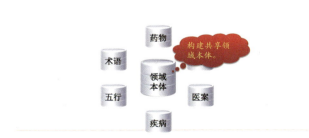

药物

术语

领域本体

五行

医案

疾病

构建共享领域本体。

知识服务平台的解决方案

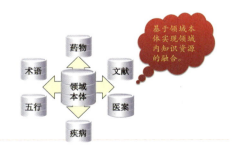

药物

术语

领域本体

文献

五行

医案

疾病

基于领域本体实现领域内知识资源的融合。

知识服务平台的解决方案

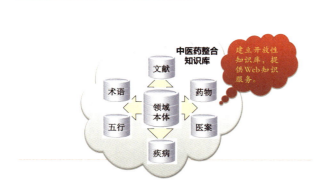

知识服务平台的解决方案

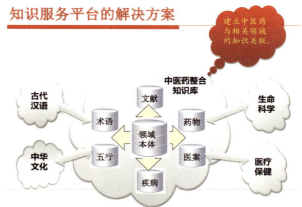

知识服务平台的解决方案

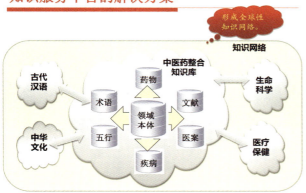

知识服务平台的解决方案

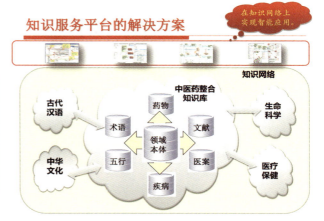

中医药知识服务平台建设中的核心科学问题

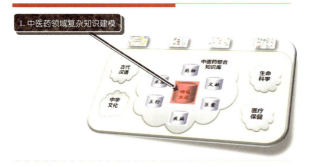

中医药知识服务平台建设中的核心科学问题

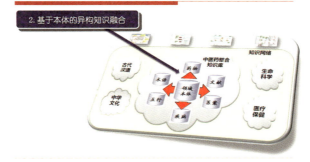

中医药知识服务平台建设中的核心科学问题

3、挖掘中医药与相关领域之间的知识关联

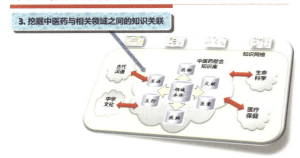

总结

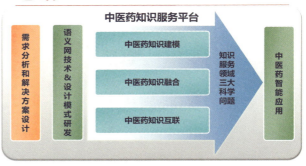

中医药3D虚拟社区Demo成果展示

☐ 将Social 3D引入到中医药知识服务中

➢以3D技术展示中医药信息
➢包含名医馆和中医学堂药材部
➢包含疾病、药方、药材等数据
➢具备多人在线交流功能

寓教于乐，辅助学习和知识的获取

中医药3D虚拟社区Demo成果展示

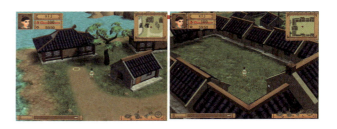

中医药3D虚拟社区Demo成果展示

名医馆

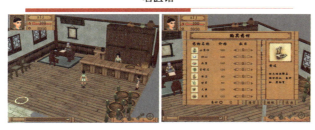

中医药3D虚拟社区Demo成果展示

药材部

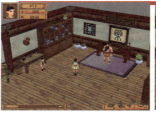
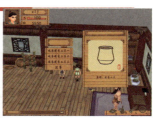

支持中医药信息学
——知识服务的模型、方法及平台

吴朝晖 博士
浙江大学 教授、博导
国家现代服务业领域总体专家组 组长
中国卫生信息学会 副会长

引子：现代中医药发展需要信息学支撑与引领

◆ 正当快速发展中国迎来全球最为规模城镇化、最为规模的老龄人口之际，正当医学治疗模式发生变革、慢性病等非传染性疾病迅猛发展，"首诊在基层、首诊在全科"的中国医疗制度变革悄然推进之时，正当医疗健康已成为现代服务业重要产业、并将造就下一个兆亿产业的拐点之时；

◆ 现代中医药将迎来新的发展机遇，中医药信息学将是其发展的关键与基础。

提纲

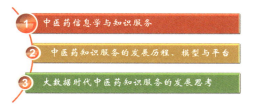

1. 中医药信息学与知识服务
2. 中医药知识服务的发展历程、模型与平台
3. 大数据时代中医药知识服务的发展思考

---

❶ 知识服务是中医药信息学的重要内容

中医药信息学：新兴交叉学科

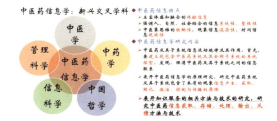

基于大数据的知识服务创新了中医药信息学研究手段

□ Wiki定义：
■ 由数量巨大、结构复杂、类型众多数据构成的结构或非结构数据集合，用传统的数据库技术、软件技术难以处理的数据，但通过数据的整合共享，交叉复用等可以形成智力资源和知识服务能力。

□ 互联网数据中心（IDC）
■ 指为了更经济更有效地从高频率、大容量、不同结构和类型的数据中获取价值而设计的新一代架构和技术，用它来描述和定义信息爆炸时代产生的海量数据，并命名与之相关的技术发展与创新。

□ 麦肯锡：
■ 社交技术与大数据将提升生产力

基于大数据的知识服务创新了中医药信息学研究手段

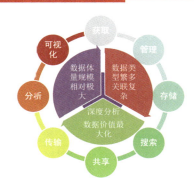

中医药信息与"大数据"知识服务：相似性分析

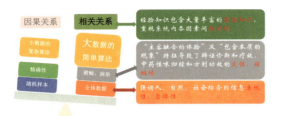

大数据时代知识服务：支撑中医药信息化

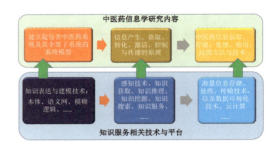

第四研究范式的革命

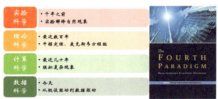

提纲

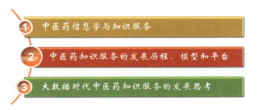

中医药信息数字化发展历程

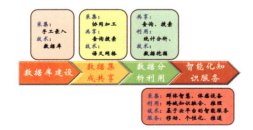

信息技术在中医药应用：信息服务→知识服务

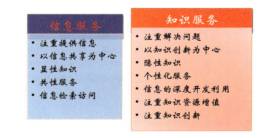

中医药知识服务平台建设实践进程

- 1998年，开始与北京中医药信息研究所合作，建设开发中医药数据库系统
- 2003年，DartGrid1.0
- 2006年，DartGrid1.4
- 2007年，语义网格 DartGrid 2.0
- 2009年，DartGrid3.0支持Web服务，并行执据
- 2010年，向知识服务平台演进

2014年，建设知识服务平台DartGrid4.0并展开应用

十七年磨一剑、构建中医药知识服务平台DartGrid

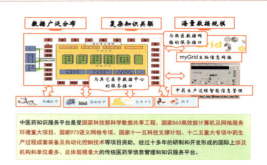

中医药知识服务平台是受国家科技部科学数据共享工程、国家863高效能计算机及网格服务环境重大项目、国家973语义网格专项、国家十一五科技支撑计划、十二五重大专项中药生产过程成套装备及自动化控制技术等项目资助，经过十多年的研制和开发形成的国际上涉及机构和单位最多、总体规模最大的传统医药学信息管理和知识服务平台。

中医药知识服务：*层次服务观*

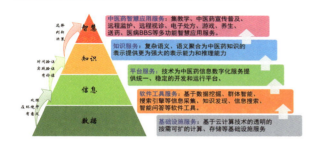

- **中医药智慧应用服务：** 集教学、中医药宣传普及、远程监护、远程视诊、电子处方、游戏、养生、送药、医病BBS等多功能智慧应用服务。
- **知识服务：** 复杂语义、语义聚合为中医药知识的表示提供更为强大的表示能力和推理能力
- **平台服务：** 技术为中医药信息数字化服务提供统一、稳定的开发和运行平台、
- **软件工具服务：** 基于数据挖掘、群体智能、搜索引擎等信息采集、知识发现、信息搜索、智能问答等软件工具。
- **基础设施服务：** 基于云计算技术的透明的按需可扩的计算、存储等基础设施服务

中医药知识服务平台：体系架构

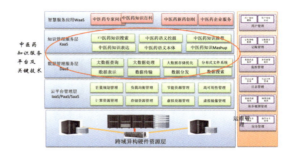

支持知识服务平台的*基础1*——DartGrid语义网格平台

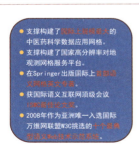
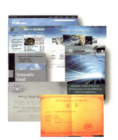

- 支撑构建了国际上规模最大的中医药科学数据应用网格。
- 支撑构建了国家高分辨率对地观测网格服务平台。
- 在Springer出版国际上首部语义网格英文专著。
- 获国际语义互联网顶级会议10年最佳论文奖。
- 2008年作为亚洲唯一入选国际万维网联盟W3C挑选的十个经典语义网技术应用案例。

支持知识服务平台的*基础2*——DartCloud云平台

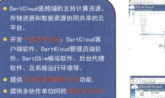
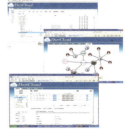

- DartCloud是跨域的支持计算资源、存储资源和数据资源协同共享的云平台。
- 开发一整套软件：DartCloud客户端软件、DartCloud管理员端软件、DartCSim模拟软件、后台代理软件、及系统运行环境等。
- 提供大规模的网络存储服务功能。
- 提供多协作单位间的网络协同共享架构。
- 提供云数据中心模拟平台DartCSim。
- 基于DartCloud支撑了一个跨单位的语言翻译云服务平台。

建设知识服务平台的智慧应用中心

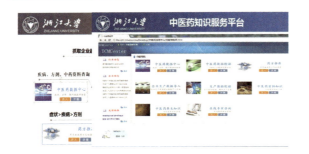

基于知识服务平台：智慧应用中心的服务概览

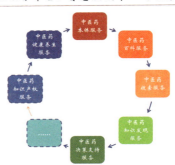

中医药本体服务

- 中医药本体服务旨在支持中医药本体的有效管理、共享和利用。
- 基于描述逻辑等技术，实现中医药术语标准和语义网络的表示和存储，并支持分布式加工。
- 表示中医药语言中的同义词、相关词、术语定义与关联关系。
- 支持概念查询、语义关联查询、概念实例查询、概念层次查询等功能，并可直接显示概念层次与语义关联图。

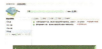

中医药知识百科服务

- 维基（Wiki）是在网络时代中涌现的大众化知识工程技术。
- 特点是允许任意网络用户对任意页面进行创建和编辑，因此能集思广益，突破了传统知识工程的知识获取瓶颈。
- 在生物医学领域，维基已被用于临床实践、医学教育和研究等领域，成为虚拟协作的有效方式

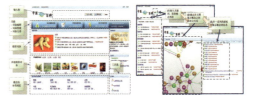

中医药搜索服务

- 用户可以围绕一个领域主题集进行高效而全面的信息检索。
- 提供多样化的智能搜索服务，
  - 基于内容的搜索。
  - 智能语义查询。
  - 语义图浏览。
  - 相关概念推荐。
  - 按主题的信息综合等

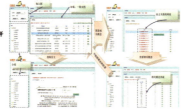

中医药知识发现服务

- 利用人工智能与数据库，通过机器学习、数据分析和挖掘技术从海量数据中获取有效、新颖、隐性知识。
- 面向中医药文献的知识发现
- 面向中医学的知识发现
- 面向中药学的知识发现
- 面向中药新药研发的知识发现

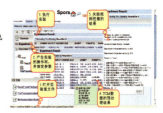

中医药决策支持服务

- 是从潜在可操作知识中实时地获取可操作的显性知识，辅助客户产生可操作的隐性知识。
- 面向中医辨证的推理决策
- 中医药智能决策系统

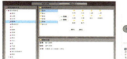

(a) 辅助诊疗界面。

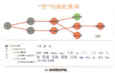

(b) 推理模型界面。

应用案例1：集成研发中医药科研知识服务系统

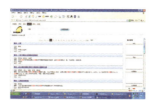
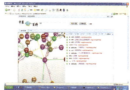

应用案例1：集成研发中医药科研知识服务系统

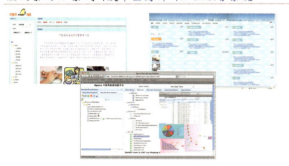

应用案例2：扩展研制中药生产知识服务系统

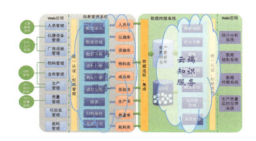

中医药知识服务：模型方法与关键技术

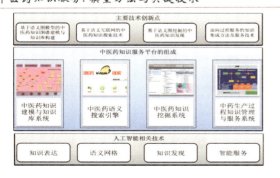

中医药知识服务面临的难点及关键技术

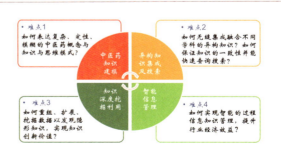

关键技术突破1
基于语义图的中医药知识图谱与知识库构建

重点突破1大难题
① 复杂中医药知识建模问题

主要提出2项关键方法
① 提出了基于多图语义的知识图谱建模方法
② 提出了唯象中医药知识建模方法。

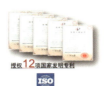

授权 **12** 项国家发明专利

Health Informatics — Semantic Network Framework of Traditional Chinese Medicine Language System

ISO国际标准 **1** 项：中医药语义网络

基于多图语义的知识图谱建模方法

□ 以"郁怒"为例的中医临床推理过程的语义图表示

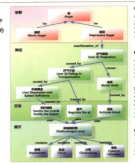

唯象中医药知识建模方法

□ 中医象思维及设计模式

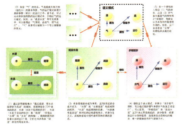

从"疏浚水流"到"肝郁疏肝"的取向比类思维过程知识表示

关键技术突破2
基于语义互联网的中医药知识搜索技术

重点突破2大难题
① 知识服务的语义一致性保证
② 海量异构知识集成搜索问题

主要提出2项关键方法
① 提出了多模型语义映射方法
② 提出了分布式语义索引方法

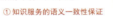

授权4项国家发明专利

国际标准1项
中医药元数据

英文专著1项　获得4项软件著作权

多模型语义映射方法

数据库到语义图的语义映射

不同模式数据到语义本体的语义映射

分布式语义索引方法

□ 单服务器体系架构中大规模数据搜索是一个潜在的性能瓶颈。
□ 我们提出并实现的分布式语义索引方法能同时满足分布于20多个中医药数据中心的数据搜索服务。

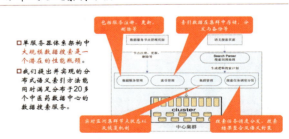

关键技术突破3：
基于语义图挖掘的中医药知识发现

重点突破1大难题
① 中医药知识的深度利用问题

主要提出3项关键方法
① 提出了复杂网络化知识的搜索挖掘方法
② 提出了基于语义图的泛化关联规则挖掘方法

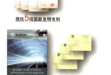

授权5项国家发明专利

英文专著1项　获得3项软件著作权

复杂网络化知识的搜索挖掘方法

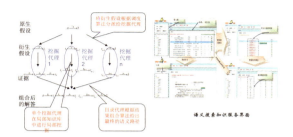

语义搜索知识服务界面

基于语义图的泛化关联规则挖掘方法

□ 基于各种语义关联发现方法，可以将各种知识碎片连接为一个整体性的知识网络，避免知识孤岛现象的发生。

□ 语义关联挖掘（Semantic Association Mining）旨在从关联数据中挖掘新颖的语义模式，从而推测和验证任意资源之间的潜在关系

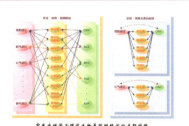

中医症候群与现代生物基因网络间的关联挖掘

关键技术突破4：
面向过程服务的知识集成方法及服务技术

重点突破1大难题
① 中药生产过程的智能信息管理问题

主要提出3项关键方法
① 提出了面向过程服务的知识集成方法及服务技术
② 提出了基于语义发布订阅的知识集成方法
③ 面向移动环境的知识服务集成方法

专著1部

授权10项国家发明专利

中医药知识服务平台建设取得的成果

□ 平台在复杂中医药知识图谱构建、中医药语义搜索、中医药语义图挖掘和过程化知识服务集成等方面取得突出的技术及应用创新。

□ 总共获得31项授权发明专利，7项软件著作权，2项ISO国际标准，4部专著（其中英文2部）。

□ 2014年获教育部技术发明一等奖

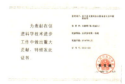

第三方评价：网格之父Ian Foster

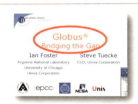

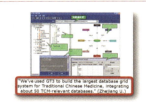

国际网格之父Ian Foster 在2005年的GlobusWorld 大会上把我们平台列为全球十大典型应用平台之一，是亚太地区唯一入选的平台。

第三方评价：语义互联网工作组主席

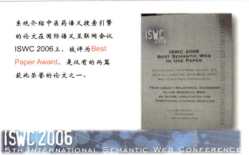

语义互联网领域国际知名学者，国际万维网联盟W3C语义互联网工作组主席Ivan Herfman先生在其公开报告和技术博客中都多次积极评价该系统。

第三方评价：国际万维网联盟W3C

基于语义的中医药搜索与查询系统方法在2008年被国际万维网联盟W3C列为国际上十个最典型的语义互联网技术示范之一。是亚洲地区唯一入选的项目。

第三方评价：最佳应用论文奖

系统介绍中医药语义搜索引擎的论文在国际语义互联网会议ISWC 2006上，被评为Best Paper Award，是仅有的两篇获此荣誉的论文之一。

提纲

1. 中医药信息学与知识服务
2. 中医药知识服务的发展历程、模型和平台
3. 大数据时代中医药知识服务的发展思考

大数据时代：生活、思维、工作大变革
改变思维模式、商业服务模式及管理模式

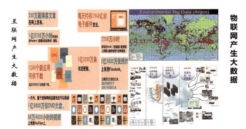

大数据时代：为信息服务行业带来发展机遇
基于知识的信息服务——传统模式→智能商务模式

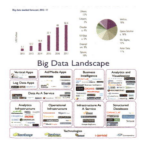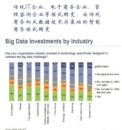

传统IT企业、电子商务企业、管理咨询企业等模式转变：由传统商务向大数据技术为基础的智能商务模式转变

大数据时代：丰富多彩的智能体感设备
围绕人的信息服务——全数据、体验数据采集成为可能

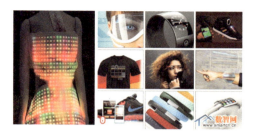

移动互联网：特众服务、数字人生
个性化的信息服务：移动化、特众定制、主动推送

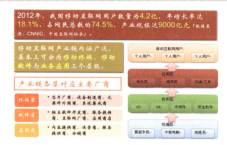

移动互联网：个人信息消费的新时代
开放互动的信息服务——面向大众、交互、基于信息价值的计费

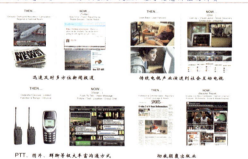

大数据时代商业模式：垂直整合、融合跨界
跨界融合的信息服务——跨行业整合服务

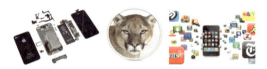

中医药科学数据共享的跨界特征

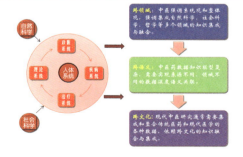

老年人健康服务——中医药信息学跨界创新？

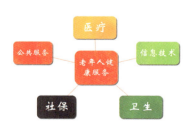

大数据时代：泛在普适信息服务时代

- 新信息观＝人类社会＋信息世界＋物理世界（iCPS）
- CPS不仅会催生出新的工业，加速信息社会发展进程；甚至会重新排列现有产业布局，推动工业与服务产品的升级换代与融合发展。

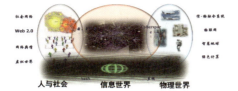

政策背景："十三五"规划纲要及25课题

- 2006年2月10日发布《国家中长期科学和技术发展规划纲要》将中医药传承与创新发展列为人口与健康领域五大优先主题之一。
- 2007年3月21日发布《国家中医药创新发展规划纲要（2006-2020）》将信息技术的应用列为中医药现代化的核心手段之一。
- 2014年1月28日发布《中国食物与营养发展纲要（2014-2020）》明确了2020年食物与营养发展目标。
- 国家"十三五"科技计划重大领域战略前期研究
  - 人口健康领域、信息技术领域、现代服务业领域

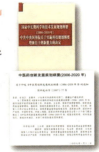

① 进一步加强中医药信息学学科建设

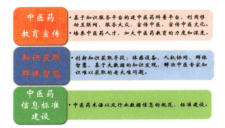

② 加强跨界知识服务大平台建设

围绕跨界服务，研究复杂服务计算技术体系，对服务复杂服务中的大规模复杂服务发现、选择、系统融合进行研究。研制支持跨界服务的知识服务平台。

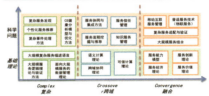

③ 研究一批中医药知识服务关键技术

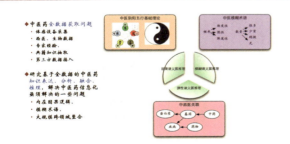

④ 设立"中医药知识服务与健康养生、养老健康"重大项目

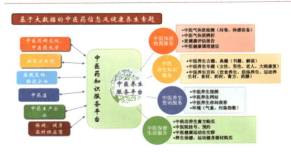

5 建立中医药跨行业跨界创新联盟

◆ 实现全数据采集
◆ 提供跨界知识服务
　➤ 中医药知识百科
　➤ 中医药文献搜索查询
　➤ 专题知识服务
　　• 养生、康复、职业病
　➤ 自发中医药社区
　　• 读者、著者群
　　• 病人群
　　• 医生群
◆ 实现跨界服务商业模式
　➤ 从领域→开放
　➤ 从免费→收费

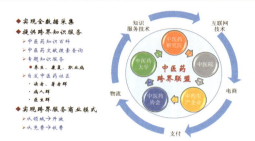

中医药行业的跨界知识服务应用展望

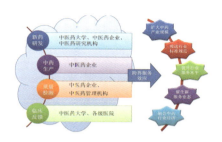

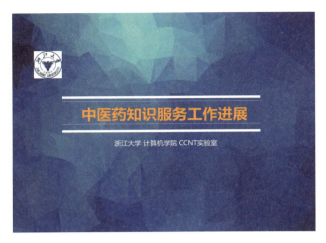

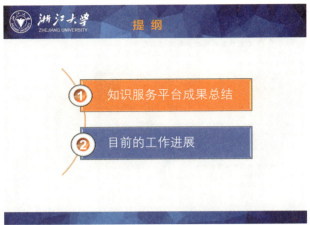

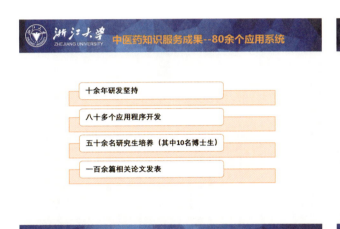

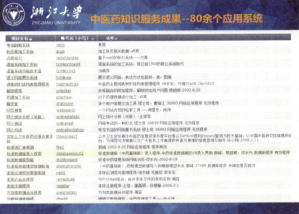

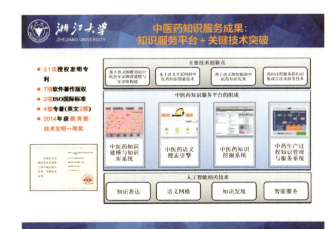

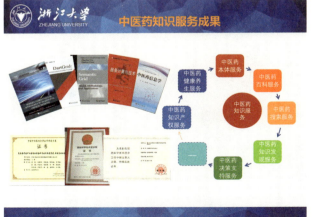

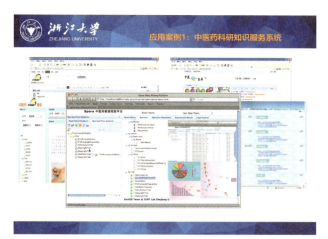

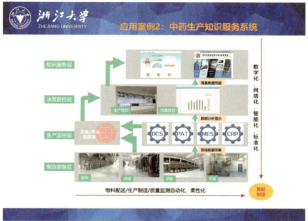

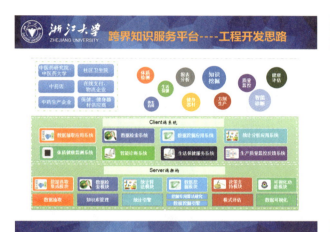

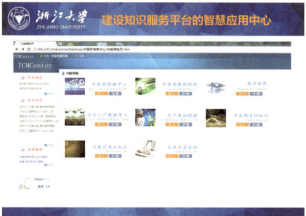

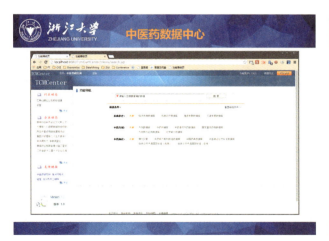

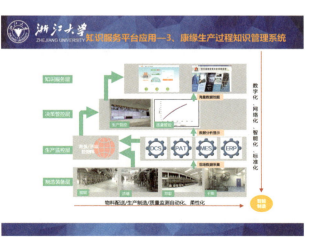

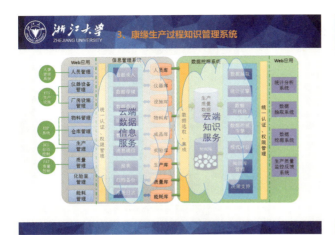

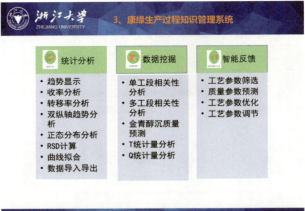

浙江大学 ZHEJIANG UNIVERSITY　3、康缘生产过程知识管理系统

统计分析
- 趋势显示
- 收率分析
- 转移率分析
- 双纵轴趋势分析
- 正态分布分析
- RSD计算
- 曲线拟合
- 数据导入导出

数据挖掘
- 单工段相关性分析
- 多工段相关性分析
- 金青醇沉质量预测
- T统计量分析
- Q统计量分析

智能反馈
- 工艺参数筛选
- 质量参数预测
- 工艺参数优化
- 工艺参数调节

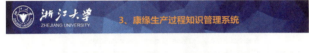

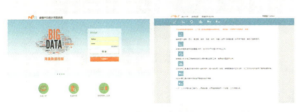

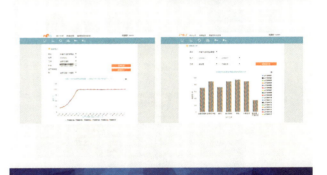

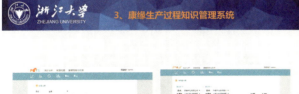

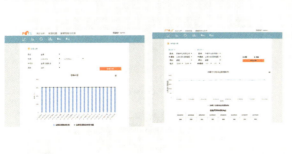

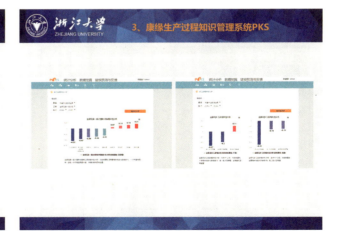

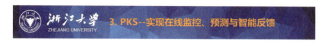

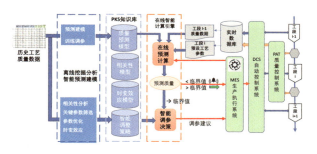

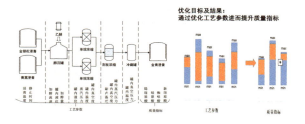

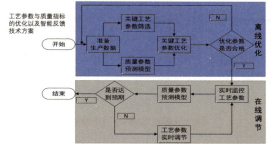

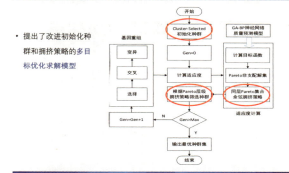

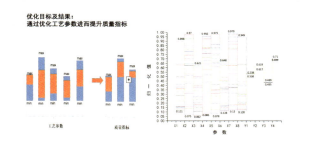

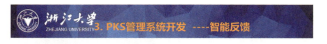

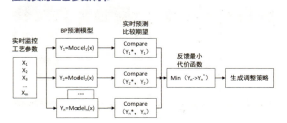

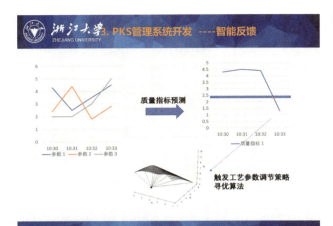

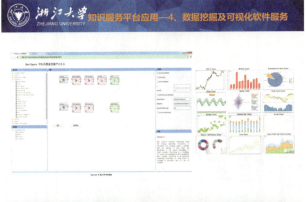

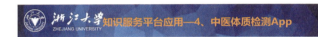

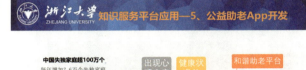

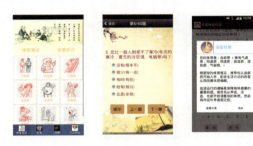

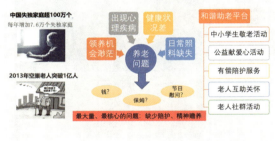

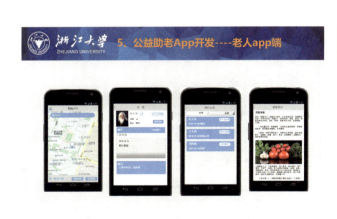

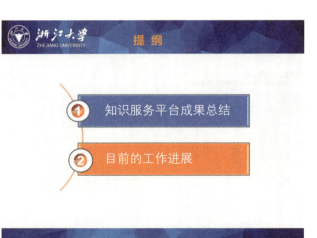

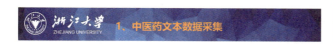

1、中医药文本数据采集

中成药
9327条

数据原始来源是各
个制药企业的药品
出厂信息

中药材
18294条

数据原始来源是《中国
药典》《全国中草药汇
编》《中药大辞典》
《中华本草》

中药方
52050条

数据原始来源是《中国药典》
《北京市中成方选集》
《医统》《医心方》《奇效
良方》《摘京年指医方》
《景岳全书》《重订通俗伤
寒论》《济阴纲目》《局方》
《普济方》等

2、基于中医药文本的症状分词与药材推荐系统

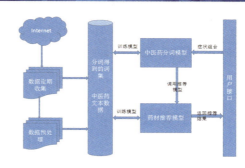

基于中医药文本的症状分词与药材推荐系统—相关技术

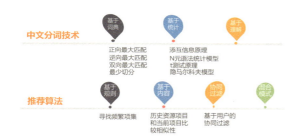

中文分词技术

基于词典 正向最大匹配 逆向最大匹配 双向最大匹配 最少切分

基于统计 添互信息原理 N元语法统计模型 t测试原理 隐马尔科夫模型

基于理解

推荐算法

基于规则 寻找频繁项集

基于内容 历史资源项目和当前项目比较相似性

协同过滤 基于用户的协同过滤

混合模式

基于双向条件概率和相对位置的症状分词算法

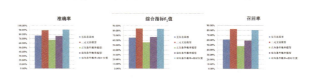

算法	准确率	召回率	F 值	运行时间
互信息原理	77.51%	61.38%	65.86%	1083ms
二元文法模型	89.08%	82.73%	84.26%	7839ms
正向条件概率模型	67.65%	47.92%	56.10%	873ms
双向条件概率模型	76.51%	59.38%	66.86%	1624ms
双向条件概率+相对位置	91.08%	80.73%	83.79%	1965ms

爬虫技术

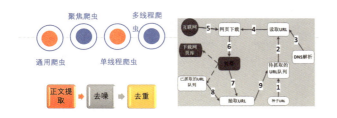

聚焦爬虫　多线程爬虫

通用爬虫　单线程爬虫

正文提取 → 去噪 → 去重

3、基于医院病历数据的智能中医辅助诊疗系统

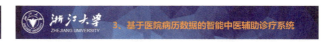

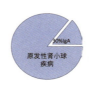

30%IgA

原发性肾小球
疾病

15%-20%的患者10年后进展至 ESRD
30%-40%的患者在20年内达到ESRD

临床、病理形态上表现多样，对治疗反应和
预后均有很大的差异，病因未明，
西医尚无理想治疗方案。
中医治疗的疗效值得肯定。

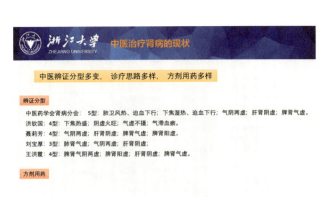

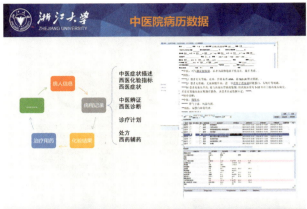

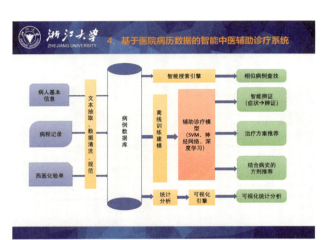

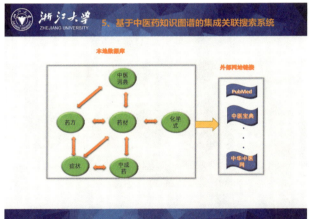

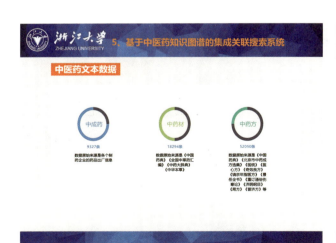

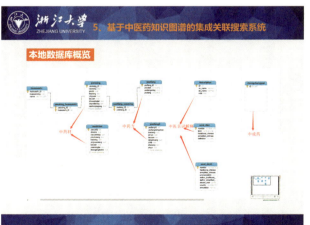

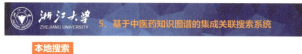

本地搜索

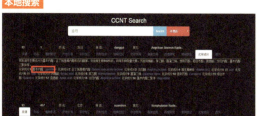

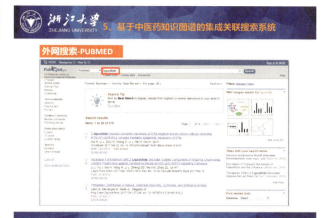

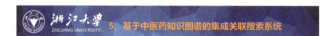

本地搜索

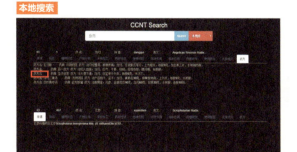

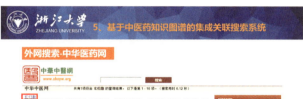

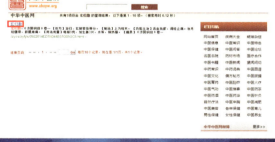

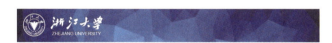

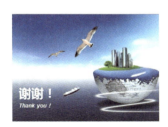

后　记

"健康中国2030"规划纲要指出,要充分发挥中医药独特优势,提高中医药服务能力,发展中医养生保健治未病服务,推进中医药继承创新。随着我国新型工业化、信息化、城镇化、农业现代化深入发展,人口老龄化进程加快,健康服务业蓬勃发展,人民群众对中医服务的需求越来越旺盛,迫切需要继承、发展、利用好中医,造福全人类健康。为了适应新形势的需要,国务院制定了《中医药发展战略规划纲要(2016—2030年)》,对新时期推进中医药事业发展做出系统部署,进一步聚焦中医药的继承、创新、现代化、国际化,明确把中医药发展上升为国家战略。

中医发展迎来新的战略机遇期,新一代信息技术、新材料、人工智能等迅速发展,为充分发挥中医优势提供了强有力的支撑。5G等新一代通信技术推动"互联网＋中医"落地,培育远程中医、移动中医、智慧中医等新型医疗服务模式。以柔性材料为代表的新兴材料支撑中医脉诊仪等关键设备取得突破。人工智能应用在"望、闻、问、切"各个环节中,为医生提供更敏锐的眼睛、更灵敏的耳朵等增强感官,赋予医生海量案例、瞬间搜索、知识链接等博记睿智的大脑。

中医传承精华、守正创新,为百姓提供普惠服务。传承精华:通过构建中医元数据库、中医知识图谱,对中医医史文献、中医基础理论、中医药文化等思想理论进行数字化、信息化、知识化全面系统继承。守正创新:借助新兴材料、创新硬件、新一代信息技术,增强医生的感知能力,提升医生的判断能力;引入数据挖掘和药物设计等方法,发现有效中药方剂,加速重大疑难疾病、慢性病等中医新药研发;依靠互联网、物联网、务联网等新型基础设施建设,积极开展中医线上线下诊疗和健康管理、中医药膳食疗科普活动,推广中医传统运动项目,加强中医药健康养生养老文化宣传;探索互联网延伸医嘱、电子处方等网络中医医疗服务应用,构建集医学影像、检验报告等健康档案于一体的医疗信息共享服务体系,利用移动互联网等信息技术提供在线预约诊疗、候诊提醒、划价缴费、诊疗报告查询、药品配送等便捷服务。

普惠中医应用前景主要体现在三个方向:一是在基层医疗机构,通过中医人工智能,在临床上大规模应用中医智能化系统,通过给基层村医、西学中医生赋能,提高基层医生的中医辨证论治水平,辅助他们看好原来不太有把握的病,尤其是一些中医有优势的特色病种;二是在中医馆,通过人工智能为中医馆年轻医生赋能,利用中医人工智能提升中医馆年轻中医医师素养,让他们拥有更高的水平,帮助中医馆打造特色专病专科,形成中医馆自己的专病特色;三是在日常养生保健,当中医形成生活化的格局后,在日常生活中通过技术化手段搜集人的基础信息,通过数据采集和中医人工智能辅助,为百姓赋能决策日常养生中医保健。

普惠中医在抗疫中展现了重要作用。西医思想着重于寻找对症药物,而中医防疫思维注重将患者病情控制在较早阶段,阻止轻症病人向重症转化。"中国方案"的一大亮点在于对新冠肺炎患者的凝血因子和炎症指标进行早期干预,这实际上体现了中医"治未病"思想。在抗击新冠肺炎疫情的关键时刻,中医人快速反应、积极应对、全面参与、全程救治,取得了令世人瞩目的成绩。中医药治疗新冠肺炎的经验正在为国际社会防控疫情提供"中国经验"和"中国智慧"。

普惠中医在新模式、新技术、新材料的赋能下不断传承创新,切实成为人民群众不断增强获得感、幸福感、安全感的重要来源。愿这一国之瑰宝在不久的将来为建设健康中国、增进人民健康福祉做出新的贡献。

图书在版编目(CIP)数据

中医药智能计算：浙江大学成果汇编 / 未来计算编委会编. —杭州：浙江大学出版社，2020.10
ISBN 978-7-308-20655-6

Ⅰ.①中…　Ⅱ.①未…　Ⅲ.①中国医药学－医学信息学　Ⅳ.①R2-03

中国版本图书馆 CIP 数据核字(2020)第 195319 号

中医药智能计算：浙江大学成果汇编

未来计算编委会　编

策　　划	许佳颖
责任编辑	金佩雯
责任校对	殷晓彤
封面设计	周　灵
出版发行	浙江大学出版社
	（杭州市天目山路 148 号　邮政编码 310007）
	（网址：http://www.zjupress.com）
排　　版	浙江时代出版服务有限公司
印　　刷	浙江海虹彩色印务有限公司
开　　本	889mm×1194mm　1/16
印　　张	20
字　　数	552 千
版 印 次	2020 年 10 月第 1 版　2020 年 10 月第 1 次印刷
书　　号	ISBN 978-7-308-20655-6
定　　价	120.00 元